Forensic cultures in modern Europe

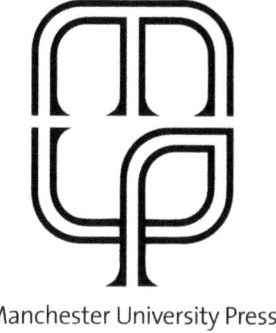

Manchester University Press

SOCIAL HISTORIES OF MEDICINE

Series editors: David Cantor, Anne Hanley and Elaine Leong

Social Histories of Medicine is concerned with all aspects of health, illness and medicine, from prehistory to the present, in every part of the world. The series covers the circumstances that promote health or illness, the ways in which people experience and explain such conditions, and what, practically, they do about them. Practitioners of all approaches to health and healing come within its scope, as do their ideas, beliefs, and practices, and the social, economic and cultural contexts in which they operate. Methodologically, the series welcomes relevant studies in social, economic, cultural, and intellectual history, as well as approaches derived from other disciplines in the arts, sciences, social sciences and humanities. The series is a collaboration between Manchester University Press and the Society for the Social History of Medicine.

To buy or to find out more about the books currently available in this series, please go to: https://manchesteruniversitypress.co.uk/series/social-histories-of-medicine/

Forensic cultures in modern Europe

Edited by

Willemijn Ruberg, Lara Bergers, Pauline Dirven
and Sara Serrano Martínez

MANCHESTER UNIVERSITY PRESS

Copyright © Manchester University Press 2023

While copyright in the volume as a whole is vested in Manchester University Press, copyright in individual chapters belongs to their respective authors.

This electronic version has been made freely available under a Creative Commons (CC BY-NC-ND) licence, thanks to the support of the European Research Council (ERC), which permits non-commercial use, distribution and reproduction provided the editor(s), author(s) and Manchester University Press are fully cited and no modifications or adaptations are made. Details of the licence can be viewed at https://creativecommons.org/licenses/by-nc-nd/4.0/

Published by Manchester University Press
Oxford Road, Manchester M13 9PL

www.manchesteruniversitypress.co.uk

British Library Cataloguing-in-Publication Data
A catalogue record for this book is available from the British Library

ISBN 978 1 5261 7233 4 hardback

First published 2023

The publisher has no responsibility for the persistence or accuracy of URLs for any external or third-party internet websites referred to in this book, and does not guarantee that any content on such websites is, or will remain, accurate or appropriate.

Typeset by Newgen Publishing UK

Contents

List of figures — vii
List of contributors — ix

Introduction – Willemijn Ruberg — 1

1 Blood will out: Blood typing, forensic culture and gender in a 1950s Scottish paternity case – Alison Adam — 25

2 A culture of testimony: The importance of 'speaking witnesses' in Dutch sexual crimes investigations and trials, 1930–1960 – Lara Bergers — 49

3 The making of evidence after mass violence: Forensics in the aftermath of the Second World War – Taline Garibian — 71

4 Teaching Grossian criminalistics in Imperial Germany – Heather Wolffram — 92

5 Sober suits, bowler hats and white lab coats: Enclothed impartiality, masculinity and the tailoring of a bourgeois expert persona in British courtrooms, 1920–1960 – Pauline Dirven — 117

6 Reassessing the legacy of Cesare Lombroso: Criminal anthropology in the expert testimony of Mario Carrara, 1910–1930 – Franco Orlandi — 147

7 Expert evidence and uncertainty in English infanticide trials, *c.* 1725–1945 – Rachel Dixon and Tony Ward — 169

8 Forensic physicians and the Francoist prosecution of infanticide, *c.* 1939–1969: The case of the haemorrhage of the umbilical cord as cause of death – Sara Serrano Martínez — 191

9 Doing law, psychiatric expertise and 'crimes of
  passion' in the Netherlands and Russia in the
  twentieth century – Volha Parfenchyk
  and Willemijn Ruberg   216
10 A culture of consensus: Organising expertise in
  Norwegian forensic psychiatry, late nineteenth to
  early twentieth century – Svein Atle Skålevåg   240
11 The 'key' to the crime: Criminal cases and the
  projection of expectations about forensic DNA
  technologies in the Portuguese press – Filipe Santos   261

Index   282

Figures

5.1 Portrait picture of Sir Sydney Alfred Smith (1883–1969), Regius Professor of Forensic Medicine at Edinburgh University from 1928 to 1953. Photograph by W. & E. Drummond Young (The University of Edinburgh, UA CA1/1 h, 'Sir Sydney Alfred Smith (1883–1969) – Our History', accessed 14 February 2022, http://ourhistory.is.ed.ac.uk/index.php/Sir_Sydney_Alfred_Smith_(1883–1969)) 124

5.2 Home Office analyst John Webster (left) and chemist William Willcox (right) as they arrive or leave at the court, 1920. (ANL/Shutterstock, accessed 16 December 2021, www.shutterstock.com/nl/editorial/image-editorial /john-webster-l-and-dr-wh-willcox-toxicologists-who-examined-the-body-of-mabel-greenwood-4735558a) 125

5.3 Pathologist Keith Simpson arriving at Westminster Coroner Court to give evidence at the inquest of the Ritz Hotel murder and suicide, 13 March 1953. (Trinity Mirror / Mirrorpix/ Alamy Stock Photo, accessed 14 February 2022, www.alamy.com /stock-photo-dr-keith-simpson-the-home-office-pathologist-arriving-at-westminster-83443376.html) 126

5.4 The jurors in the Dr Ruxton murder trial as they return to court to return their verdict of guilty, 1935. (Photo by Mirrorpix/Mirrorpix via Getty

Images, accessed 14 February 2022, www.gettyimages.nl/detail/nieuwsfoto%27s/dr-ruxton-murder-case-members-of-the-jury-at-he-trial-who-nieuwsfotos/591974956) 129

5.5 Team of expert witnesses who worked on the *Ruxton* case. (ANL/Shutterstock, accessed 14 February 2022, www.shutterstock.com/editorial/image-editorial/forensic-experts-working-on-the-ravine-murders-lr-prof-js-brash-prof-sydney-smith-prof-john-glaister-dr-wg-millar-and-dr-cl-godfrey-box-651–2407121527-ajpg-5727859a) 129

5.6 Bernard Spilsbury in post-mortem garment. (Wellcome Images / Wikimedia, CC BY-SA 4.0: Library reference: ICV No 11802, Photo number: V0011537, accessed 14 October 2022, https://commons.wikimedia.org/wiki/File:Sir_Bernard_Spilsbury,_a_famous_pathologist._Reproduction_of_Wellcome_V0011537.jpg) 131

5.7 Photograph of Sir Bernard Spilsbury posing in the laboratory wearing a white lab coat, 1920s. (Photograph by Edward Cahen, National Portrait Gallery, London, accessed 16 December 2021, www.npg.org.uk/collections/search/use-this-image/?mkey=mw189943) 133

5.8 Photograph of Sydney Smith in white lab coat posing as a scientist, used on the cover of his autobiography *Mostly Murder*. (Accessed through Royal College of Physicians of Edinburgh) 134

5.9 (Cedric) Keith Simpson posing with murder weapon, skull and flask in 1978. (Photograph by Judith Aronson, 1978, National Portrait Gallery, London, accessed 19 August 2022, www.npg.org.uk/collections/search/portrait/mw62365/Cedric-Keith-Simpson?LinkID=mp61813&role=sit&rNo=6) 135

Contributors

Alison Adam is professor emerita of Science, Technology and Society at Sheffield Hallam University and has also worked at the universities of Lancaster, Manchester and Salford. Her earlier research centred on gender and technology, especially AI, critical information systems and computer ethics where her major works include *Artificial Knowing: Gender and the Thinking Machine* (Routledge, 1998) and *Gender, Ethics and Information Technology* (Palgrave, 2005). From 2008 to the present day she has researched the history of forensic science in the UK in the mid-twentieth century. Her main works include *A History of Forensic Science: British Beginnings in the Twentieth Century* (Routledge, 2016) and an edited collection: *Crime and the Construction of Forensic Objectivity from 1850* (Palgrave, 2020). She is currently researching the development of forensic science in twentieth-century Scotland.

Lara Bergers is a PhD candidate at Utrecht University, where she researches how criminality and victimhood are constructed in twentieth-century Dutch forensic-scientific, judicial and policing practices. She obtained her research master's degree in History and Philosophy of Science at Utrecht University, writing her master's thesis on the (absence) of lie detection in the Netherlands. This research formed the basis for an article in *Wonderkamer* 2 (2020). With Didi van Trijp, she has co-authored an article on science museums in *Isis* 108:2 (2017).

Pauline Dirven is a PhD candidate at Utrecht University. Her research interests are gender, the body, performance and knowledge practices. She has published on embodiment and dance, including 'Ballet, an Empowering Embodied Experience: A Feminist Phenomenological Analysis of Ballerinas' Bodies', *Locus* (2020). Her doctoral research focuses on forensic culture in twentieth-century England, in particular on embodied performances of forensic expertise. She analyses how forensic scientists and doctors used and experienced their bodies in examination practices and how they displayed themselves before a lay audience. She studies how expertise was enacted in gestures, sensory practices, emotional experiences and dress culture. On this topic she recently published in *Wonderkamer* 3 (2021).

Rachel Dixon is a lecturer in Law at the University of Hull, England, where she teaches Criminal Law and Criminal Justice. Her research interests lie in English medico-legal history and in particular in infanticide. She is the author of *Infanticide: Expert Evidence and Testimony in Child Murder Cases, 1688–1955* (Routledge, 2022).

Taline Garibian is a lecturer in Modern History at the University of Geneva. She is also an associate researcher at the Institute of Humanities in Medicine (University of Lausanne) and a visiting fellow at the Wellcome Centre for Ethics and Humanities (University of Oxford). Her areas of interest include the history of medicine and science, the history of wars, violence and genocide, and the history of gender and sexualities.

Franco Orlandi is a doctoral fellow of the Research Foundation – Flanders (FWO) at KU Leuven, where he is attached to the Cultural History since 1750 Research Group. His current research project investigates the legacy of Cesare Lombroso and the global impact of Italian criminal anthropology in the age of totalitarianism.

Volha Parfenchyk was a postdoctoral researcher at Utrecht University until 2021. She received her LL.M at the University of Amsterdam and defended her doctoral dissertation at Tilburg University. She worked on her PhD within the framework of the Joint Doctoral Programme in Law, Science and Technology. Her research interests include the relations between science, technology and law and the influence of local culture on techno-scientific and legal practices.

Willemijn Ruberg is associate professor of Cultural History at Utrecht University. Her research interests include the modern history of gender, knowledge, forensic expertise and the body, as well as cultural theory. She recently published *History of the Body* in the History and Theory series of Red Globe Press (2020); 'Hysteria as a Shape-Shifting Forensic Psychiatric Diagnosis in the Netherlands ca. 1885–1960', *Gender and History* (2022); and 'Infanticide and the Influence of Psychoanalysis on Dutch Forensic Psychiatry in the Mid-Twentieth Century', *History of Psychiatry*, 32:2 (2021). She is the principal investigator of the research project 'Forensic Culture. A Comparative Analysis of Forensic Practices in Europe, 1930–2000 (FORCE)', funded by an ERC Consolidator Grant (2018–2024).

Filipe Santos has a PhD in Sociology and is currently co-coordinator and researcher of the Science, Economy and Society Research Group (NECES). His research interests are focused on the intersections between criminal justice and forensic science, privileging theoretical approaches from Science, Technology and Society Studies. Filipe's latest publications include *Da cena de crime ao tribunal. Trajetórias e culturas forenses* (Pactor, 2020), 'The Social Life of Forensic Evidence and the Epistemic Sub-Cultures in an Inquisitorial Justice System: Analysis of Saltão Case', *Science & Justice* 59:5 (2019), and 'Patterns of Exchange of Forensic DNA Data in the European Union through the Prüm System', *Science & Justice* 57:4 (2017). His current research project (CLINIC) focuses on the execution of security measures by mentally disordered offenders in Portugal.

Sara Serrano Martínez is a PhD candidate at Utrecht University. In her PhD research she traces how the crime of infanticide was interpreted and prosecuted in the Francoist dictatorship, focusing on the role of psychiatry and legal medicine in the proceedings. She holds a BA in Philosophy from the University of Barcelona (2016), and an MA in History of Science from the Autonomous University of Barcelona (2017). In her master's thesis she studied the history of medical and psychological conceptualisations of suicide in Spain in the 1920s and 1930s. Her master's thesis received a prize *ex aequo* from the Catalan Society for the History of Science and Technology in 2019 and, based on this thesis, she published the article 'Concepciones médicas y psicológicas del suicidio en España (1926–1936)', *Actes d'Història de la Ciència i de la Tècnica* (2019).

Svein Atle Skålevåg is professor in the History of Sciences at the University of Bergen, Norway, and has written a book-length study of the history of criminal responsibility in Norway in the nineteenth and twentieth centuries: *Utilregnelighet. En historie om rett og medisin* (Pax, 2016) and the article 'The Matter of Forensic Psychiatry', *Medical History* (2006).

Tony Ward is professor of Law at Northumbria University, Newcastle upon Tyne, UK. His PhD thesis (1996) was on the development of insanity and other mental condition defences, including infanticide, from 1843 to 1939. He has published numerous articles and book chapters on these subjects and on the present-day law relating to forensic science and other forms of expert evidence. He also researches in criminology with a focus on governmental crimes. He is co-author of *Privatization and the Penal System* (with Mick Ryan, Palgrave Macmillan, 1989), *State Crime* (with Penny Green, 2004), *Law and Crime* (with Gerry Johnstone, SAGE Publications, 2010) and *State Crime and Civil Activism* (with Penny Green, Routledge, 2018).

Heather Wolffram is associate professor of History at the University of Canterbury, New Zealand. She has written on forensic psychology in Germany: *Forensic Psychology in Germany: Witnessing Crime 1880–1939* (Palgrave Macmillan, 2018), and recently published 'Forensic Knowledge and Forensic Networks in Britain's Empire: The Case of Sydney Smith' in Ian Burney and Christopher Hamlin (eds), *Global Forensic Cultures: Making Fact and Justice in the Modern Era* (Johns Hopkins University Press, 2019) and '"Children's Lies": The Weimar Press as Psychological Expert in Child Sex Abuse Trials' in Alison Adam (ed.), *Crime and the Construction of Forensic Objectivity from 1850* (Palgrave, 2020)

Introduction

Willemijn Ruberg

The eleven chapters in this volume together discuss the ways scientific expertise was used in modern European courtrooms and pretrial investigations. They present the different practices of making scientific knowledge specifically adapted to the legal context and show how doctors, psychiatrists and other specialists played their part in investigations and trials in Scotland, England, Germany, Spain, Italy, Russia, Portugal, Norway and the Netherlands in the nineteenth and twentieth centuries. These case studies show how forensic practices in modern times were not only shaped by scientific developments, but also – perhaps even more importantly – by major changes in political, legal and cultural contexts, especially by the rise of authoritarian regimes, war crimes and their prosecution, and shifting ideas on nation, class and gender. In this introduction, I will explore new insights in the history of forensic science and address how the chapters in this volume both complement this history and point to new avenues in the research on forensic culture.

The turns to practice and culture in the historiography of forensic science

For a long time, the history of forensic science and medicine was mostly written by historians of law and historians of medicine. Legal historians were concerned with deciphering intricate contemporary discussions between legal scholars about what constituted evidence and who could act as (expert) witness. Historians of medicine explored the application of medical knowledge in physicians' court testimonies. In the first historical narratives of legal or forensic medicine, these two elements – the formations of procedural law regarding evidence and the role of expert witnesses in particular legal systems and countries on the one hand, and the role of medicine in trials and police investigations on the other – formed the basis of a generally progressivist story, in which scientists as expert witnesses gained more authority in the courtroom and legal procedures, supposedly, became more rational. Hallmarks on this road to modern forensic expertise were the advance of medicine, science and technology, specifically the medieval discovery of autopsy, the development of new technologies such as fingerprinting and blood tests as part of the new scientific branch of criminalistics in the early twentieth century, the use of DNA in court cases from the 1990s, but also the emergence of a whole new field of (forensic) psychiatry from the nineteenth century onwards.[1]

The entanglement of the histories of law, medicine and science already made the writing of forensic history complicated. New theoretical perspectives in the humanities and social sciences added layers of analysis and thus also new themes to be scrutinised. Of these theoretical perspectives, two had an especially noticeable impact on the study of forensic history: firstly, new approaches in the history of science, informed by insights from Science and Technology Studies (STS) and a turn to the history of knowledge; secondly, the cultural turn in the humanities.

From the 1970s STS brought a new focus on science in action and the social embedding of the use of technology. As part of a broader practice turn, Bruno Latour, Sheila Jasanoff and numerous other scholars unpacked how science was made in everyday practices and in specific contexts such as the laboratory and the courtroom.[2] Objects and technologies, especially the ways these were socially embedded, were central to this approach. Moreover, expertise came to be regarded as socially constructed: what type of knowledge was seen as expert knowledge depended on the institutional and cultural setting and was continuously shifting. At the same time, historians of science were increasingly taking account of the social and cultural contexts in which science was produced, as well as of the varying boundaries between expert and lay knowledge.[3] For example, Lorraine Daston and Peter Galison famously showed how the notion of objectivity was differently defined between the mid-eighteenth and early twentieth centuries.[4]

Moreover, the cultural turn in the humanities in the 1980s and 1990s highlighted semiotics, the power of discourse, symbols, texts, images and media through which meaning was made. From this perspective, the production and performance of class, race and gender identities gained centre stage. The role of ordinary people had already been stressed in the 1970s, as part of socio-economic history and historical anthropology, but influenced by the cultural turn, historians now became interested in how these people contributed to making knowledge and the ways they were excluded (via medical or psychiatric discourses on normality, for instance).[5] A new attention to performances was also part of the cultural turn, triggering interest into the performance of experts.[6]

These two new approaches – STS and the cultural turn – have in recent years also impacted on the directions the history of forensic science and medicine has taken. More attention has been paid to experts' performances in the courtroom, to medical and psychiatric discourses on gender, race or the body, to the role of the media in reporting on court cases and scientific experts, to the spaces in which knowledge was made (e.g. the crime scene, the media, the laboratory) and to the various actors, including non-human actors such as objects or animals, involved in this process. In 2013 a special issue of the journal *Studies in History and Philosophy of Biological and Biomedical Sciences* was devoted to the notion of 'forensic culture'. In this issue, Christopher Hamlin took 'forensic culture' to be the 'history of forensic science in terms of ideologies and institutions rather than developing technique',[7] thus contrasting this new approach with a more traditional focus on a progressivist history of science and technology. Hamlin presented an 'analytic' for comparing forensic cultures, including four elements: exemplary forensic methods and techniques; foremost forensic professions (varying from midwives to chemists); dominant juridical institutions (e.g. inquisitorial, adversarial and the 'colonial rule of incomprehensible others'); and prevailing anxieties. In the same issue, Simon Cole qualified the notion of forensic culture as a flexible one 'to mean a variety of things ranging from race and ethnicity to cultural (or media) representations of forensic science to the impact of forensic science on popular culture'.[8] These two articles by Hamlin and Cole, scholars who have been central to defining the field of the history of forensic science and medicine, both indicate the novelty of a focus on forensic culture and the difficulty of defining this notion.

Two recent edited volumes testify to the increasing influence of this paradigm of forensic culture. The first book was edited by Ian Burney and Christopher Hamlin: *Global Forensic Cultures: Making Fact and Justice in the Modern Era* (2019). Its chapters discussed forensic institutions and practices in several countries and regions (Germany, France, Spain, the British empire, Palestine, Siam/Thailand, the United States) even though the volume as a whole did not aim to trace global or transnational knowledge formations. The book featured 'the entanglement of techniques, professions, and systems of jurisprudence/governmentality' in regard to forensic science and medicine (not addressing forensic psychiatry) and acknowledged race or ethnicity as 'differentiator of forensic practices'.[9] In addition, in his introduction to the volume Hamlin reflected on what exactly was 'cultural' when locating forensic practices: 'we find them everywhere rooted in what is unambiguously cultural: with ideas of what kinds of persons the world includes; of what dangers it and they pose; and, at an even deeper level, of why things happen.'[10]

The second recent volume considering forensic cultures is the one edited by Alison Adam, *Crime and the Construction of Forensic Objectivity from 1850* (2020). Rather than the notion of forensic culture per se, the central concept in this volume is 'forensic objectivity', regarded as 'a kind of emergent property, developing from professional practices and media commentary, systems of representation of crimes and crime artefacts'.[11] The book 'decentres' the professional expert, instead focusing on how forensic objectivity is constructed through 'a web of interests', e.g. via 'the vectors of criminal, victim, class, gender, place, crime scene, experts, media and the public woven together in the performance of forensic objectivity'.[12] Concretely, the chapters in this book cover practices of representation from the mid-nineteenth century to the present day, such as crime photography, the techniques through which jurors could be made 'virtual witnesses', the professional networks of medical and scientific witnesses, the role of the media and the ways criminal records were recorded and developed.[13]

Comparing these two recent edited volumes, it can be concluded that *Global Forensic Cultures* highlights experts, governance and institutions somewhat more than *Crime and the Construction of Forensic Objectivity from 1850*, which revolves around cultural representations and conceptualisations of objectivity. However, both volumes have one important claim in common: forensics are shaped by local circumstances. Hamlin identified as one common theme in *Global Forensic Cultures* that the chapters regarded forensic science as 'a fabric of contingencies'[14] and Adam downplayed the image of 'warring experts', arguing for a 'more subtle and more complex' construction of forensic objectivity, including attention for differing institutional arrangements and state support: 'Local, contingent arrangements do more than influence the trajectory of knowledge; they make it.'[15] By highlighting local conditions and contingencies, both volumes also underscore that technologies, institutions and ideas are entangled.

This overall foregrounding of local differences between forensic cultures has been illuminating since it has shown that technology or legal systems alone cannot explain the daily functioning of forensic experts. It has also provided us with interesting questions to explore: How do the different elements of forensic cultures (such as the availability of technology, the legal system, politics or the media) influence the impact of scientific expertise? And how do expert performances relate to different spaces and audiences, to specific crimes and to historically and culturally variable norms on class, race or gender? If local circumstances play such an important role in shaping forensics, what impact did national, global and transnational knowledge exchanges have on the development of these local practices? And what are the specific hallmarks of *modern* forensic cultures?[16]

The chapters in this volume point to some directions the answers to these questions could take. Overall, this book has three aims. Firstly, it highlights the concept of modernity[17] and its ramifications on forensic culture. Recent research has started to pay more attention to forensics in the twentieth century, the period that has witnessed major changes in regard to science, politics and culture. Historians of science and medicine have looked for the modern character of forensic cultures as expressed in the institutionalisation, technologies and social impact of science; in the political development of totalitarian and democratic regimes and disciplinary power; and in changing cultural norms and roles, for instance with regard to gender, epistemic values and the role of the media. The chapters in this volume provide reflection on these particularly modern hallmarks, as well as on the ways they coexist with older, unchanging, elements. This can help us grasp the conceptions of modernity and how these ideas corresponded with the experiences of the actors who enacted these 'modern' forensic practices.

Secondly, this volume highlights the importance of forensic *practices*, in contrast to forensic institutions or scientific discourses. Following the practice turn in the humanities and social sciences, several of the chapters demonstrate that practices have their own powerful dynamics and inform discourses and institutions, as well as being influenced by the latter. A focus on practice can, in fact, inform us on the entanglements of scientific and political discourses, the legal system and other institutions, as well as enactments of gender, nation or class. The agency and interactions central to forensic practices also help us to understand how forensic cultures can change over time.

Thirdly, the chapters in this book explore the notion of 'forensic culture' in more detail, for instance in regard to the units of analysis that are used: whereas earlier research mostly took the type of legal system (inquisitorial/accusatorial) or nation as a unit of analysis, increasingly more local systems of knowledge, or at the opposite end, global networks, are beginning to be studied. A more specific explanation of this notion can aid us in comparing different forensic cultures.

The notion of 'forensic culture'

Most scholars agree that the notion of 'forensic culture' may help us to go beyond the perspective of institutional rules and scientific discourse, towards a study of the practices of forensic medicine. More problematic, however, is defining what a forensic culture further entails. Important elements, in addition to technology and the professionalisation of experts, may include ideology (political ideology, but also ideas on religion, class, race and gender), the role of the media, legal systems and the formulation of criminal and procedural law. We need to ask how these factors are practically enacted and mutually entangled. Also, are the boundaries of a forensic culture national or do they correspond to other geographical or cultural units such as (former) colonial empires exchanging knowledge between metropole and colonies? Or should we rather regard these boundaries as determined by the distinction between accusatorial or inquisitorial systems?

Historical research has provided some robust evidence that has helped us to understand how forensic cultures function. It is increasingly becoming clear that the division between accusatorial and inquisitorial systems does not have such an unequivocal, unilateral relationship with the role and impact of scientific experts as assumed in the literature that has been limited to the ways legal systems function in theory. For instance, the American and English legal systems, based on common law, a jury and two parties as opponents (the accusatorial or adversarial system) is often contrasted with inquisitorial systems based on Roman law, in which the judge leads the examination. Legal historians regard these differences as having resulted in a flourishing discipline of forensic science in Scotland and the European Continent, and in a failing profession in the Anglo-American world from the eighteenth century onwards. They have suggested that the accusatorial system, in which each party hires its own expert, is detrimental to scientific expertise, each expert fighting the other. Controversy regarding scientific evidence is thought to be less frequent in the continental law systems than in adversarial systems.[18] Although undoubtedly the type of legal system shapes the role and impact of forensic science to some extent, in practice many legal systems combine elements of the inquisitorial and adversarial systems. Moreover, in modern history several countries have witnessed changes in their judicial systems. In addition, as the chapters in this volume show, ideology and national political culture – consensual, authoritarian, liberal or conservative – frequently shape the impact of forensic experts equally, if not more, than the broad difference between inquisitorial and adversarial systems.

Thus, it seems convenient to speak of a 'legal system' as more than accusatorial or inquisitorial: it entails institutions, often steered by the state, and rules such as procedural law. These may differ per country, state or region. These important building blocks, are, however, not sufficient to qualify as a specific forensic culture. This qualification also needs to include political and cultural ideology as well as social contexts, that – in turn – influence science and knowledge, and vice versa. Thus, we might speak of the 'formal role of forensic doctors in the Spanish legal system', but this is only shaped in the 'Francoist forensic culture', characterised by a certain political, social and ideological context. The chapters in this volume indeed show how in Europe national ideologies and contexts strongly impact the form of forensic cultures.

At the same time, it is no longer self-evident to take the national framework as the main unit of analysis. For instance, recent research has established that often the colonies acted as a laboratory for experimenting with new forensic techniques before they were implemented in the motherland, partly in response to specific cultural circumstances or anxieties.[19] This has made us aware that not all forensic technological or organisational innovation took place in the context of the nation, but also in the context of empire. However, this expansion of the unit of analysis beyond the nation state has also raised questions about the exact entanglement of global forensic cultures. Even though authors widely acknowledge that forensic-medical texts were circulated internationally, hardly any research has been done into the international networks of forensic scientists, their exchange of knowledge or their animosities. Furthermore, more structural comparative analysis of forensic cultures in different regions, countries and localities still needs to be performed. The chapters in this volume present one step in this direction by comparing different forensic cultures in Europe in the modern period. They highlight that *within* Europe, as well, there were centres and peripheries, presumed forerunners and stragglers, sometimes framed in discourses on civilisation and backwardness.

Modernity and the 'forensic turn': a shift to material evidence?

This book aims to explore the modern character of forensic science, medicine and psychiatry. Primarily, the increasingly advanced technology and the expanding institutionalisation have been regarded as the hallmarks of modern forensics. Specifically, the rise of criminalistics in the first decades of the twentieth century, revolving around material trace evidence – the so-called 'silent witnesses' – such as fingerprints, the discovery of hair and blood analysis by the mid-twentieth century and the use of DNA as evidence from around 1990 stand out as technological innovations. In their study of England in the first half of the twentieth century, Ian Burney and Neil Pemberton trace a new forensic regime, which saw the rise of criminalistics, centring around the meticulous analysis of traces on the crime scene and the corpse in the laboratory. This regime replaced an older forensic regime that revolved around the pathologist who examined the victim's body and performed the autopsy.[20] At the same time, national discussions on the development of forensic science often revolved around a comparison with other countries that were showcased as more advanced in terms of technology or organisation and institutionalisation. Especially Germany, France and Austria were presented as innovative and having taken the lead in forensic science and psychiatry around 1900 (after the Second World War the United States would become the point of reference).[21] Ironically, in her chapter in this volume Heather Wolffram writes that in Germany, by the second decade of the twentieth century criminologists and jurists complained that – in contrast to other countries – German universities rarely offered lectures on forensic psychology, criminalistics, forensic chemistry and other scientific aids to legal praxis. These German advocates of innovation thus practised what Wolffram terms 'forensic patriotism', encouraging Germany to catch up with the leading countries regarding teaching forensic science. Although in some cases these comparative images of forerunners and backward countries may have been a correct reflection of the state of criminalistics, they probably mostly served to stimulate governmental funding to establish national forensic institutes and education on forensic science in addition to creating a modern professional self-image and reflecting nationalism.

Progressivist narratives of the march of forensic science have been challenged in other respects as well. Research has traced the rising significance of forensic anthropologists and pathologists in the reconstructions of mass violence and their role as expert witnesses in courts of international criminal and human rights, accompanied by an emphasis on material evidence, bodies and objects, particularly in relation to the Holocaust and concentration camps. This has been coined the 'forensic turn', which supposedly ended the 'era of witness', the prominent value put on the testimony of human eyewitnesses. The Eichmann trial in 1961 is considered as heralding the age of the witness or the turn towards testimony as the basis for prosecuting and possibly healing crimes against humanity. The identification of the bodily remains of Mengele in 1985, by contrast, and in particular the use of different scientific techniques, is seen to exemplify the turn towards material evidence, bodies and objects. Thomas Keenan and Eyal Weizman argue that forensic investigation is also a stage of public persuasion, using 'scientific, rhetorical, theatrical and visual mechanisms' to make things appear to speak for themselves to convince a non-specialist audience.[22] However, the chronology of this shift from the era of witness to the era of forensics has been complicated.[23] As Taline Garibian points out in her chapter in this volume, the evidentiary paradigms of testimonies and forensics often overlap, moreover this opposition was already thematised before the 1960s. While the Americans mostly used documents, British war crime trials relied on testimonies, hence testifying to the coexistence of different judicial cultures at the same time. Garibian furthermore shows that the forensic turn occurring in the 1980s was characterised more by a shift in the evidential paradigm – and the popularisation of specific techniques – than by scientific advances.

Other chapters in this volume also complicate a narrative that describes a complete shift from the use of eyewitnesses and an emphasis on confessions to value attached to expert testimony and material evidence. On the one hand Heather Wolffram's chapter confirms this shift for the forensic culture of Imperial Germany, which came to attach more value to expert testimony and physical evidence left at crime scenes than to confessions and witnesses. On the other hand, Lara Bergers, in her chapter on cases of sexual assault in the Netherlands in 1930–1960, finds a continuing emphasis placed on witnesses and a remarkable neglect of material evidence and expertise. Thus, the relative valuation of witnesses, experts and the so-called material 'silent witnesses' as evidence reveals both change and continuity.

In other respects, as well, continuities can be found in the history of forensic science. For example, medico-legal structures have particularly since the early modern period been inextricably connected with the state and political ideology.[24] This comes to the fore in the coroner system, which in the United Kingdom has been present since the Middle Ages. Although differences exist on national, state and local level, the coroner in Anglo-American countries is generally a state officer tasked with the public investigation of sudden or unnatural death, in contrast to the Continent, where police or judiciary only decide which suspicious deaths will be subject to medico-legal investigation. The function of the coroner was, moreover, regarded as a 'bulwark of democracy' in England. The English appreciated the practice of public enquiry of judicial decisions through an elected coroner, including a lay jury.[25] The coroner system thus not only exemplifies a medico-legal structure with a long and venerable history, but also testifies to the entanglement of science, law and politics.

The history of forensic science and medicine, which came to be more separated in the twentieth century, has therefore testified to continuities, for example in regard to procedural law, but also to ruptures such as new institutions and techniques. The introduction and acceptance of modern forensic techniques has moreover not been straightforward and has differed per country, depending on the legal system and a broader cultural and political context.[26]

Modern forensic cultures and authoritarian regimes

A particular hallmark of twentieth-century European forensic culture is the influence of state ideology in authoritarian regimes on forensic medicine. Research on the functioning of forensic medicine and psychiatry in authoritarian systems has demonstrated how the role of these experts could be strongly restricted. An infamous example is the abuse of Russian and Soviet (forensic) psychiatry for political purposes.[27] Still, historians have warned that state ideology in authoritarian countries such as Soviet Russia was not the only factor defining the shape of laws and forensic expertise; legal and medical professionals also participated in this process.[28]

Several chapters in this volume engage with these debates. Franco Orlandi places his chapter on the influence of criminal anthropology in the courtroom in Liberal and Fascist Italy (1910–1930) in a broader discussion on the legitimising role of criminology in the repression and systematic elimination of alleged enemies of the state in authoritarian regimes.[29] According to Mary Gibson, the Lombrosian school contributed to 'an intellectual environment conducive to the dictatorship' in Fascist Italy.[30] However, both Gibson and Orlandi conclude that the ideas of Cesare Lombroso on the 'born criminal' were not appreciated when expressed in court by medical expert witnesses during the Fascist dictatorship in the 1920s. Similarly, Volha Parfenchyk and Willemijn Ruberg, who compare (Soviet) Russian and Dutch 'crimes of passion', demonstrate that although the Russian and Soviet criminal codes were suffused with socialist ideology, in practice legal actors and psychiatrists could participate in shaping central notions such as 'pathological jealousy' and 'unaccountability'. A focus on forensic *practices* can thus prove that authoritarian systems need not completely steer the role and conclusions of scientific experts. Nevertheless, as Sara Serrano Martínez argues in her chapter on Spanish medical experts in infanticide cases during the Franco regime, even in trials that at first sight do not seem to deal with politics directly, doctors could also act as 'crucial agents of Francoist justice'. Whereas historians of Francoist forensic practices have mostly been preoccupied with scientific practices and theories in military trials and in the so-called special jurisdictions for political repression, Serrano Martínez calls for attention to how physicians in ordinary jurisdictions, such as criminal law courts, as well, could contribute to repression. In short, several chapters in this volume propose that authoritarian regimes shape modern forensic cultures, but sometimes in unexpected ways.

Modern epistemic values, gender and the media

The entanglements of power, culture and science also come to the fore in other historical studies of forensic expertise. Foucauldian approaches have, for instance, highlighted how a modern form of disciplinary power targeted at the body took shape from the nineteenth century, in which law, medicine and psychiatry became inextricably connected, together giving rise to a discourse on criminal bodies and personalities.[31] Not only the bodies of criminals could be the target of disciplinary power, the embodied habitus of the expert was also moulded according to certain professional and cultural expectations. Here the concept of 'epistemic virtues' may be applied. Recent research on epistemic virtues has highlighted the importance of modern scientific values, for instance, objectivity and impartiality. Corinna Kruze has remarked that contemporary forensic culture has become increasingly probabilistic, in the face of acknowledgement of the inherent uncertainty of materials or technologies. Probabilistic reasoning and representation facilitate standardisation and the exchangeability of experts, thus also encouraging impartiality.[32] Overall, trust in experts is regarded as a principal hallmark of modern societies.[33] These epistemic values were also strategically appealed to in the modern courtroom. Stephanie Wright has, for example, shown how in sexual assault cases in Francoist Spain the prestige of modernity and objectivity surrounding medical evidence was strategically used by both the defence and victims, who regarded medical evidence as a potential shield against the notoriously arbitrary nature of the Francoist justice system.[34] And Pauline Dirven in her chapter in this volume describes how English forensic experts by means of wearing sober suits literally fashioned themselves as impartial, credible personae. Thus, she explores how epistemic virtues are fused with ideals of masculinity.

Dirven's work also demonstrates that cultural ideas and practices relating to the body and gender have undergone vast changes in the twentieth century, related to the rise of feminism, the sexual revolution, and the disciplining and mediatisation of bodies. These deserve to be further explored in historical research on forensic cultures. For example, the increasing participation of women in the police force, as lawyers, but also as forensic doctors, pathologists, chemists, psychiatrists and psychologists has so far hardly been addressed. Recent research has examined the relationship between forensic science and medicine and gender images in court cases,[35] but this focus can be extended to other types of cases. In her chapter in this volume, for instance, Alison Adam discusses the role of blood group evidence in a Scottish paternity case in 1957–1958, arguing that the rejection of the scientific evidence can be explained by considering the wider socio-cultural context of divorce, illegitimacy and the role of mothers in mid-twentieth century Britain, in addition to the mother's perceived unreliability as a witness.

The power of images is often played out in the media. Media reporting on crime and forensics have recently become themes in research on the history of modern forensic science.[36] The term 'CSI effect' started to appear in the US media in 2002, shortly after the TV series *CSI* was first broadcast. It refers to the concern that the jury members would expect more scientific evidence, as presented in the series, and hence have too high expectations of forensic expertise, which in turn might lead to unjustified acquittals. In his chapter to this volume, Filipe Santos explores the representation of forensic science and technology in Portuguese media, both tabloid and quality press. Santos found two dominant types of discourse regarding DNA technologies in specific: a more popular discourse celebrating DNA technology as 'truth machine' assisting justice, and a more critical discourse in quality newspapers that scrutinises actual forensic practices and resources. Again, we see that the reception of forensic science depends on a cultural context, which in modern times is shaped to a large extent by the media. Santos moreover underlines how the Portuguese projection of more sophisticated forensic techniques and scientific methods onto the United States by means of *CSI*, exemplifies the 'cultural effectiveness' of the imagination of a centre-periphery relationship in the media.

Practical dynamics and historical transformations of forensic cultures

The chapters in this volume engage with the above-mentioned elements of modern forensic culture: advanced technology and institutionalisation, but more importantly, novel epistemic virtues like objectivity, the impact of authoritarian regimes on forensic practices, gender images and the increasing importance of modern media in the representation of forensic science. Moreover, the chapters explore the relationship between the formal elements of forensic cultures and their practices, as well as their development.

The notion of forensic culture not only refers to a static culture, but also triggers questions about how a forensic culture changes and how forensic knowledge is transferred between different national or cultural contexts. In her chapter on Imperial Germany

Heather Wolffram traces the attempts to reform the curriculum of legal education (practitioners of criminal law) to include more attention to science, particularly criminalistics, in all parts of the criminal justice process, including investigation and prosecution. Wolffram prefers the notion of 'forensic culture' over 'forensic regime', since she regards the latter as limited to (attitudes towards) concrete forensic work in the mortuary or laboratory, whereas the former concept has an eye for 'all those ideas and values in circulation about the problem of crime and its investigation, not just among investigators, pathologists and scientists, but also among others involved in the criminal justice process as well as the public'. Applying this conception of forensic culture, Wolffram argues that in Imperial Germany the increasing use of expert witnesses and testimony of material evidence replaced a forensic culture in which judicial truth-finding was bound tightly by formal rules of evidence and dependent on confessions and witnesses. These innovative criminal justice practitioners sought to share forensic knowledge nationally, but also drew inspiration from foreign institutional models and practices, using the latter to encourage systematic change by appealing to patriotic anxieties of Germany lagging behind in comparison to other countries. This case study demonstrates that transitions to newer forensic cultures can take time and may be frustrated by state institutions and by debate over which professionals should lead the transition. Localised initiatives, for instance short instructional courses, can be the start of attempts at systematic innovation.

That it may take many years to change a forensic culture is demonstrated in Franco Orlandi's chapter on criminal anthropologists as expert witnesses in the Italian courtroom during the Liberal and Fascist regime (1910–1930). Criminal anthropologists such as Mario Carrara carried the legacy of the now infamous Cesare Lombroso (1835–1909) and still followed his theories. Carrara's 1940 *Handbook of Forensic Medicine* continued to stress Lombroso's link between body and criminal behaviour. Partially contradicting previous historians' claims that the Fascist regime used criminal anthropology to repress deviance by adopting its scientific racism, Orlandi argues that the Fascist judiciary was not necessarily benevolent towards Lombrosian medical witnesses. Perhaps more importantly, Orlandi shows that the theory of a forensic culture can contrast with its practice: Carrara was reluctant to employ explicitly Lombrosian language and methods in his psychiatric evaluations since he was aware that Lombroso's ideas had lost their scientific reputation in the interwar period. The contrast between forensic theory and its practice in the courtroom is addressed in other chapters as well. Volha Parfenchyk and Willemijn Ruberg compare forensic cultures in (Soviet) Russia and the Netherlands in the twentieth century in regard to 'crimes of passion' or 'jealousy crimes'. Using cultural historian Rebekka Habermas's method of 'doing law', which entails looking at justice as a 'process of negotiation involving many participants rather than a process of assignment', the authors aim to show that the nature of the 'crime of passion' was continually debated and negotiated by multiple actors: the legislature, the judiciary and psychiatrists. In their cross-cultural comparison, Parfenchyk and Ruberg conclude that both in Russia and the Netherlands the cultural discourse of 'crimes of passion' revolved around 'othering': these crimes were seen as typical of other countries or classes, thus confirming a certain self-image. The Soviet socialist discourse framed 'capitalist' jealousy as its opposite and the 'moderate' and 'rational' Dutch contrasted themselves with the passionate French and Italians who were seen as more lenient towards perpetrators trying to uphold their honour. In both countries perpetrators of this crime were regarded as backwards. However, legal practice did not always correspond to this cultural-political imagery, and sometimes even contradicted it.

That forensic practices can have their own dynamics comes to the fore in the chapter by Lara Bergers too. Bergers contrasts forensic medical practice in Dutch cases of sexual assault to medico-legal writings and thereby takes issue with common understandings in the historiography on rape regarding the distrust of the victims' testimonies and the importance of medical expertise. Qualifying the Dutch culture regarding the prosecution of sexual crimes in the period 1930–1960 as 'a culture of testimony', Bergers points to the absence of a jury, the slow professionalisation of defence attorneys and the lack of interest in witness psychology as factors that explain its features, but also warns that these do not automatically hold true for other types of crimes. Importantly, a forensic culture may thus only be functioning as such for specific crimes, not necessarily for a national system of criminal justice.

Bergers' chapter, as well as the chapters by Wolffram and Serrano Martínez, furthermore call for attention to the phase of the pretrial investigation and to cases that were dismissed by police or prosecutors. While due to a lack of available source material a historical analysis of such cases is challenging, a fuller understanding of forensic culture would benefit from a closer inspection of the mechanisms that underly dismissals. Also, the local police may selectively shape the narrative of a certain crime they encounter, possibly directing the further trajectory of the case, as Santos describes for the Portuguese urban and rural police forces in the period 1995–2010. Santos also remarks how during this initial phase of the investigation, Portuguese media were already highlighting forensic science as an explanatory factor for success or failure, thus moulding the narrative of the crime and potentially influencing the course of justice.

All chapters in this volume underline this entanglement of legal systems, procedural law and cultural images of science, victims and perpetrators. Svein Atle Skålevåg in his chapter highlights how legal systems, procedures and ideas on unaccountability came together in the local organisation of forensic psychiatry in Norway around 1900, arguing that the Norwegian forensic psychiatric culture had evolved towards consensus, both within the psychiatric community and between psychiatrists and lawyers. Skålevåg defines forensic culture as the working relationship between representatives of medicine and law, including everyone who took part in the legal process, both in courts of law and in parliament: lawyers, judges, forensic experts, writers on legal issues and politicians. This working relation was shaped both by inherent features of law and medicine and by more local characteristics in Norway. The criminal procedure, which did not encourage divergent medical opinions to be articulated in court, and the restructuring of forensic psychiatry, which led to the creation of a central commission for forensic medicine that oversaw the practice, produced a consensus-based forensic culture, seeking to generate uniformity of medical judgment.

The Norwegian focus on consensus underlines the importance of (epistemic) values and virtues, which are discussed in several chapters in this volume. Rachel Dixon and Tony Ward trace the prosecution of cases of infanticide in England in *c.* 1725–1945 and in particular the role of medical evidence. As the only authors in this volume to take a much larger timeframe into consideration, they illustrate how both uncertainty and certainty could be valuable resources for lawyers and the courts. Despite the advances in forensic pathology over this long period, doctors continued to express their uncertainties regarding the evidence. Dixon and Ward point to the context of the adversarial jury trial, to argue that jurors could use this medical uncertainty when they sympathised with the unmarried mother who killed her baby. For defendants it offered a line of defence. Interestingly, Dixon and Ward prove that – at least in cases of infanticide – there was a 'cautious forensic culture' that was different from the picture often painted by historians, who sketch uncertainty being produced by experts publicly disagreeing during the adversarial trial.

Whereas in the English infanticide cases the court performance of the medical experts could lead to leniency, the chapter by Sara Serrano Martínez shows that, by contrast, in the first two decades of the Franco regime, in practice Spanish forensic doctors made crucial contributions to the indictment and conviction of women who had committed infanticide, even when this contradicted the ideas and prescriptions expressed in textbooks on forensic medicine. From their medical standpoint, some medical experts framed the death of the baby as 'lack of care' – establishing the haemorrhage of the umbilical cord as cause of death – and thus as a criminal act. Serrano Martínez argues that both ideas about motherhood and the particular shape of the Francoist forensic culture allowed for the hypothesis of the umbilical haemorrhage to become typical in cases of suspected infanticide and provided the pretext for many convictions. Both chapters on infanticide thus highlight the (lack of) agency of the forensic experts, and how their findings, as presented in the courtroom or in pre-trial written reports, are also connected to their performance of epistemic values.

Equally or even more important than values such as consensus and certainty, has been the quality of objectivity. In her chapter, Pauline Dirven zooms in on a notion closely related to objectivity, namely that of impartiality. Perhaps surprisingly, Dirven takes as a case study the practice of dress by English forensic experts in 1920–1960 to show that these experts adopted a sober middle-class look, thus enacting a sense of trust and authority and suggesting impartiality. By wearing sober, dark-coloured, three-piece lounge suits and matching overcoats, they conformed to the modern, masculine, middle-class fashion trend of the 1920s–1950s. Dirven argues that in this way they could convince the jury that they were impartial, objective witnesses, whose testimony could not be 'bought' by the prosecution or defence party, a fear that often surfaced in the adversarial system. Thus, Dirven also proposes that historians concentrate more on the practices through which experts fashioned themselves as impartial, credible personae, rather than on how historical actors have shaped forensic evidence as objective knowledge. This focus on the embodiment of epistemic virtues is an important part of the cultural and performative turn that promises to make original contributions to histories of forensic cultures.

Conclusion

To conclude, this book aims to dissect the notion of 'forensic culture', showing how the production of forensic knowledge in practice is inextricably connected with ideological and cultural norms, national legal and political institutions, procedural law and local legal, scientific and medical practices. It calls for a more thorough analysis of the connections between science, culture and politics, at the same time as underscoring how the performance of experts is shaped by epistemic virtues and the bodily fashioning of experts' personae. As I have argued, this volume calls for exploring the notion of 'forensic culture' in more detail, particularly in regard to distinguishing features of modernity, while highlighting forensic *practices*.

Future research can hopefully build on the directions taken by the chapters in this volume, but may also delve into new themes. Firstly, studies of forensic culture should broaden the units of analysis: from the nation state to regions as well as international, perhaps global, connections. A truly transnational or global history of forensic practices remains to be written. And although this volume contains several steps towards comparison, we still need more systematic comparative histories of forensic science. This book also underlines the shifting boundaries of forensic cultures at the same time as pointing to the importance of studying the transfer of knowledge. As Wolffram argues in her chapter in this volume, the interplay of national and international (educational) systems of forensic knowledge and expertise deserves much more attention. Secondly, whereas forensic culture so far has mostly been studied in relation to criminal law, future research should connect this field with forensic cultures surrounding civil law and international criminal and human rights law, including forensic anthropology. In addition, it may excavate how these fields have come to be studied apart from each other and how that relates to discipline formation. Thirdly, a novel adoption of phenomenological approaches may inform us better about what happens in the encounter between forensic doctors and victims or perpetrators.[37] In any case, the chapters in this volume point towards the many ways in which science, legal systems, politics and ideas, together with individual people – experts, perpetrators, victims, judges, prosecutors, lawyers, reporters – make up forensic cultures in practice.

Notes

This project has received funding from the European Research Council (ERC) under the European Union's Horizon 2020 research and innovation programme (grant agreement No 770402). I would like to thank Lara Bergers, Anne van Dam, Pauline Dirven, Sara Serrano Martínez and Ido de Haan for their excellent feedback on previous versions of this introduction, and Anne van Dam for also helping with the index to this volume.

1 For an overview see Katherine D. Watson, *Forensic Medicine in Western Society. A History* (London and New York: Routledge, 2011); see also Francesco Paolo de Ceglia (ed.), *The Body of Evidence: Corpses and Proofs in Early Modern European Medicine* (Leiden and Boston: Brill, 2020); Michael Clark and Catherine Crawford (eds), *Legal Medicine in History* (Cambridge: Cambridge University Press, 1994); Wendy J. Turner and Sara M. Butler (eds), *Medicine and the Law in the Middle Ages* (Leiden and Boston: Brill, 2014).
2 For an overview see Simon A. Cole and Alyse Bertenthal, 'Science, Technology, Society, and Law', *Annual Review of Social Science* 13 (2017), pp. 351–371.
3 Reiner Grundmann, 'The Problem of Expertise in Knowledge Societies', *Minerva* 55 (2017), pp. 25–48.
4 Lorraine Daston and Peter Galison, *Objectivity* (New York: Zone Books, 2010 [2007]).

5 Simone Lässig, 'The History of Knowledge and the Expansion of the Historical Research Agenda', *Bulletin of the German Historical Institute* 59 (Fall 2016), pp. 29–58; Harry Oosterhuis, 'Sexual Modernity in the Works of Richard von Krafft-Ebing and Albert Moll', *Medical History* 56:2 (2012), pp. 133–155.
6 E. Summerson Carr, 'Enactments of Expertise', *Annual Review of Anthropology* 39 (2010), pp. 17–32; Stephen Hilgartner, *Science on Stage: Expert Advice as Public Drama* (Stanford, CA: Stanford University Press, 2000).
7 Christopher Hamlin, 'Forensic Cultures in Historical Perspective: Technologies of Witness, Testimony, Judgment (and Justice?)', *Studies in History and Philosophy of Biological and Biomedical Sciences* Part C 44 (2013), pp. 4–15, here p. 4.
8 Simon Cole, 'Forensic Culture as Epistemic Culture: The Sociology of Forensic Science', *Studies in History and Philosophy of Biological and Biomedical Sciences* Part C 44 (2013), pp. 36–46, here p. 36.
9 Christopher Hamlin, 'Introduction', in Ian Burney and Christopher Hamlin (eds), *Global Forensic Cultures. Making Fact and Justice in the Modern Era* (Baltimore: Johns Hopkins University Press, 2019), pp. 1–33, here pp. 17–18.
10 Hamlin, 'Introduction', p. 3.
11 Alison Adam, 'Crime and the Construction of Forensic Objectivity from 1850: Introduction', in Alison Adam (ed.), *Crime and the Construction of Forensic Objectivity from 1850* (London: Palgrave, 2020), pp. 1–13, here p. 3.
12 Adam, 'Crime and the Construction of Forensic Objectivity', p. 5.
13 *Ibid*., p. 3.
14 Hamlin, 'Introduction', p. 17.
15 Adam, 'Crime and the Construction of Forensic Objectivity', pp. 2–3.
16 Neither of the two aforementioned edited volumes reflects on the notion of modernity as a concept that refers to more than a period. Bruno Bertherat, 'Cleaning Out the Mortuary and the Medicolegal Text: Ambroise Tardieu's Modernizing Enterprise', in Burney and Hamlin, *Global Forensic Cultures*, pp. 257–278 discusses 'Tardieu's progression' (p. 271) and focuses on the advancement of forensic medicine, while also placing Tardieu in a social context.
17 Joris van Eijnatten, Ed Jonker, Willemijn Ruberg and Joes Segal, 'Shaping the Discourse on Modernity', *International Journal for History, Culture and Modernity* 1:1 (2013), pp. 3–20.
18 Catherine Crawford, 'Legalizing Medicine: Early Modern Legal Systems and the Growth of Medico-Legal Knowledge', in Clark and Crawford (eds), *Legal Medicine in History*, pp. 89–116; Watson,

Forensic Medicine in Western Society; Tal Golan, *Laws of Man and Laws of Nature: A History of Scientific Expert Testimony* (Cambridge, MA: Harvard University Press, 2004). Katherine Watson, *Medicine and Justice: Medico-legal Practice in England and Wales, 1700–1914* (London: Routledge, 2020). Roland Bal, 'How to Kill with a Ballpoint: Credibility in Dutch Forensic Science', *Science, Technology, & Human Values* 30:1 (2005), pp. 52–75.

19 Jeffrey Jentzen, 'Death and Empire: Medicolegal Investigations and Practice across the British Empire', in Burney and Hamlin, *Global Forensic Cultures*, pp. 149–173; Mitra Sharafi, 'The Imperial Serologist and Punitive Self-Harm: Bloodstains and Legal Pluralism in British India', in Burney and Hamlin, *Global Forensic Cultures*, pp. 60–85; Binyamin Blum, 'From Bedouin Trackers to Doberman Pinschers: The Rise of Dog Tracking as Forensic Evidence in Palestine', in Burney and Hamlin, *Global Forensic Cultures*, pp. 205–234. Simon Cole, *Suspect Identities: A History of Fingerprinting and Criminal Identification* (Harvard: Harvard University Press, 2002).

20 Ian Burney and Neil Pemberton, *Murder and the Making of English CSI* (Baltimore: Johns Hopkins University Press, 2016).

21 Burney and Pemberton, *Murder and the Making of English CSI*; Willemijn Ruberg and Nathanje Dijkstra, 'De forensische wetenschap in Nederland (1800–1930): een terreinverkenning', *Studium* 9:3 (2016), pp. 121–143; José Martínez Pérez, 'Restableciendo la salud del Estado. Medicina y regeneración nacional en torno a un proceso judicial en la encrucijada de los siglos XIX al XX', *Dynamis* 18 (1998), pp. 127–156.

22 Thomas Keenan and Eyal Weizman, *Mengele's Skull: The Advent of a Forensic Aesthetics* (Sternberg Press: Frankfurt am Main, 2012), p. 67.

23 Francesco Mazzucchelli, 'From the "Era of the Witness" to an Era of Traces Memorialisation as a Process of Iconisation?' in Zuzanna Dziuban (ed.), *Mapping the 'Forensic Turn': Engagements with Materialities of Mass Death in Holocaust Studies and Beyond* (Vienna: New Academic Press, 2017), pp. 169–191; Roma Sendyka, 'Posthuman Memorialisations, Memorials After the Forensic Turn', in Dziuban (ed.), *Mapping the 'Forensic Turn'*, pp. 291–308.

24 Watson, *Forensic Medicine*, pp. 54, 149; Ian Burney, *Bodies of Evidence: Medicine and the Politics of the English Inquest, 1830–1926* (Baltimore: Johns Hopkins University Press, 2000).

25 Jentzen, 'Death and Empire', p. 153. The coroner system existed in Scotland only between 1400 and 1800.

26 See José Ramón Bertomeu Sánchez, 'Fingerprints and the Politics of Scientific Policing in Early Twentieth-Century Spain', in Burney and Hamlin, *Global Forensic Cultures*, pp. 174–204.

27 Dan Healey, 'Russian and Soviet Forensic Psychiatry: Troubled and Troubling', *International Journal of Law and Psychiatry* 37:1 (2014), pp. 71–81. See also Dan Healey, *Bolshevik Sexual Forensics: Diagnosing Disorder in the Clinic and Courtroom, 1917–1939* (DeKalb, IL: Cornell University Press, 2009) and Kateřina Lišková, ' "Now You See Them, Now You Don't": Sexual Deviants and Sexological Expertise in Communist Czechoslovakia', *History of the Human Sciences* 29:1 (2016), pp. 49–74.
28 P. H. Solomon, *Soviet Criminologists and Criminal Policy: Specialists in Policy-Making* (New York: Columbia University Press, 1978).
29 Cyrille Fijnaut, *Criminology and the Criminal Justice System: A Historical and Transatlantic Introduction* (Cambridge: Intersentia, 2007), pp. 325–354.
30 Mary Gibson, *Born to Crime: Cesare Lombroso and the Origins of Biological Criminology* (Westport: Praeger, 2002).
31 Michel Foucault, 'About the Concept of the "Dangerous Individual" in 19th Century Legal Psychiatry', *International Journal of Law and Psychiatry* 1 (1978), pp. 1–18; Michel Foucault, *Les anormaux: cours au Collège de France, 1974–1975* (Paris, Gallimard; Seuil, 1999). Michel Foucault, *Surveiller et punir: naissance de la prison* (Paris, Gallimard, 1975); Svein Atle Skålevåg, 'The Matter of Forensic Psychiatry: A Historical Enquiry', *Medical History* 50:1 (2006), pp. 49–68.
32 Adam, 'Crime and the Construction of Forensic Objectivity from 1850', pp. 7–8; Corinna Kruze, 'Making Forensic Evaluations: Forensic Objectivity in the Swedish Criminal Justice System', in Adam (ed.), *Crime and the Construction of Forensic Objectivity from 1850*, pp. 99–121.
33 Kerstin Brückweh, Dirk Schumann, Richard Wetzell and Benjamin Ziemann (eds), *Engineering Society: The Role of the Human and Social Sciences in Modern Societies, 1880–1980* (Basingstoke: Palgrave Macmillan, 2012); Joris Vandendriessche, Evert Peeters and Kaat Wils (eds), *Scientists' Expertise as Performance: Between State and Society, 1860–1960* (London: Routledge, 2015).
34 Stephanie Wright, ' "Facts that are Declared Proven": Francoism, Forensic Medicine, and the Policing of Sexual Violence in Twentieth-Century Spain', paper given at the conference 'Forensic Cultures', Utrecht University, 26–28 August 2021. See also Stephanie Wright, ' "Caballeros mutilados" y mujeres "deshonradas": cuerpo, género y privilegio en la posguerra española', *Historia y Política* 47 (2022), pp. 163–192, here p. 182.
35 J. Du Mont and D. Parnis, 'Sexual Assault and Legal Resolution: Querying the Medical Collection of Forensic Evidence',

Medicine and Law 19:4 (2000), pp. 779–792; Victoria Bates, *Sexual Forensics in Victorian and Edwardian England: Age, Crime and Consent in the Court* (Basingstoke: Palgrave Macmillan, 2016); Heather R. Hlavka and Sameena Mulla, *Bodies in Evidence. Race, Gender, and Science in Sexual Assault Adjudication* (New York: NYU Press, 2021).

36 See Heather Wolffram, ' "Children's Lies": The Weimar Press as Psychological Expert in Child Sex Abuse Trials', in Adam (ed.), *Crime and the Construction of Forensic Objectivity from 1850*, pp. 257–278; Lindsay Steenberg, *Forensic Science in Contemporary American Popular Culture: Gender, Crime, and Science* (London and New York: Routledge, 2013).

37 See Joanna Bourke, 'Police Surgeons and Victims of Rape: Cultures of Harm and Care', *Social History of Medicine* 31:4 (2018), pp. 711–731.

1

Blood will out: Blood typing, forensic culture and gender in a 1950s Scottish paternity case

Alison Adam

Introduction

By the late 1950s a number of techniques from forensic science were well accepted in the repertoire of crime analysis around the world, hence criminal and civil courts were familiar with dealing with expert scientific evidence.[1] By the 1950s the significance of blood typing and laws of inheritance of blood types were well understood and scientifically accepted; paternity cases had already been decided on their basis as, of course, had murder cases.[2] At first sight, it is difficult to understand why the judges in the appeal stage of the paternity case described in this chapter were able to reject blood-typing evidence based on seemingly incontrovertible scientific analyses. However, I argue that a range of factors should be considered in order to understand why a court could deny conclusive scientific evidence. These include the historical treatment of women in relation to forensic evidence, especially in relation to their perceived unreliability, coupled with the wider cultural context of divorce, illegitimacy and the role of mothers in mid-twentieth century Britain. It is also clear that there was considerable variation, even to the point of inconsistency, in the acceptance of scientific evidence in court in the middle of the twentieth century.

The case considered here was an unusual paternity case from Scotland that was heard in the Court of Session (civil court) in Edinburgh in 1957 and 1958.[3] Blood group evidence which demonstrated conclusively that the putative father was not the child's biological father, although accepted in the initial case, was subsequently rejected by the judges in the appeal hearing. It is an important case in Scots law and has attracted a considerable amount of legal attention largely because of the rejection of widely accepted, conclusive scientific analyses. The case is listed in the canonical *Law of Evidence in Scotland* and it is referenced in a number of articles and dissertations.[4]

Broader cultural concerns must be set alongside the particular legal matters which contributed towards the rejection of the scientific evidence in this case. These include the requirement for the mother to produce a high standard of proof (beyond reasonable doubt) that the putative father was *not* the biological father and the strong presumption in Scots law that a man who married a woman after a child is born must be the child's father. Although scientific evidence was admissible in Scottish courts in the mid-twentieth century, in practice there was considerable variation in its acceptance. Indeed, as this case demonstrates, the (same) scientific evidence was accepted in the initial hearing but rejected in the appeal, although on the grounds of admissibility in this case; there was no argument against the validity of blood typing as a scientific technique. There are examples in Scots law, in this period, of cases where a well-accepted forensic analysis was rejected despite the implicit arrangement whereby Scottish courts admitted accepted scientific analysis as evidence. Conversely, there are also cases where a far from well-accepted scientific technique was held to be admissible. Examples of both are discussed later in this chapter. The considerable variation in the acceptance of scientific findings and the closure which was apparently offered by forensic evidence was contingent on legal and cultural circumstances. In particular, the scientific objectivity of forensic evidence in paternity cases rested on a complex entanglement of factors including the use of blood grouping and views on marriage, the proper way to raise children, the moral character of the mother and legal standards for evidence.

This chapter attempts to add to the burgeoning literature where cultural factors including gender are used to explain how forensic evidence is shaped.[5] This literature primarily focuses on criminal cases, mainly infanticide, sexual assault and rape. Nevertheless, there are clear parallels between the way that women have historically been treated in criminal cases in relation to forensic medical evidence and the treatment of the main actor in this case study in terms of the characterisation of women as not 'respectable', as unreliable witnesses and prone to lying. For instance, Judith Rowbotham, writing on Victorian sexual offences, argues that the perceived virtue of 'respectability' was central to the performance of women as 'victims' and to cultural stereotypes of 'victimhood' in court.[6] Victoria Bates contends that medical evidence was an important part of the cultural construction or denial of women as victims. Many women were denied the right to be seen as victims because they were not regarded as respectable.[7] In relation to infanticide, Daniel Grey has shown that in England and Wales in the twentieth century and beyond, forensic expertise was central in infanticide trials. Yet such evidence could be selectively applied and was subject to significant challenge by juries and even the media and public opinion when findings were not in keeping with preconceptions of women's respectability.[8] Indeed, in the paternity case described below, the perception of the woman's respectability appears to have been a significant factor facilitating the judges' rejection of scientific analyses in the appeal hearing.

Such views are reinforced by a wider literature on family life, discussed below, that focuses on the unreliability of women, especially women who were mothers.[9] This chapter adds to the literature by demonstrating the importance of understanding how forensic evidence may be used, or denied, to reinforce stereotypes of appropriate female behaviour, even in civil cases not concerned with sexual assaults.

In the following section the use of scientific evidence in the Scottish legal system in the mid-twentieth century is described, noting considerable variation in the acceptance of scientific evidence. The development of blood typing and its use and limitations in paternity testing is considered in the next section and this provides the scientific context for the present case. The discussion is then broadened to the wider context of parenthood, illegitimacy and the role of the mother. It is against this backcloth that the paternity case described here, *Imre v Mitchell*, is considered.

Scientific evidence and Scottish courts

Forensic medicine flourished in Scotland through the nineteenth and into the twentieth century in medical schools and forensic experts were widely used by the Scottish Courts.[10] However, the balance of forensic excellence began to change in the UK by the 1930s. Evidence suggests that officials in the Scottish Home and Health Department, the UK government department responsible for Scottish affairs including policing, looked with envy at the newly instituted network of forensic science laboratories set up by the Home Office in England and Wales and found the situation in Scotland with regard to forensic science to be wanting.[11] Hence, from a position of pre-eminence in forensic medicine in the early years of the twentieth century there was a perception that Scotland was lagging behind in its use of scientific evidence in courts in the post-war period.

The Scottish legal system is separate to that of England and Wales, with a separate legislation and court structure although both are adversarial systems. In Scotland, serious criminal cases are heard before a jury. Most civil cases (except for personal injury claims) do not involve a jury and are decided by a judge or judges. The paternity case considered here was heard by one judge in the initial hearing and a bench of four judges in the appeal hearing. As in other legal jurisdictions no formal legal test of scientific acceptability existed in the UK, in this period. Maher points out: 'the traditional, though largely implicit, approach of Scots law [is] that admissibility of expert evidence depended upon it being based on generally accepted methodology ... there was no special role for the court to be satisfied that the methodology was sound.'[12]

Indeed the oft-quoted case law which demarcates the role of expert evidence in Scots law is a civil case which was heard in the Court of Session in 1953.[13] In relation to this case, the judge, Lord Justice Cooper, stated: 'The scientific opinion evidence, if intelligible, convincing and tested, becomes a factor (and often an important factor) for consideration along with the whole other evidence in the case, but the decision is for the Judge or jury.'[14] Although this case was based on a very different scientific area from the paternity case considered in this chapter, it is nevertheless important in understanding the use of scientific evidence in Scots law because it demarcates the admissibility of scientific evidence in Scots law and has become the canonical case on this topic. The case involved a claim for damage to houses in Edinburgh where the pursuer argued that blasting activities, which had been undertaken in the course of constructing new sewers, had damaged his house and neighbouring properties. The city authorities produced civil engineering expert witnesses who gave evidence as to the mathematical relationship between the destructive capabilities of an explosive blast and the distance from a property indicating that the blasting could not have caused the damage. Paradoxically, while accepting the credentials and competence of the evidence of the main expert witness, the judge, Lord Justice Cooper, found *against* the city authorities and awarded damages to the pursuer, apparently believing that houses do not sustain structural damage without reason so the city authorities' blasting activities must have been responsible.[15] Arguably the judge was making a 'common sense' decision. As he stated, the scientific evidence must not usurp the decision of judge or jury, who may come to a decision which opposes the evidence, which was the decision here.[16]

The civil engineering case set the standard for expert scientific evidence in general in Scots law, however, it is fingerprinting which has often been held to set the gold standard of forensic infallibility. A case from 1934, where the only identification evidence was a set of fingerprints which police experts confirmed was a complete match on sixteen points, established what Scottish courts came to understand by 'infallible means of identification' thereafter.[17] In this case the appeal court heard that fingerprinting as a means of identification had been widely used around the world and there had never been an example of identical prints identified from two different people. Here the court produced a definition of the expert view of infallibility by arguing that it was a question of *practical* rather than *absolute* infallibility and the reliability of the evidence (both in legal and scientific terms) could be accepted, 'not because it is irrebuttable in its own nature, but because long and extensive experience is shown to prove no instance in which it has ever been successfully rebutted'.[18]

Conversely, there were important cases in Scotland in a similar period where less than solid scientific techniques were accepted with relatively little discussion. An example of this is a much-quoted murder case from 1967 where a conviction was secured by the evidence of a bite-mark on a murdered girl's body as there were no witnesses and no other trace evidence to link the perpetrator to the crime. At the time this was hailed as 'a triumph for forensic odontology' despite forensic odontology being an embryonic discipline.

Indeed, it was a discipline whose ability to provide objective evidence would come into question in subsequent years.[19]

The judge in the civil engineering case went against the findings of the experts on damage due to blasting. In the bite-mark case a youth from a special school for young offenders was convicted on the evidence of photographs of a single bite-mark matching dental impressions at a time when forensic odontology had only been used in a handful of cases in the UK. These three examples from civil engineering, fingerprinting and bite-mark identification added to case law which helped define and delineate the admissibility of scientific evidence in Scots law. Coupled with the paternity case described below, where the appeal court judges dismissed incontrovertible blood type evidence, these four cases demonstrate that there was considerable variation in the interpretation of admissibility of generally accepted science in the Scottish legal system in the mid-twentieth century.

The development of blood typing for paternity testing

Before the advent of blood typing, if there was no other evidence available, one of the main ways of attempting to ascribe disputed paternity was through family resemblance.[20] However, the whole landscape for paternity claims changed with the discovery of blood types and the laws for the inheritance of blood types which depend on the blood types of the parents. The human ABO blood groups, MNS system and the inheritance of blood groups were discovered in the early part of the twentieth century; the Rhesus system in 1940. Blood typing can never offer certainty of positive identification, only the possibility in some cases. However, it can provide certainty of negative identification, i.e. exclusion, but, again, only in some circumstances. As the red cell antigens are inherited a child cannot have a blood group antigen that is not present in one or both parents. For example, if the child belongs to group A and both the mother and the putative father are group O, the man is excluded from paternity.

If a potential father was not excluded by a test under the ABO system, the serologist could test whether the father was excluded under the MNS system and could also consider Rhesus status. Such tests were well accepted in many legal jurisdictions by the 1950s, which suggests that, although one could potentially challenge the way that a test had been carried out if, for instance, there was evidence of poor procedure or contamination, if the tests were carried out properly then the results should be regarded as conclusive.[21]

Possibly the most famous paternity case of this period was that of the film star, Charlie Chaplin. Astonishingly, in 1943 a US court ruled that Charlie Chaplin was the father of a child where a blood test had shown that he was definitely excluded.[22] Although the circumstances and fame of the main characters in the *Chaplin* case were very different from the case described later in this chapter, nevertheless there are similarities in terms of the denigration of the mother's character and accusations of promiscuity. Despite the result of the *Chaplin* case, a legal conclusion which overturned blood type evidence was becoming harder to uphold in the USA in the late 1940s and 1950s. For instance, in *Ross v Marx* (1952) although other evidence pointed to the defendant being the father of the child, he was nevertheless excluded on the evidence of blood tests. The court took the view that the results of the blood tests were not opinions on which experts could differ but were scientifically established facts where 'for a court to declare that these tests are not conclusive would be as unrealistic as it would be for a court to declare that the world is flat'.[23] Although decisions such as these had no legal force in Scotland, they were nevertheless well known and the science behind them was well accepted.[24]

The wider context for paternity cases in the 1940s and 1950s

When it comes to admissibility of blood-typing evidence it is clear that the issues involved in establishing paternity claims were broader than just the determination of blood types. In many societies, until relatively recently, a level of stigma surrounded birth to parents who were not married. For the aristocracy, so-called illegitimate children could not inherit titles, wealth or land.[25] The language surrounding this is important. The terms 'bastard', 'bastardise' and 'bastardy' were in legal use at the time of this court case. Although these are indeed legal terms, at the same time they are highly pejorative terms which still assault contemporary sensibilities. The terms 'illegitimate' in relation to the birth of children, 'bastard' and 'bastardise' were removed from Scots law in 1986; 'declarator of bastardy' or 'illegitimacy' was changed to 'declarator of parentage or non-parentage' reflecting a welcome relaxation of views on marriage and parenting in the UK from the fourth quarter of the twentieth century.[26]

Although the mother, and to some extent the father, might bear the stigma of a child born outside marriage, the full weight of stigma was held to fall on the child, who had no choice as to its birth.[27] 'Through the late Victorian period to World War II and even beyond, bastardy was a serious stigma legally, socially and emotionally.'[28] Attitudes towards sexuality and legitimacy did not begin to relax until the 1960s with the advent of the so-called 'permissive society', but it is fair to say that the permissive society was still a long way over the horizon in 1950s Scotland.[29]

Hence, when the judges made much of the stigma of illegitimacy in the legal judgment in this case's appeal hearing they were reflecting widely held contemporary views which were reinforced by legal language. In paternity cases there are implications for the maintenance and upkeep of a child, considerations as to whether the child would be maintained by the mother, father, the family or even by the state. Indeed, in the appeal hearing in the case described below, the judges accused the mother of potentially trying to 'saddle' another man with the paternity of her child with the implication that another man could be made responsible for the child's maintenance as a result of her potentially fraudulent claim.[30] This reinforced negative views of women as devious and deceptive where they were seen as potentially perpetrating fraud against a man, and also fed on a pejorative view of women as promiscuous.[31]

Paternity cases were quite often related to divorce petitions. From 1937 in England and Wales, and 1938 in Scotland, it was possible to obtain a divorce for matrimonial offences including adultery yet it was not particularly easy to get a divorce and it was not common in mid-twentieth century Britain.[32] High levels of divorce were regarded as a social welfare issue, particularly for the children of divorcing parents.[33] Additionally, the war years were seen as having placed particular strain on family life. After the Second World War the rebuilding of the nuclear family was seen as central to the reconstruction of the country in social and economic terms.[34] The war had affected not just physical aspects of family life but also the social and moral fabric of family life with worries about illegitimate births in the war years and divorces, many of which were on the grounds of adultery. There was a widespread view that family life and marriage had been undermined by promiscuity and infidelity.[35] However, as Pat Thane argues, rather than extramarital sexual relations being 'invented' later on in the 1960s, they were commonplace through the nineteenth and twentieth centuries and a substantial percentage of children were born to parents who were not married.[36] It was attitudes rather than behaviour which began to change in the 1960s. Concern over promiscuity and the potential for the breakdown of family life during and after the war years can be seen as a form of 'moral panic', despite relatively low rates of marriage break-up. Indeed, as Pat Thane suggests, there is a lengthy history of moral panics about the disintegration of the family. Moral panics over family life have regularly surfaced over the last century or more, suggesting that these ought to be treated with some scepticism.[37] In post-war Britain, problem families and neglected children were largely blamed on the mother.

Although there was criticism of fathers – as in the trope of 'absent fathers' – there seems little doubt that it was the women, the mothers, who were subject to far more condemnation in relation to the perceived threat of family break-up. Separated mothers were said to take up with new partners, committing adultery, and giving birth to illegitimate children, exposing children to 'the gravest moral danger'.[38] The 'feckless mother' or problem mother was the ideal construction of a blame figure on which to project anxieties about class and even eugenics.[39] The next section discusses how this played out in the current case where the judges appeared to largely subscribe to the stereotypical view of women as directly responsible for problem families. The story reflects legal views on the stigma of illegitimacy and the role of one particular 'feckless mother' who was unreliable to the point of lying in court, possibly promiscuous and, therefore, in the eyes of the court an unsuitable person to gain custody of her child.

Imre v Mitchell (1958)

The bare facts of the *Imre v Mitchell* 'declarator of bastardy' case are as follows.[40] The 'pursuer', Betsy Imre, wished to have her daughter legally declared a bastard. Imre, the mother of the child in question, had married the 'father' of the child, Alexander Mitchell, in January 1949, a few weeks after the child's birth in December 1948. Less than three years after the marriage the child's father divorced her on the grounds of her adultery (she left Mitchell for another man, Imre, in 1951 and had subsequently married him after the divorce) and the 'father' had been granted custody of the child since then. The mother did not contest the custody at the time of the divorce and access arrangements were made.[41]

A year or so later Betsy Imre started legal proceedings for a 'declarator of bastardy' claim in order to pursue a legal case to prove that Mitchell was not the child's father. She maintained that the father of the child was another man, a Polish soldier, who had been based in a camp in Perthshire near her house, after the war. She asserted that she had sexual relations with the soldier after dances held in the Polish soldiers' camp in April 1948. She said she met Mitchell in August 1948 when he had asked her to marry him and she agreed. Meanwhile, the soldier was repatriated to Poland, now under communist rule, and he could not be contacted. Betsy Imre's aim in bringing the declarator of bastardy claim was to have the child legally declared illegitimate so that it would be recognised that Mitchell was not the child's father. The court case was unable to authorise custody directly, nevertheless she believed this was the route by which she could ultimately gain custody of her child.

Blood tests from the mother (Imre), 'father' (Mitchell) and child (Rosemary) were made and analysed by three serologists (lecturers in forensic medicine from the University of Glasgow); these tests excluded Mitchell from being the natural father of the child. In the original court proceedings Betsy Imre's claim was upheld and the child was declared illegitimate.[42] However, Mitchell immediately appealed and the original ruling was overturned in the appeal hearing where the court rejected the scientific evidence and Imre's evidence and found Mitchell to be the father. It was held that blood group evidence alone was insufficient to enable the court to displace legitimation of a child whose parents had married after its birth. Furthermore, it was held that the blood group evidence had been obtained improperly, that there was a very small chance of mutation in a blood group and that Betsy Imre's evidence was not sufficient to uphold her claim.[43]

Even though proper permissions had not apparently been obtained (a serious matter in itself), the rejection of the scientific evidence from the blood tests excluding Mitchell from being the father of the child could appear akin to declaring the earth to be flat. Hence it is unsurprising that the case has attracted attention.[44] Nevertheless, there is considerably more to this case than a seemingly inexplicable rejection of incontrovertible scientific evidence as the following sections discuss.

Reasons for the appeal hearing decision

Under Scots law there is a strong presumption that a man is the legitimate father of a child if he is married to the mother at the time of birth or if he marries her after the birth of a child. The appeal court judges also held the view that having declared a child legitimate, the legitimacy could not readily be removed later. The legal presumption that a man is the father of a child if he subsequently marries the mother after the birth is of longer standing in Scots law than in English law where there was a change to illegitimacy law in 1926. Hence, although by the time of this court case Scots and English law were aligned with respect to legitimacy conferred by subsequent marriage, this legal point had a much longer pedigree in Scots law. The long-standing aspect of this legal point may have added weight to the seriousness with which the judges pronounced the 'almost irresistible presumption of legitimacy'.[45] In Scots law, the meaning of this legal expression is that a child is presumed legitimate by being born to married parents or to parents who subsequently marry such that the presumption of legitimacy cannot be 'resisted' and should not be subsequently removed. Hence, although this is primarily a legal presumption, it is also implicitly a biological assumption in that Scots law presumes that a man would not marry a woman unless he knew himself to be the father of the child. Until the advent of blood typing, it could be argued that the biological presumption was immaterial as it would not have been possible to prove whether the man was the biological father or not. Furthermore, Lord President Clyde, one of the appeal court judges, pointed out:

> It is an agreed point by all writers, that if either of the two (parents) have ... acknowledged the child as lawful, there is a right acquired to him by that acknowledgment which is not to be taken away by any posterior testimony to the contrary. In my opinion this principle applies in the present case and renders the testimony of the pursuer in the present case of no avail for the purpose of establishing her case of illegitimacy.[46]

Hence, the legal point, based on long-standing Scots law, is not just that marriage gives an 'irresistible presumption of legitimacy', it is also that a parent could not go back later and declare the child illegitimate. However, at least in this case, blood testing threatened to undermine the long-established law which held that a child should not have its legitimacy removed. Understandably, under the circumstances where scientific evidence threatened long-standing law, which mapped out how a child was to be treated within the family, a judge might wish to reject the science. Indeed, Lord Clyde was quoting from a book of Scots law written in 1785. His argument was echoed forcefully by his colleague, Lord Sorn, who stated in the appeal hearing: 'there is something abhorrent in the idea that spouses should acknowledge a child and yet be allowed to keep it up their sleeves at any time to revoke this decision and take away the status of legitimacy they have ostensibly bestowed upon the child.'[47]

Competence of the legal action

A major issue which was raised in the appeal was whether or not the original legal action was 'competent', i.e. whether it was legally permissible, focusing on how the blood test evidence had been acquired. Although the original legal hearing had accepted the blood tests as admissible evidence, two of the appeal court judges, Lords Carmont and Russell, subsequently held that the blood test evidence was inadmissible as proper consent to the tests had not been granted either by the second defender, Mitchell, or on behalf of the child, Rosemary (the first defender). The putative father, Mitchell, although an adult and therefore able to consent to blood tests, had not understood what the tests were for and so had been put into a position which was potentially disadvantageous to him. Permission for the child's test had been given by a *curator ad litem* (a legal representative appointed by the court to represent the interests of the child) who made no representation in court. The lack of in-person representation was criticised by the judges who also held that the *curator ad litem* was not an appropriate person to give such permission in the first place. Rosemary was legally a 'pupil' child, in other words a child under the age of twelve, so it was necessary for a legal guardian to give permission for the blood tests.[48]

In the appeal case, four judges were sitting (not including Lord Wheatley who presided over the original case); one of these judges was Lord Clyde, who was the most senior judge of the Scottish judiciary (Lord President) and who demonstrated a clear antipathy towards scientific evidence. Even though the scientific and other evidence was unchanged from the initial hearing, the court reversed the original decision, holding that the pursuer had failed to overcome the 'almost irresistible presumption' of the paternity of a child whose mother has married a man who knew her to be pregnant.[49] By a majority, the appeal court judges rejected the blood test because Mitchell had not appreciated what he was doing when he gave a sample of blood, and also because consent for taking the child's blood sample was not given by the appropriate person. In a recent Scottish paternity case there had been a ruling that no one could be compelled to take a blood test.[50] Although the child had not been forced to take the blood test, the fact that consent was not given by the right person made the precedent case relevant. Importantly, it was emphasised that 'the advisers of a child whose blood is to be so tested should hesitate before they allow a course to be taken which may have a devastating and lasting effect on that child's whole life, especially when it is a course which the Court will not compel anyone to adopt'.[51]

For the original court proceedings, blood samples were taken from Imre, Mitchell – via his solicitors – and from the child, Rosemary, via the *curator ad litem*. The blood groups of the parties on the ABO system are not detailed in the legal report hence it can be inferred that it was not possible to exclude Mitchell on the ABO system. However, on the MNS system the results were:[52]

Imre MM
Rosemary MM
Mitchell NN.

In the original hearing, under the presiding judge, Lord Wheatley, the results of the blood tests were held to demonstrate that Mitchell could not have been the father as he would have had to pass an N factor to the child which was not present. In terms of possible errors, there was a very small chance of a mutation which could invalidate the tests; the serologists undertaking the blood tests stated that such mutations were no more frequent than 1 in 100,000 cases. There was also a very small chance of a weaker N2 factor which could be read as an M which had recently occurred in a Danish case. However, the expert witnesses knew about this possibility and were especially careful to look for it (the blood tests were undertaken in triplicate) so it seems extremely unlikely that the N2 factor was present.[53]

Nevertheless, Lord Wheatley had stressed the potential unreliability of the tests emphasising in particular the possibility of a mutation and of non-detection of a weak N2 antigen, refusing to accept the proposition that the evidence could be regarded as completely conclusive. On the other hand, his lordship had also pointed out that:

> The fact that there is 100,000 to one chance of error in a test does not rob that test of all evidential value. On the contrary, if the proposition is stated the other way, namely that the odds are 100,000 to one on the test being accurate and proving the non-paternity of Mitchell, it can be said that the high degree of probability is sufficient to discharge the onus of proof which the law requires for the establishment of the pursuer's case.[54]

On this basis Lord Wheatley held that the pursuer had proved her case to the required high standard of proof. He accepted that the scientific evidence was sufficiently conclusive, exhaustive and accurate, and also, given the possibility of mutation rated by the experts was about 1 in 100,000 (likely to be an expression of a very low probability rather than a calculated probability), this was held to be sufficient in law to discharge the onus of proof required for the establishment of non-paternity.[55]

In terms of whether the pursuer had succeeded in establishing that her child was illegitimate: 'our law has always regarded the label of illegitimacy as involving a taint which the Courts will be slow to attach to any child unless the circumstances clearly warrant it. For once the label is attached it will almost certainly accompany that child to the grave.'[56]

The appeal court judges were insistent that it would have formed a dangerous precedent if Imre were allowed to bastardise her child. The judges regarded the onus of proof on the pursuer, Imre, to be extremely heavy and they held that she had *not* proved that Mitchell was not the father. It is important to note that before the law in Scotland was changed in 1976, illegitimacy cases were held to a higher standard of proof than the 'balance of probabilities' standard normally used in civil cases. 'The presumption against illegitimacy, when it arose, could be rebutted only by proof beyond reasonable doubt.'[57] The expected standard of proof was, therefore, equivalent to that of criminal cases and was, therefore, much harder for Imre to achieve. Despite this, in the initial case, heard before Lord Wheatley, it was held that this high standard of proof *had* been achieved by the scientific evidence, yet this was overturned on appeal. Even before considering the court's negative view of Imre a number of factors were stacked against her claim in terms of the presumption of legitimacy, given she had married Mitchell after Rosemary's birth, the higher standard of proof required, the question of consent to the blood tests and the very small chance of a mutation, hence the scientific evidence was crucial.

Fallibility of scientific evidence

Imre's evidence was not accepted by the appeal judges largely because they believed she lied and was of unreliable character; numerous imputations as to her lying and feckless character were peppered through the legal reports. In the initial hearing, the judge effectively decoupled the unreliability of Imre's evidence, the 'irresistible presumption of legitimacy' and the question of whether the blood tests had been legitimately obtained from the incontrovertible scientific evidence. The appeal court judges settled on the very small chance of error, arguing that the tests were not reliable given the small chance that there was an error. They also argued that Imre had not proved her case beyond reasonable doubt. The appeal court judges were not prepared to accept that the scientific evidence proved Imre's case; indeed they did not accept that the scientific evidence was conclusive.

Arguing against accepting the blood-typing evidence, one of the appeal court judges, Lord Sorn, stated that the appeal court was asked to treat the blood test evidence in the same way that fingerprint evidence is treated in terms of its certainty; 'the finger print system is not a system based upon theory and it has been so well tested over many years that it can claim, as nearly as may be, to be infallible ... But in this case, and especially in view of the strong presumption in favour of legitimacy [because the 'putative' father had married the mother], I am not prepared to bastardise the child on the strength of the blood test alone.' Lord Sorn continued:

> it is clear from the evidence that on present scientific and medical knowledge this test is not infallible. It is in quite a different category therefore from the finger print test the basis of reliability of which is its never having been proved wrong. In contrast to this the M.N. test has been shown to fail, and its essential basis (namely that the child's blood must contain one or more of the factors disclosed in the sample of a father's blood) has been shown not to be universally true ... In the first place, it has recently been ascertained that the factors in a child's blood may change... The infallibility of the test is destroyed. In the second place, a misleading result may be obtained owing to the presence of a factor in a weak form which the test did not disclose [the N2 factor].[58]

It is difficult to appreciate why Lord Sorn believed that the fact that fingerprinting was not based on theory made it superior to blood typing in terms of fallibility.[59] Alistair Brownlie, the solicitor for the pursuer, Betsy Imre, commented in a later article that the fingerprint comparison was unfortunate. Just because no two fingerprints had been shown to be alike does not mean it is impossible; rather it is a question of probabilities. Writing in 1965, Brownlie argued:

> It is ... hardly correct to say that blood groups contrast unfavourably with fingerprints because the former 'have been shown to fail' when the fingerprint system is similarly 'fallible'. The truth is surely that

fingerprints and blood groups both now afford a sufficiently reliable basis for the decision of ordinary human affairs.[60]

As Brownlie pointed out, the upshot of this case was that, for two decades Scottish courts were wary of blood group evidence – 'blood grouping was regarded as unsatisfactory and not to be touched by solicitors'.[61] However, the situation quietly and gradually changed and by the 1980s Scottish courts were accepting blood group exclusion evidence. There was no sudden revolution, rather it appears to have been a gradual acceptance of this type of scientific evidence which had already become well accepted in England and elsewhere.

Gender and scientific evidence

In terms of the balance between scientific research and the question of the legitimacy of a child, Lord Sorn argued in the appeal case: 'the Court should have regard to the non-medical evidence in the case to see to what extent the scientific evidence is confirmed or confuted by such other evidence.'[62] There is little doubt that the evidence she gave, and the manner in which she gave it, cast Betsy Imre in a bad light and all the judges, both in the original case and in the appeal, had a low opinion of her character. She was only eighteen when her child was born and she married Mitchell, and it seems that very little allowance was made for the transgressions of youth, the fact that she may have been quite a vulnerable person herself rather than being the calculating, promiscuous woman portrayed by the legal profession. The attempt to show that Mitchell was not the father and to progress the case took place over a period of five or more years. Clearly, Betsy Imre had been persistent in her attempts to gain custody of the child and was prepared to put herself through a stressful court case where her private life was put on very public display. None of this seemed to work in her favour. It is hard to escape the conclusion that the language used to describe her in the legal reports portrayed her in such a negative light that it facilitated the rejection of her evidence. There are so many negative nuances used in the legal reports and the appeal that there is space to detail only the most striking of these here.

> Since 1951 the child has in fact remained in the custody of Mitchell ... The pursuer however now seeks to go back on all this. According to her evidence, she had been having sexual relations with a Pole in April and the following months of 1948 ... As a result of this association ... she became pregnant ... She did not scruple therefore to take advantage of so timely an offer of marriage, nor did she hesitate to deceive the man who had offered to marry her [Mitchell]. She states that she never had any affection for him at all, and indeed it was not long after the marriage that she became party to a course of adultery which led to its termination. Her object in this present action is to get round the decree of custody ... so as presumably to represent herself as a fit and proper person to have the custody of the child herself. The means ... an action in which she seeks to brand her own child as an illegitimate ... her endeavour to saddle the Pole with paternity ... does not exclude the possibility of the Pole, or for that matter some other man, being the father, since the pursuer might well have been indulging in promiscuous intercourse with different men at the time ... if she had been a truthful, acceptable, and reliable witness her identification of the father would have carried great evidential weight. As I concluded that she was lying in certain instances, and she had an avowed and selfish motive in seeking to bastardise the child.[63]

The judge went on to state: '[T]he pursuer was quite willing to let the divorce action go undefended in order to facilitate her marriage to her present husband, who was then her current paramour, even if it meant foregoing custody of the child at the time...'[64] In the space of a few paragraphs, the pejorative language of the judge was clear and had the effect of completely undermining Betsy Imre's character.

Conclusion

The verdict on Betsy Imre's character was damning enough to undermine the evidence she gave, which was then held to be unable to outweigh the scientific evidence. Imre was classified as a 'feckless mother', a promiscuous woman who had lied to her former husband and had lied to the court. The judges argued that she could have potentially damaged her child in her attempts to 'bastardise' her and hence to gain custody. The aspersions which were cast on

Imre's character align with the stereotypical view of women often found in the literature on gender and forensic medicine.[65] In addition to the view of Imre as lying and selfish this also included the view that she was promiscuous, and although this was not strictly relevant to the case it served to further undermine her character. Ironically, Betsy Imre appears to have lived with her second husband, her 'current paramour' for at least the next fifty years in a quiet suburb of Edinburgh until her death.[66] The court proceedings reveal little sympathy for Imre with no suggestion that she may have been taken advantage of by the men in her life at a young and impressionable age. Daniel Grey, Judith Rowbotham and Kim Stevenson emphasise the importance of the perception of women as respectable in order to be seen as victims in infanticide and sexual assault cases.[67] Any 'respectability' that Betsy Imre had was undermined by the negative light in which she was portrayed.

The appeal court was not prepared to abandon many years of legal precedent in Scots law which states that a child born to parents who marry is the child of the father. In addition, they were not willing to see this long-standing law undermined by scientific evidence. There was clear antipathy to scientific evidence from the most senior judge in the appeal case, Lord Clyde, who spoke sternly about solicitors 'who dabbled in scientific stuff'.[68] In any case the appeal judges were not prepared to grant that Imre had proved that Mitchell was not the father beyond reasonable doubt which was the evidence standard then required in illegitimacy cases. Given the 'beyond reasonable doubt' standard the only way that Imre could have proved that Mitchell was not the father of her child, given that she was unable to contact the child's real father and given that her other evidence was a matter of her word against Mitchell's word, was through the blood-typing evidence. When a majority of the judges rejected the blood-typing evidence in the appeal hearing, Imre's case was fatally undermined.

The irregularity of Betsy Imre's evidence, the unreliability of her character and the question of whether obtaining the blood test evidence was legally valid, reinforced the unfavourable comparison between potentially fallible blood testing and supposedly infallible fingerprinting as forensic techniques. Yet, at the same time, the scientific and other evidence was unchanged from the first hearing to the appeal hearing. Rather it was the judges' interpretation of the scientific evidence read against their belief that Imre had not proved her case beyond reasonable doubt, which was different from the original hearing. This echoes Grey's point that forensic evidence can be selectively applied if not in keeping with preconceptions as to women's behaviour.[69] This case demonstrates the ways in which forensic fallibility or infallibility of scientific techniques, even those such as this technique which was widely accepted in this period, is interwoven with legal norms and cultural and social concerns, in particular relating to gender and views on how women ought to behave.

Notes

1 See Alison Adam, *A History of Forensic Science: British Beginnings in the Twentieth Century* (Abingdon: Routledge, 2016), pp. 118–154.
2 Alistair R. Brownlie 'Blood and the Blood Groups: A Developing Field for Expert Evidence', *Journal of the Forensic Science Society* 5 (1965), pp. 124–174.
3 The original case was *Imre v Mitchell* 1958 SLT 57 heard on 12 July 1957 where it was held that the blood group evidence proved Imre's case. The original case was heard before Lord Wheatley at the Court of Session, Edinburgh. *Imre v Mitchell* 1958 SC 439 and *Imre v Mitchell* 1959 SLT 13 are the main documents for the appeal hearing heard on 23 March 1958. The appeal was heard before Lord President Clyde and Lords Carmont, Russell and Sorn.
4 Margaret L. Ross and James P. Chalmers, *Walker and Walker: The Law of Evidence*, Third Edition (Haywards Heath, West Sussex: Tottel, 2009), p. 96; Susan V. Hartshorne, 'Proof of Paternity: the History' (M.Phil. dissertation, University of Manchester), p. 64; Brownlie, 'Blood and the Blood Groups', pp. 170–171; Nicholaos E. Kotsifakis, 'Towards a New Perspective in the Parent Child Relationship' (LLM thesis, University of Glasgow, 1981), pp. 47, 58; Geoffrey W. Bartholomew, 'The Nature and Use of Blood-Group Evidence', *Modern Law Review* 24:3 (1961), pp. 319–330; Alistair R. Brownlie, *The Treasured Years: An Enhanced Autobiography* (Kilmarnock: ICS books, 2006), pp. 227–922.
5 Victoria Bates, 'Forensic Medicine and Female Victimhood in Victorian and Edwardian England, *Past and Present* 245:1 (2019), pp. 117–151; Daniel Grey, 'The Lady Vanishes? Forensic Culture, "Common Sense" and the Ongoing Problem of Infanticide in

England and Wales, 1900–2020', Forensic Cultures Conference, 26–28 August, 2021, Utrecht; Ivan Crozier and Gethin Rees, 'Making a Space for Medical Expertise: Medical Knowledge of Sexual Assault and the Construction of Boundaries between Forensic Medicine and the Law in late Nineteenth-Century England', *Law, Culture and the Humanities* 8:2 (2012), pp. 285–304; Judith Rowbotham and Kim Stevenson (eds), *Criminal Conversations: Victorian Crimes, Social Panic, and Moral Outrage* (Columbus OH: Ohio State University Press, 2005).

6 Judith Rowbotham, 'Criminal Savages? Or "Civilizing" the Legal Process', in Rowbotham and Stevenson (eds), *Criminal Conversations*, pp. 91–105.
7 Bates, 'Forensic Medicine and Female Victimhood', p. 130.
8 Grey, 'The Lady Vanishes?'.
9 Rosemary Elliot, 'Suffer the Children? Divorce and Child Welfare in Postwar Britain', *Journal of Family History*, 46:4 (2021), pp. 433–459; Pat Starkey, 'The Feckless Mother: Women, Poverty and Social Workers in Wartime and Post-War England', *Women's History Review* 9:3 (2000), pp. 539–557.
10 M. Anne Crowther and Brenda White, *On Soul and Conscience: The Medical Expert and Crime* (Aberdeen: Aberdeen University Press, 1988).
11 See National Records of Scotland (NRS) File HH55/711 Identification of Criminals: Laboratory assistance in connection with criminal investigation in Scotland, 1939–1967; Brownlie, *The Treasured Years*, p. 229.
12 Gerry Maher, 'Guarding the Gate: Some Problems in Expert Evidence in Scots Law' (Edinburgh Law School Working Papers; No. 2015/07, University of Edinburgh) p. 5.
13 Craig Adam, *Forensic Evidence in Court: Evaluation and Scientific Opinion* (Chichester: Wiley, 2016), p. 59.
14 *Davie v Magistrates of Edinburgh* 1953 SC 34, p. 40. Scots law cases are available via the Westlaw database.
15 *Ibid*.
16 Maher, 'Guarding the Gate', p. 2.
17 *Hamilton v HM Advocate* 1934 JC 1. This is a leading case establishing the competence of fingerprinting in Scots law. See Ross and Chalmers, *Walker and Walker: The Law of Evidence*, p. 96. This case is cited in Maher, 'Guarding the Gate', p. 4.
18 *Hamilton v HM Advocate* 1934 JC 1, pp. 3–4; Maher, 'Guarding the Gate', p. 4.
19 Alison Adam, 'The Biggar Murder: 'A Triumph for Forensic Odontology', in Alison Adam (ed.), *Crime and the Construction*

of *Forensic Objectivity from 1850* (Cham, Switzerland: Palgrave Macmillan, 2020), pp. 69–98. It is notable that bitemark evidence is now regarded as unreliable. See Michael J. Saks *et al.*, 'Forensic Bitemark Identification: Weak Foundations, Exaggerated Claims', *Journal of Law and the Biosciences* 3:3 (2016), pp. 538–575.
20 Nara B. Milanich, *Paternity: The Elusive Quest for the Father* (Cambridge MA: Harvard University Press), pp. 98–104.
21 The most widely used blood group system is the ABO system but there are many others including the MNS system. The ABO blood group system is used to classify blood types according to different types of antibodies in blood plasma and antigens in the blood cells. For a detailed description of blood group systems, including the identification of thirty-three blood grouping systems (as of 2014) see Ranadhir Mitra, Nitasha Mishra and Girija Prasad Rath, 'Blood Group Systems', *Indian Journal of Anaesthesia* 58: 5 (2014), pp. 524–528. For a discussion of the significance of blood group systems to paternity cases in this period see Brownlie, 'Blood and the Blood Groups', pp. 129–133.
22 Milanich, *Paternity*, pp. 1–5, 326.
23 *Ross v Marx* 90 A. 2d 545 (1952); Bartholomew, 'The Nature and Use of Blood-Group Evidence', p. 319.
24 Crowther and White, *On Soul and Conscience*, pp. 108–110.
25 Milanich, *Paternity*, p. 3.
26 See Family Law (Scotland) Act 2005 Section 15B for abolition of illegitimacy which also made it no longer possible to bring a declarator of illegitimacy action (pp. 11–12). The Law Reform (Parent and Child) (Scotland) Act 1986 repealed earlier legislation on declarator of bastardy or illegitimacy on the recommendation of the Scottish Law Commission's Report on Illegitimacy (1983) which recommended the removal of differences between legitimate and illegitimate people and the removal of declarators of bastardy and illegitimacy. The report found the term 'declarator of bastardy' was 'needlessly offensive' (p. 42) and recommended the terms 'declarator of parentage or non-parentage' instead (p. 43).
27 Ginger Frost, ' "The Black Lamb of the Black Sheep": Illegitimacy in the English Working Class, 1850–1939', *Journal of Social History* 37:2 (2003), pp. 293–322.
28 *Ibid.*, p. 293.
29 Frank Mort, 'Victorian Afterlives: Sexuality and Identity in the 1960s and 1970s', *History Workshop Journal* 82:1 (2016), pp. 199–212.
30 *Imre v Mitchell* 1958 SC 439; *Imre v Mitchell* 1959 SLT 13.
31 Starkey, 'The Feckless Mother'.

32 Elliot, 'Suffer the Children?'.
33 *Ibid.*
34 Janet Fink, 'Natural Mothers, Putative Fathers, and Innocent Children: The Definition and Regulation of Parental Relationships outside Marriage in England, 1945–1959', *Journal of Family History* 25:2 (2000), pp. 178–195.
35 *Ibid.*, pp. 178–179.
36 Pat Thane, 'Happy Families, History and Family Policy', A Report prepared for the British Academy, British Academy, 2011, Available at www.thebritishacademy.ac.uk/publications/happy-families-history-family-policy/, accessed 20 July 2022, p. 7.
37 *Ibid.*, p. 67.
38 Elliot, 'Suffer the Children?', p. 7.
39 Starkey, 'The Feckless Mother'.
40 *Imre v Mitchell* 1958 SC 439; see note 26 for the evolution of the term: 'declarator of bastardy'.
41 *Ibid.*, p. 1.
42 *Imre v Mitchell* 1958 SLT 57.
43 *Imre v Mitchell* 1958 SC 439.
44 See note 4 above.
45 *Imre v Mitchell* 1958 SC 439, p. 15. Refers to John Erskine, *An Institute of the Law of Scotland* (Edinburgh: Bell, 1785). For the change in English law in 1926 see Frost, ' "The Black Lamb of the Black Sheep" ', p. 293 and Fink, 'Natural Mothers', p. 190.
46 *Imre v Mitchell* 1958 SC 439, p. 17.
47 *Ibid.*, p. 23.
48 *Ibid.*, p. 1.
49 *Ibid.*, p. 16 and see note 67.
50 *Whitehall v Whitehall* 1958 SC 252.
51 *Imre v Mitchell* 1958 SC 439, p. 18.
52 Brownlie, *The Treasured Years*, p. 228.
53 *Imre v Mitchell* 1958 SC 439, p. 8.
54 *Ibid.*, p. 9.
55 *Imre v Mitchell* 1958 SLT 57, p. 3.
56 *Ibid.*, p. 15.
57 Ross and Chalmers, *The Law of Evidence*, p. 60 points to the historical exceptions to the Scots civil law evidence standard of the 'balance of probabilities' where the presumption against illegitimacy could be rebutted only by proof beyond reasonable doubt. *Imre v Mitchell* is cited as one of the precedent cases. 'All of these exceptions are now superseded by the general application of the general civil standard to all family proceedings regardless of the issues raised', p. 60.

58 *Ibid.*, p. 17.
59 *Hamilton v HM Advocate* 1934 JC 1.
60 Brownlie, *The Treasured Years*, p. 229.
61 *Ibid.*, p. 229.
62 *Imre v Mitchell* 1958 SLT 57, p. 9.
63 *Imre v Mitchell* 1958 SC 439, pp. 2–3.
64 *Ibid.*, p. 12.
65 Bates, 'Forensic Medicine and Female Victimhood', p. 130.
66 I have inferred this from a death notice in a newspaper. No reference is given in order to protect the privacy of Mrs Imre's family members.
67 Grey, 'The Lady Vanishes?'; Rowbotham and Stevenson, *Criminal Conversations*.
68 Interview between Alison Adam and Alistair Brownlie OBE, 29 September 2016. Mr Brownlie was the solicitor who prepared Mrs Imre's case. He recalled being warned off using this type of scientific evidence by the judiciary and that it was Lord Clyde who was particularly keen to exclude the scientific evidence in the appeal hearing.
69 Grey, 'The Lady Vanishes?'.

2

A culture of testimony: The importance of 'speaking witnesses' in Dutch sexual crimes investigations and trials, 1930–1960

Lara Bergers

Introduction

In 1949, a family returning home after a springtime outing encountered the eighteen-year-old nanny 'crying and in a totally excited state'. Worried, her employers asked her what had happened. She explained that she had been out enjoying the weather when she was sexually assaulted by a stranger. Upon hearing this, her employer drove to the local police station and brought back an officer. After a quick recounting of the story, the officer, the employer and the victim hopped in the employer's car and drove around town in an attempt to find the perpetrator. On the main road from Soest to Utrecht the girl spotted her attacker riding a bike. After a confrontation with the victim and a brief interrogation, right there on the side of the road, the suspect confessed. Police also interviewed a number of witnesses, who had encountered the distraught victim and returned her to her employers' home. More extensive questioning of the victim and the suspect followed, after which the suspect was examined by a psychiatrist, convicted and sentenced to one year in prison.[1]

While many cases of sexual violence tried between 1930 and 1960 by the court in Utrecht were more complicated, in this chapter I show that this 1949 case is typical in its dependence on testimony and concomitant neglect of physical evidence. In fact, I argue that the investigations and trials of sexual crimes in this period were marked by a 'culture of testimony,' with the evidence provided by 'speaking witnesses', including victims, occupying a central role. This claim runs counter to what has been found in other national contexts, with historians of forensic science showing that the 'testimony of people' had become increasingly de-emphasised in favour of the 'testimony of things' since the turn of the nineteenth century.[2] In some forensic cultures – including in the United States, England, France and German-speaking Europe – a number of developments coincided to create a 'crisis of confidence around witness credibility'.[3] In Germany, for example, the formal rules excluding some specific types of 'incompetent' witnesses were gradually abandoned in favour of the principle of 'free evaluation of evidence' by judges, resulting in new eligibility to testify for witnesses, including women and children, who had previously been excluded.[4] At the same time, new psychological research into human perception and memory called the reliability of witnesses into question – a finding exploited by newly professionalising defence attorneys.[5] According to historians of forensic science Ian Burney and Neil Pemberton, this crisis had two interrelated consequences. Firstly, it created an increasing realisation that those involved in criminal investigations and prosecutions needed to deepen their understanding of the fallibility of witness testimony and to 'adjust their strategies for eliciting and interpreting witness statements' to avoid being led astray. Secondly, 'commentators elevated material over human testimony, seeking out "mute witnesses" wherever possible to short-circuit the evident dangers of relying on the human alternative'.[6]

The realisation that witness testimony was central to Dutch sexual violence investigations in the early and middle part of the twentieth century is also surprising in light of research by historians of sexual violence, who have found that the testimony of victims has seemingly been perpetually distrusted. Confronted with overwhelming evidence that rape was a severely underreported crime and that women who came forward often had to go through a gruelling and invasive process, only for the case to be dismissed or for the offender to be acquitted, activists and sociologists have sought to explain these injustices since the 1970s. They have concluded that pervasive, wrongheaded attitudes about rape – 'rape myths' – are a major contributing factor.[7] Historians interested in sexual violence have established that these same myths are pervasive in their historical material as well. The evidence for the persistence and consistency of these ideas in medico-legal literature is especially plentiful.[8]

The mismatch between the empirical findings presented in this chapter and the existing historiography points to some of the idiosyncrasies of early and mid-twentieth century Dutch forensic culture generally, and early and mid-twentieth-century Dutch sexual violence investigations and trials in particular. As shown in the next section, the content of Dutch medico-legal literature was largely in line with international literature about the reliability of victims and witnesses of (sexual) crime; it is in its examination of investigative and trial practices, then, that this chapter exposes some of these particularly Dutch characteristics. In centring forensic practices in my analysis, I have heeded the advice and followed the examples of scholars such as Stephen Robertson, Louise Jackson, Victoria Bates and Willemijn Ruberg.[9]

The chapter is based on an examination of thirty-three case files, as well as 128 verdicts of sexual violence cases tried at the Utrecht criminal court between 1930 and 1960. They include extramarital rapes (article 242 of the Dutch criminal code), sexual assaults (article 246), instances of sexual intercourse with underaged girls (articles 244 and 245), indecency [*ontucht*] with a child under the age of sixteen (247) and indecency with a minor under one's education or care (249). In the period under examination, the crimes listed under articles 242 and 246 were committed with the use of violence or under the threat of violence, while sexual acts with a minor were illegal regardless of the level of threat or violence. Dutch case files are meant to contain all documentation drawn up during the course of the investigation and are sent, in their entirety, to the trial judge(s). It is on the basis of the case file and additional testimony at trial that a verdict is reached. Unfortunately, some of the case files in my sample are incomplete, especially those tried in the 1950s. Verdicts, meanwhile, list the minimum amount of evidence necessary for a conviction.[10] The cases in this sample were randomly selected with the aim of revealing the day-to-day goings-on of sexual crimes investigations and trials. I have supplemented my analysis with an examination of the prosecutors' registers from the period 1960–1969, as well as medico-legal and police literature.

Internationally circulated ideas about the reliability of witnesses

Doubts about the reliability of women and children who reported sexual violence were consistently discussed in medico-legal textbooks in the nineteenth and twentieth centuries. Both in original Dutch works and in translations of works by international authors, the claim that allegations of sexual violence were often made up was repeated as an undisputed fact.[11] Whether for the purpose of blackmail, to protect their honour and the reputation of the men who fathered their illegitimate children, or because they were hysterical, women who accused men of rape were considered particularly likely to lie. The Dutch judge W. E. T. M. van der Does de Willebois phrased it pointedly in his 1904 handbook for investigators:

> The danger for the prosecution to be led astray is perhaps nowhere as large as precisely in these types of crimes ... It occurs that a hysterical woman or girl proclaims all sorts of evil things about an entirely innocent man. To extort money from him, he is sometimes threatened with a police complaint about a crime against the morals, and if the case is investigated, the accusation is maintained against better judgement. It has also happened that a girl, who had a molar pulled by a doctor, made the entirely false claim that he, after sedating her, had sexual intercourse with her. Later it became clear that the girl was pregnant by a boy ... and to protect his and her own honour and name, had resolved to place the blame of her pregnancy on the doctor. The possibility of a false accusation, then, ... will often need to be taken into account.[12]

Authors like van der Does de Willebois warned that children – particularly girls – should likewise be treated with suspicion; impressionable as they were, they could easily be taught to deliver a well-rehearsed story to aid in a blackmail-scheme or revenge-plot. Besides, children were fantasists: they might simply have imagined that something inappropriate had happened.[13]

From the turn of the nineteenth century, pre-existing ideas about the reliability of victims of sexual violence were supported by German and French findings in the new field of witness psychology. The new science had found that 'women forget less, but fabricate more'. It was also argued that too much credence was given to children's statements, that children under the age of seven were entirely unsuited to give testimony and that no one should be convicted on the basis of children's testimony alone.[14] Witness psychology, of course, went beyond doubting accusations by would-be victims of sex crimes, but called into question the reliability of witness testimony in general – based on evidence of the fallibility of human perception and memory – and offered practical solutions to avoid being misled. The findings of the new science were circulated in the Netherlands, for example when they were printed, apparently with approval, in *Het Weekblad van het Regt* (The Weekly Journal of Law) in 1905; like their German and French colleagues, then, Dutch legal practitioners encountered new calls to be careful about the use of 'speaking witnesses'.

Pemberton and Burney have argued that the loss of faith in the witness was connected to the elevation of 'the testimony of things'. In the Netherlands, too, investigators became more interested in physical evidence from the turn of the century. This is apparent from the establishment of private criminalistics laboratories – most notably by Co van Ledden Hulsebosch in 1910 – the rise of crime scene photography and fingerprinting in police departments, and the publication of police handbooks summarising the work of Hans Gross. A more complete institutionalisation of forensic science in the Netherlands would arrive in the late 1940s and early 1950s with the establishment of national institutes for criminalistics, forensic psychiatry and psychology, and forensic pathology.[15]

Even as there was an increasing interest in the 'testimony of things', however, the level of concern about witness testimony in the early to middle part of the century seems to have been limited: there was little original Dutch research on the subject, and when the newly scientifically established unreliability of witnesses was acknowledged, commentators resisted the idea that psychologists should be brought into the courtroom to address the issue.[16] In 1935, the attorney S. J. M. van Geuns noted that Dutch judges displayed good psychological insight and were able to question witnesses in such a way as to avoid suggestion and to value witness statements appropriately: 'Most of the time the judge will be able to assess the reliability for himself.'[17]

In what follows, I show that Dutch forensic practice in cases of sexual violence proceeded from a base-level of trust in the statements of 'speaking witnesses'. Before delving into the case files and verdicts that make up my sample, however, I must contend with a challenge that plagues the historiography on rape: interpreting acquittals and dismissals.

Making sense of dismissals

An acquittal or dismissal may be an indication that the victim's accusation was not believed. Indeed, feminist activists and sociologists who raised alarm over the treatment of victims of sexual violence in the 1970s pointed to high dismissal and acquittal rates to underwrite survivors' harrowing tales of scepticism and ill-treatment by law enforcement and the judiciary. Due to limitations of the source material, it can be difficult to gain an insight into the reasoning behind dismissals and acquittals; in my sample, verdicts relating to acquittals contain no information indicating why the court found the suspect not guilty. In any event, if a case went to trial, acquittal was unlikely: there are only four such cases in my sample (3 per cent). Dutch prosecutors had discretion to decide whether any given case was to be prosecuted and brought to trial; indeed, dismissals by prosecutors were far more common than acquittals and left little documentation behind.[18] While I did not have access to information about the number of cases dismissed before trial in the period 1930–1960, I was able to study the prosecutors' registers for the 1960s, which shows that a substantial number of sexual violence cases did not make it to trial (44 per cent).[19] I have no reason to believe that the dismissal rate would have been significantly different in the preceding period.[20]

The prosecutors' registers often contain a two-word explanation of why a given case was dismissed. Though limited, this information can shed some light onto the proportion of cases in which distrust of victims may have played a role. Among the reasons given in the prosecutors' registers, two classes are most likely to involve doubts about the truth of an allegation: 19 per cent of dismissals resulted from the facts of the allegation not being a crime under Dutch law. It is clearly possible that such dismissals resulted from the prosecutor *not believing* crucial details of the allegation. Specifically, a prosecutor and other legal actors might have thought that sexual acts had indeed occurred, but that the would-be victim had actually consented. Additionally, concerns about false accusations may have played a role in those dismissals that resulted from a lack of evidence (21 per cent).

However, a dismissal did not *necessarily* mean that the truth of an allegation was doubted. Indeed, in the types of dismissal just described, it is possible that the complainant's statement was believed in its entirety, but either simply did not fit the formal definition of a crime under Dutch law or was not supported by any other evidence. As the Dutch Code of Criminal Procedure specified that judges could not declare a suspect guilty on the basis of the statement of one witness only, there could be insufficient evidence even when police and prosecutor deemed the victim totally reliable.

Moreover, in a significant number of dismissals, the truth of the allegation was irrelevant, not doubted or assumed. Some cases were dismissed due to the youthful age of the suspect (19 per cent); in such cases the prosecutor judged that prosecution or punishment would not be in the best interest of the young suspect or, indeed, society at large. Prosecutors also had discretion to dismiss cases conditionally; they agreed to not pursue the case so long as the suspect did not reoffend and fulfilled a number of pre-agreed conditions. The majority of cases dismissed by the prosecutor in the 1960s was of this type (29 per cent). In such cases, too, it appears the victim was, at core, believed.

The dismissal of a case of sexual violence would likely have felt like an injustice to many victims. There is insufficient evidence, however, to suggest that such injustice necessarily or even typically resulted from distrust of victims, even as ideas about the unreliability of sexual crimes victims were familiar to prosecutors and other actors involved. Based on data from the prosecutors' registers of the 1960s, I have found that a portion of dismissals – 40 per cent, or some 18 per cent of the total number of cases reported to the prosecutor – *may have* resulted from the victim's allegation being called into question. The number of cases among them where distrust of the victim *actually* resulted in dismissal is unknowable. In what follows I examine casefiles and verdicts from the period 1930–1960. Given the Dutch Procedural Code's insistence on two pieces of independent evidence, I will examine the ways that the second piece of evidence – the first being the complainant's statement – was typically furnished.

The curious absence of doctors

The first notable finding is that medical testimony played a negligible role in sexual crimes investigations. Among the 161 cases examined, I found evidence of a medical practitioner being involved in only four (2 per cent). To be sure; it is possible – even likely – that doctors were involved in other cases for which no complete case file exists. Remarkably, however, even in cases where a medical witness would have been in a position, according to medical textbooks, to provide clarity – e.g. in cases where the suspect confessed to indecency, but not to sexual intercourse – verdicts made no mention of medical testimony.

In the four cases in which there is evidence of a medical examination, the issue that ostensibly needed to be resolved was indeed whether sexual intercourse had taken place. The examinations were done by general practitioners, who may or may not have had a pre-existing relationship with local police; so-called police-doctors treated officers and their families, and were called upon to treat suspects in police custody or to weigh in on forensic medical issues. Police-doctors were not, however, required to have a specialist education, nor did they perform this role full-time. In each case the doctor's report was minimal – scribbled on a prescription note, or verbally given to police – underscoring the lack of standardisation.

Regarding the descriptions of injuries and the conclusions they drew, the doctors' writings also differed. Police-doctor W. van der Giesen, who examined a twelve-year-old victim in 1939, described the girl's injuries, but left his conclusions about whether penetration had occurred entirely unspoken. His sticky-note-sized report read simply: 'During the examination of the 12-year-old [victim], residing in Woerden, it became clear to me that the hymen was no longer intact. Other injuries were not perceptible.'[21] By contrast, the general practitioner Dr M. G. Pannekoek, who examined a twenty-year-old victim in 1937, expressed his conclusions in terms of how likely he considered it that penetration had taken place, finding it was as good as certain that the victim had had intercourse with a man shortly before the examination. He provided no indication of how he had reached this conclusion.[22]

Beyond the limited number of cases in which a doctor was involved or the lack of standardisation of the reports, it is striking how little impact the medical findings had on the court's verdict. In three of the four cases, the court did not mention the medical reports and, in fact, in each case came to the opposite conclusion regarding penetration. Only the 1953 statement by Dr W. J. van der Hooft, director of the Amersfoort municipal health service, was mentioned in the verdict, though not in reference to the issue of whether sexual intercourse had occurred. Instead, his description of the four-year-old victim's injuries served to motivate the severity of the sentence.[23]

Trusting witnesses

Given that medical evidence played such a limited role, and criminalistics evidence, moreover, is virtually absent from my sample, it is clear that sexual violence investigations and trials revolved almost exclusively around the testimony of victims, third-party witnesses and suspects. The roles of eyewitnesses and confessions in sexual crimes cases have gone almost entirely unexplored in the history of sexual violence, presumably due to the – rather intuitive – assumption that suspects of crimes generally deny their involvement and that sexual crimes are typically committed in the absence of witnesses.

However, even taking into account that this sample is biased towards cases with strong evidence, given that they would otherwise have been dismissed by the prosecutor, the characterisation of sexual crimes as particularly shrouded in secrecy does not seem to apply to Dutch forensic culture in the period 1930–1960. Indeed, eyewitnesses were involved in many cases. In a number of instances in my sample a passer-by directly witnessed something untoward in a public space, such as a park, a bicycle parking area, or a swimming pool, but even when a witness had not directly observed the crime, their testimony could occasionally play an important role. This was true, for example, in a case of 1949, in which the suspect confessed to having sexually assaulted an eighteen-year-old man who was unconscious due to excessive drinking. As the Dutch Code of Criminal Procedure stipulated that a court could not convict on the basis of a confession only and the victim had no memory of the assault, the circumstantial evidence provided by a witness who had seen the suspect exiting the victim's tent in the early hours of the morning was crucial for obtaining a conviction.[24]

Even when sexual crimes were committed in private residences, eyewitnesses were sometimes involved. In 1940, for example, a man, having become suspicious of his downstairs neighbour's relationship with the teenager who cleaned his home, made a hole in the floor of his apartment. Through that hole he then watched his neighbour pressing his face against the girl's 'femininity'.[25] The suspect denied everything, but was convicted on the strength of the victim's statement and that of his spying neighbour.

In cases of childhood sexual abuse, the victim's siblings were sometimes witnesses.[26] Besides, perpetrators often had more than one victim. Thus, victims could regularly confirm each other's stories. Sometimes perpetrators molested multiple kids on the same occasion, thereby making each a direct eyewitness to the violation of the other(s). In other instances, the testimony of multiple victims served to establish a pattern of behaviour. In a 1952 case the court made this logic explicit, noting that the statements of the witnesses supported each other 'in their coherence'.[27]

Thus, it is clear that the testimony of eyewitnesses could be used to provide that all-important second piece of evidence that, together with the statement of the victim, could lead to a conviction. Despite the circulation of insights from witness psychology, I have found no evidence to indicate that police officers, prosecutors or judges were worried about the reliability of eyewitness testimony, not even when the witness was a child. Never once was a psychiatrist or psychologist called on to assess a witness's or victim's credibility or reliability. In fact, if a sex crime had been witnessed by a third party, the case was as good as resolved in the eyes of the law. By extension, the statements of victims in such cases were never doubted.

Calling victims into doubt?

In cases where there were no third-party witnesses, a victim's credibility was occasionally called into question, although almost exclusively by the suspect. Thus, in 1938, a man accused of sexually abusing his two daughters claimed: 'My children told you lies. They conspire against me; I cannot understand that one would think something like this of me. Do you think me capable?'[28]

Such unequivocal claims of false accusations, however, were rare. Some suspects instead argued that victims were somehow mistaken. Perhaps they had accidentally identified the wrong person, as a nineteen-year-old suspect suggested in 1940. Claiming his initial confession to a violent sexual assault was coerced, he was reluctant to declare the victim a liar, writing to his family: 'If the lady still positively says I am the person … I won't say that she would make a false [statement], but that she is honestly mistaken'.[29] Other suspects claimed victims had misinterpreted their actions as sexual, when they had, in fact, been innocent.[30] Indeed, the above-mentioned 1938 suspect did not persist with his claim that his children had lied. During successive interviews he landed on the argument that he had indeed touched them, but accidentally during play-fights or 'as a joke, not to be dirty'.[31] By prevaricating about his actions and by claiming he had no ill motives, the suspect avoided calling the victims unreliable. After his initial statement, he seems to have understood this to be an ineffective strategy, even as the girls' supervisory guardian – their uncle – sided with the suspect.

The largest group of suspects who called the credibility of their accusers into question did so by suggesting the victims had lied about the circumstances of the crime or exaggerated the details. In some cases, this took the form of pointing to victims' seductiveness. This strategy appears to have had some minor potential for success. My sample contains two examples of psychiatrists tasked with examining the suspects who were at least willing to entertain the possibility that the victims had precipitated the crimes.[32] Thus, in a 1952 case of incest involving an adult victim, the psychiatrist P. A. H. Baan was willing to give credence to the suspect's claims about his daughter: 'In addition, one wonders … whether the … daughter … showed sufficient resistance and whether she didn't even act in a provocative manner – perhaps unknowingly.'[33] The possibility of complicity by victims was also underwritten by police officer Lien van Nie, who served the Amsterdam vice department between 1935 and 1958 and who wrote about her experiences in a 1964 book. She stated that it sometimes happened that a boy or girl occasioned the crime committed against them: 'While this does not excuse a suspect, it can impact the sentence.'[34]

Thus, on the one hand, there is some limited evidence that professional participants in sex crimes investigations were occasionally willing to entertain the idea that the victim had in some way acted provocatively. On the other hand, claims of complicity by victims could also be used against the suspect, as is illustrated by a 1932 molestation case involving three victims aged ten, twelve and thirteen. During a discussion about whether the suspect should be released from pre-arrest, the prosecutor pointed precisely to the suspect's claim to have been seduced by the girls in order to argue that he should await his trial in jail and should, moreover, be examined psychiatrically. The prosecutor gave the distinct impression that he considered the claim entirely preposterous.[35]

In sum, while suspects rarely argued that the allegation against them was entirely made up, many of them called their accusers' credibility into question in one way or another. The professional participants in sex crimes investigations, by contrast, were not particularly concerned about victims giving incorrect statements. Even in the rare cases in which a psychiatrist entertained the idea that the victim had been – unknowingly – complicit in some way, the facts of the allegations were not doubted. In my sample, moreover, police officers openly questioned the facts alleged by a would-be victim only when they denied having been victimised, after having been identified as a victim by someone else, or if their version of events was milder than that of another victim. Thus, when two seventeen-year-old twin girls were interviewed in 1949 about the abuse they had suffered at the hands of their father, it was the fact that one of them told a less horrifying version of the story that made the investigators doubtful. Confirming the officers' suspicion, the young woman later admitted that she felt embarrassed to provide all the sordid details and that she had altered the story to protect her father.[36] Likewise, in a 1939 case in which a man was prosecuted for sexually abusing three eleven- or twelve-year-olds, police noted that they suspected that one of the girls was not telling all she knew, because she was afraid of her parents, who were 'very rough'.[37] Van Nie wrote about such cases: 'I very often encountered stupid parents, who, as soon as they heard what had happened, gave the children a beating. They did not understand that the child would not dare tell them if something else ever happened ... Beatings and especially threats are to be resolutely condemned.'[38]

Van Nie and Klaas Groen – van Nie's colleague at the Amsterdam vice department and writer of several books about his experiences for a general audience – were explicit about the trust they placed in children's statements. Showing himself familiar with internationally circulated cautions, Groen wrote: 'There are jurists who don't like children's stories. They say that children are fantasists. But don't adult witnesses suffer from the same ailment? Added to that, they more than once lie on purpose, which I have rarely observed in children's statements.'[39] Van Nie further noted that 'the power of observation in children is generally great, often much greater than in us, adults. Children often notice *small* details, that we are wont to overlook.'[40]

Beyond underwriting a general confidence in children's statements, Groen and van Nie both expressed great confidence in their own ability to extract truthful statements from children. In Groen's words: 'What I think is important is this: the police officer must tell the children, with seriousness, that what they say can have a deciding influence on the fate of a human. If one does this, it is remarkable to experience how well children sense the import of their words.'[41] Making sure that the child knew the seriousness of their statement was a practice applied in court too; in lieu of an oath, which children under the age of sixteen could not take, young witnesses were instructed by a judge that what they were about to do was very serious. The verdict would include a note along the lines of: 'the witness understood the gravity of her statements and appeared reliable', thereby complying with article 360 of the Code of Criminal Procedure which required a judge to motivate his decision to accept evidence provided by a witness below the age of sixteen.

It is important to note that adults here provide a negative contrast to children: while children are painted as particularly reliable, in spite of the literature on the psychology of witnesses, the idea that adult victims in sexual crimes cases might be lying about their assault is maintained. Still, none of the case files or verdicts indicate that the – relatively few – adult victims in my sample were distrusted.[42]

Confessions

Despite the general trust in children's statements, police officer Groen said, 'we were very careful with [them] but we always had a beautiful corroboration in the person of the suspect himself, because almost always, the confession of the suspect was in line with what the children had declared'.[43] This is something that I have found in my sample as well; the overwhelming majority of these cases were resolved by the suspect's confession. In fact, out of the 161 cases examined, the suspect outright denied involvement in only fourteen (9 per cent), while a further twenty-six (18 per cent) only partially confessed or retracted earlier statements.

While it is hard to know exactly how police officers went about obtaining confessions, here and there we get glimpses of their tactics, which seem to have revolved around, either, playing on the suspects' feelings of guilt, or, alternatively, making him feel that the evidence against him was overwhelming. A common practice was the confrontation between victim and suspect. Ostensibly intended to enable the victim to positively identify the suspect, it clearly served to put pressure on the suspect to confess. Van Nie explained that

> when a suspect continued to deny, it was useful to place the [child] across from him and to ask the child to answer the questions that *we* asked. It repeatedly happened that a suspect's demeanour changed upon *seeing* his victim. He was ashamed, showed remorse, when he saw an innocent child in front of him, who told him what he had done to her.[44]

At times, the threat of confrontation was enough; in 1937 a police officer wrote to the investigative judge: 'Because he initially did not want to talk, I told him that I would fetch the girl. He said "don't bother" and then began talking of his own accord.'[45]

Confessions often came bit by bit; while a suspect might initially confess only to having been near or at the crime scene, or to knowing the victim, by the time the trial happened he had admitted to most, if not all, details. In a few cases, the opposite happened; after an initial full confession, the suspect proclaimed his innocence at trial. This, however, did not matter; if the suspect declined to confess at trial, after having admitted to the crime at an earlier stage in the investigation, the verdict simply referenced as evidence a police report or report of the prosecutor or investigative judge containing a write-up of that previously made statement.[46] In one 1949 case the verdict included a note that stated: 'suspect retracted the statement made to police – which he confirmed to the investigative judge – but he gave no reasonable explanation, so that the court does not accept his retraction'.[47] I have not found evidence of concerns that suspects might be compelled to falsely confess, even in a case where a suspect retracted a confession, saying at trial that he had 'been very nervous' when he gave his initial statement confessing to a violent sexual assault.[48] Thus, the testimony of suspects, like that of other 'speaking witnesses', was understood to be reasonably unproblematic; suspects would often confess and confessions were understood to be true.

Conclusion: A culture of testimony?

From the preceding, it is clear that Dutch sexual violence cases in the period 1930–1960 revolved around testimony, despite the presence of a long-established discourse on the supposed unreliability of sex crimes victims and a familiarity with newer German and French literature on the subject of the psychology of witnesses. There is little evidence in the source material that victims' statements were especially distrusted. Neither medical evidence nor other physical evidence played a significant part in the cases that went to trial, contrary to what has been shown to be the case in other forensic cultures. Historian of medicine Victoria Bates, for example, in her practice-focused account of Victorian and Edwardian trials of sexual violence, showed that the attitudes expressed by medical experts in their academic writings also featured in their courtroom testimony. Moreover, the important role granted to such experts in trials ensured that rape myths were a major factor impacting the proceedings and outcome of rape trials in that period.[49]

While Dutch medical practitioners were notable only by their absence from sexual crimes cases, third-party witnesses had a remarkably significant role to play. Their evidence was not questioned. Instead, the weight of distrust was placed squarely on those suspects who denied having been involved. If suspects gave multiple conflicting statements, the court took the truest statement to be whichever one was most damning. Most cases resulted in a conviction on the basis of the victim's statement and the suspect's confession.

Thus, the results in this chapter paint a different picture than previous histories, which have demonstrated that, in other forensic cultures, victims' testimony was roundly distrusted, while suspects were given the benefit of the doubt, and that medical evidence was both central to sexual crimes cases and detrimental to victims' ability to get justice. It is therefore important to examine the features of Dutch forensic culture in the early and mid-twentieth century that may have given rise to this incongruity with existing studies. Why did neither the long-established discourse on the unreliability of victims in sexual crimes cases, nor the internationally circulated findings of the psychology of witness seem to have made much of an impact on policing and trial practice in Dutch sexual crimes cases between 1930 and 1960? Wolffram has suggested that interest in the psychology of witness may have arisen in Germany and France due to changes to the legal systems in those countries. Though the Dutch legal system was also subject to much change in the period around the turn of the century, the changes were of a different nature. For example, Wolffram has pointed out that, as the German legal system shifted towards the free evaluation of evidence, it faced new witnesses that had previously been excluded.[50] In the Netherlands, by contrast, there was no change in terms of groups eligible to testify, so the evaluation of their evidence did not raise new questions.

Moreover, while the rights of the defence were expanded with the introduction of the new Code of Criminal Procedure in 1926, in practice the understanding of defence attorneys as radical advocates of their clients' interests only very slowly developed in the Netherlands.[51] This, again, provides an interesting contrast with Germany, where, as Wolffram argues, newly professionalising defence attorneys were keen to exploit the various means available to them for championing their client's cause, including presenting scientific findings calling witness testimony into doubt.

Because the Netherlands did not have a jury system, concerns about the ability of lay people to assess the reliability of witnesses were irrelevant. Meanwhile, although the age-old rape myths and the findings of the newly established field of the psychology of witnesses were widely circulated, professional participants in investigations and trials – including police officers, prosecutors and judges – appear to have had confidence in their own and others' capacity to separate truth from untruth. Given that Dutch investigators seem to have understood victims and witnesses as reliable, or at the very least transparent, it is perhaps not surprising that there was no particular emphasis on the evidence of 'mute witnesses'.

Another issue that deserves consideration is the question of why so many suspects confessed despite having a right to remain silent. Here, too, the understanding of the role of the defence provides an important partial explanation. As mentioned, during the period under examination, Dutch defence attorneys did not yet inhabit their role of providing a one-sided defence of their client. Instead, there was a persisting sense that all the participants in the legal process, including defendants and their attorneys, had a role to play in getting the truth out in the open. This ideology encouraged confessions. More concretely, attorneys were typically not present during police interrogations – the right to have an attorney present on these occasions was finally established through a 2015 decision by the Dutch Supreme Court – and thus could not assist the suspect in a situation that, as we have seen, was crucial for evidence gathering and obtaining convictions. It is also relevant to note that, while suspects had a right to remain silent, between 1937 and 1973 police had no obligation to *inform* suspects of this right.

Thus, the specificities of the Dutch legal system go some way towards explaining why sexual violence cases tried between 1930 and 1960 revolve so strongly around witness testimony. This explanation, however, is incomplete. For one, I have not given consideration to features of the Dutch forensic culture that were external to the legal system, for example the framing of sexual crime in newspapers or evolving views on gender. Moreover, it is important to realise that medical and criminalistics evidence, in the same period, played a much larger role in other types of cases, for example homicides, where the victim was necessarily mute.[52] Thus, while the slice of the legal system that concerned itself with sexual crime in the period 1930–1960 can be described as having a culture of testimony, this term cannot in good conscience be applied to Dutch early and mid-twentieth-century forensic culture as a whole.

Notes

This chapter has received funding from the European Research Council (ERC) under the European Union's Horizon 2020 research and innovation programme (grant agreement No 770402).

1 Utrechts Archief, Utrecht (hereafter UA), 1234 Arrondissementsrechtbank Utrecht 1930–1949 (hereafter 1234 ARU), 389/416, 1868 'Processtukken', 1949 and 2041 'Vonnis', 1 November 1949.
2 Ian Burney and Neil Pemberton, *Murder and the Making of English CSI* (Baltimore: Johns Hopkins University Press, 2016), pp. 9–38; for the rising importance of trace evidence in the Netherlands, see Willemijn Ruberg and Nathanje Dijkstra, 'De forensische wetenschap in Nederland (1800–1930): een terreinverkenning', *Studium* 9:3 (2016), pp. 131–137. A parallel claim is made by scholars investigating the aftermath of mass violence events – the Holocaust, in particular – for a much later period; see Taline Garibian's contribution to this volume.
3 Heather Wolffram, 'Forensic Psychology in Historical Perspective', in Oliver Braddick (ed.), *Oxford Research Encyclopedia of Psychology* (Oxford: Oxford University Press, 2020), article published 30 January 2020, accessed 12 February 2020, https://doi.org/10.1093/acrefore/9780190236557.013.639
4 See Heather Wolffram's contribution to this volume and Heather Wolffram, *Forensic Psychology in Germany: Witnessing Crime, 1880–1939* (London: Palgrave Macmillan, 2018), pp. 46, 61; Marcus B. Carrier, 'The Value(s) of Methods: Method Selection in German Forensic Toxicology in the Second Half of the Nineteenth Century', in Ian Burney and Christopher Hamlin (eds), *Global Forensic Cultures. Making Fact and Justice in the Modern Era* (Baltimore: Johns Hopkins University Press, 2019), pp. 40–42.
5 Wolffram, *Forensic Psychology in Germany*, pp. 43–48.
6 Burney and Pemberton, *Murder and the Making of English CSI*, p. 15; see also Raluca Enescu and Leonie Benker, 'The Birth of Criminalistics and the Transition from Lay to Expert Witnesses in German Courts', *Journal on European History of Law* 9:2 (2018), pp. 59–66; Wolffram, *Forensic Psychology*, pp. 44–45; Miloš Vec, *Die Spur des Täters: Methoden der Identifikation in der Kriminalistik (1879–1933)* (Baden-Baden: Nomos, 2002), pp. 12–15.
7 The term was first defined by Martha R. Burt, 'Cultural Myths and Supports for Rape', *Journal of Personality and Social Psychology* 38:2 (1980), pp. 217–230; see also Kimberly A. Lonsway and Louise

F. Fitzgerald, 'Rape Myths: In Review', *Psychology of Women Quarterly* 18:2 (1994), pp. 133–164.
8 Joanna Bourke, *Rape: Sex, Violence, History* (Emeryville, CA: Shoemaker & Hoard, 2007); Willemijn Ruberg, 'Trauma, Body, and Mind: Forensic Medicine in Nineteenth-Century Dutch Rape Cases', *Journal of the History of Sexuality* 22:1 (2013), pp. 94, 96–98; Victoria Bates, 'Forensic Medicine and Female Victimhood in Victorian and Edwardian England', *Past and Present* 245:1 (2019), pp. 117–151; Victoria Bates, *Sexual Forensics in Victorian and Edwardian England. Age, Crime and Consent in the Courts* (London: Palgrave Macmillan, 2016); Ivan Crozier and Gethin Rees, 'Making a Space for Medical Expertise: Medical Knowledge of Sexual Assault and the Construction of Boundaries Between Forensic Medicine and the Law in late Nineteenth-Century England', *Law, Culture and the Humanities* 8:2 (2012), pp. 285–304; Louise A. Jackson, *Child Sexual Abuse in Victorian England* (New York, NY: Routledge, 2000), pp. 71–89.
9 Stephen Robertson, 'Signs, Marks and Private Parts: Doctors, Legal Discourses, and Evidence of Rape in the United States, 1823–1930', *Journal for the History of Sexuality* 8:3 (1998), pp. 345–388; Jackson warned that 'While [medico-legal texts] may be considered as representative of the views of medical specialists, it is unclear to what extent their arguments either influenced or reflected the minds of the vast rank of general practitioners'; Jackson, *Child Sexual Abuse in Victorian England*, p. 72; Willemijn Ruberg, 'Onzekere kennis. De rol van forensische geneeskunde en psychiatrie in Nederlandse verkrachtingszaken (1811–1920)', *Tijdschrift voor Sociale en Economische Geschiedenis* 9:1 (2012), pp. 87–110; Bates, *Sexual Forensics*.
10 Articles 338–344 of the *Wetboek van Strafvordering* (Code of Criminal Procedure) deal with evidence at trial.
11 For examples from the nineteenth century, see Ruberg, 'Trauma, Body, and Mind', pp. 94–97. Twentieth-century examples include A. I. Oerlemans, *Beknopte opsporingsleer* (Velp: J.A. Reeskink, 1939), p. 104; W. E. T. M. van der Does de Willebois, *De nasporing van het strafbaar feit: een leidraad voor ambtenaren en beambten van justitie en politie* (Heusden: L.J. Veermans, 1903), p. 228; H. F. Roll, *Leerboek der gerechtelijke geneeskunde, IIIde deel* (*'s-Gravenhage*: Algemeene Landsdrukkerij, 1912), pp. 368, 404; Henri van der Hoeven, *Psychiatrie: Een handleiding voor juristen en maatschappelijk werkers, deel III* (Rotterdam: W. L. & J. Brusse's Uitgeversmaatschappij, 1936), p. 37; G. C. Bolton, *Een rechterlijke*

dwaling? *Medisch-forensische beschouwingen over eene belangrijke strafzaak* (The Hague: G. Naeff, 1928), pp. 182–206. These concerns conformed with more general notions of women as duplicitous and impacted investigations other than those into sexual violence, including civil suits about disputed paternity; see Alison Adam's contribution to this volume.

12 Van der Does de Willebois, *De nasporing*, pp. 228–229. All quoted text from primary source material has been translated from Dutch by the author.

13 *Ibid.*, p. 22; Bolton, *Een rechterlijke dwaling?*, p. 183. Roll, *Gerechtelijke geneeskunde*, p. 368; Van Oerlemans, *Opsporingsleer*, p. 104.

14 'Regels omtrent het getuigenbewijs en de betrouwbaarheid van getuigen', *Weekblad van het Regt* 8210 (17 May 1905), p. 4; the source of the eighteen rules reprinted here was William Stern, 'Leitsätze über die Bedeutung der Aussagepsychologie für das gerichtliche Verfahren', *Beiträge zur Psychologie der Aussage* 2:2 (1904), p. 73; For a discussion of this text, see Wolffram, *Forensic Psychology in Germany*, pp. 74–77.

15 See Ruberg and Dijkstra, 'Forensische wetenschap in Nederland'.

16 Exceptions are H. E. L. Vos, 'Bijdrage tot de psychologie van het getuigenis van schoolkinderen: analyse der uitspraken over een door hen aangehoord verhaal' (PhD thesis, University of Amsterdam, 1909) and Dirk Johannes Beck, 'Over suggestie. Een proefondervindelijke studie' (PhD thesis, University of Groningen, 1917).

17 S. J. M. Geuns, 'Het psychiatrisch psychologisch element in de strafrechtspraak' (Verslag van de bijeenkomst op 6 April 1935 te Amsterdam, Psychiatrisch-Juridisch Gezelschap), p. 5, https://resolver.kb.nl/resolve?urn=MMUBVU05:000000315:pdf

18 See Sibo van Ruller and Sjoerd Faber, *Afdoening van strafzaken in Nederland sinds 1813. Ontwikkelingen in wetgeving, beleid en praktijk* (Amsterdam: VU Uitgeverij, 1995).

19 I counted a total of 1,547 sexual violence cases listed in the Utrecht prosecutors' register in the period 1960–1969. UA, 1348 Arrondissementsrechtbank Utrecht 1950–1979 (hereafter 1348 ARU) 4682–742.

20 It is important to acknowledge that there is no data available about the number of sexual crimes that failed to reach the prosecutor's desk. Writing in the 1970s, feminist jurist and journalist Jeanne Doomen noted:

> according to the law the police is obliged to draw up a police report [*process-verbaal*] about every reported crime. In practice, this does

not always happen, especially if they expect the prosecutor won't proceed with a prosecution anyway. In many police departments there is a kind of internal policy in which only the strongest cases are sent to the prosecutor's office. A sympathetic prosecutor, in this way, does not even get the chance to present a less strong (that is, less stereotypical) rape to a judge.

Jeanne Doomen, *Heb je soms aanleiding gegeven? Handleiding voor slachtoffers van verkrachting bij de confrontatie met politie en justitie* (Amsterdam: Feministische Uitgeverij Sara, 1978), p. 20.
21 UA, 1234 ARU 1930–1949, 457, 95 'Processtukken', 1939.
22 UA, 1234 ARU, 151, 504 'Processtukken', 1937.
23 UA, 1348 ARU, 1168, 1629 'Vonnis', 18 September 1953.
24 UA, 1234 ARU, 559, 2078 'Vonnis', 4 November 1949.
25 UA, 1234 ARU, 468, 1693 'Vonnis', 24 September 1940; the case decided in UA, 1234 ARU, 559, 2197 'Vonnis', 17 December 1949 proceeded in a similar way.
26 For example in UA, 1234 ARU, 468, 1687 'Vonnis', 24 September 1940; UA, 1234 ARU, 465, 822 'Vonnis', 14 May 1940; and UA, 1234 ARU, 176, 1261 'Processtukken', 1938.
27 UA, 1348 ARU, 1236, 279 'Verdict', 12 February 1959.
28 UA, 1234 ARU, 176, 1261 'Processtukken', 1938.
29 UA, 1234 ARU, 209, 705 'Processtukken', 1940.
30 UA, 1348 ARU, 1147, 482 'Verdict', 4 March 1952.
31 UA, 1348 ARU, 135, 1459 'Procesdossier', 1959.
32 Psychiatrists were commonly asked to draw up a report about the suspect's mental state: in at least 87 out of 162 cases in my sample.
33 UA, 1348 ARU, 130, 389 'Procesdossier', 1952.
34 Lien van Nie, *Recherche zedenpolitie: Ervaringen van een vrouwelijke rechercheur bij de kinder- en zedenpolitie* (Amsterdam: A. J. G. Strengholt, 1964), p. 134.
35 UA, 1234 ARU, 65, 284 'Processtukken', 1932.
36 UA, 1234 ARU, 384, 1459 'Processtukken', 1949.
37 UA, 1234 ARU, 195, 959 'Processtukken', 1939.
38 Van Nie, *Recherche zedenpolitie*, p. 134.
39 Klaas Groen, *Kamer 13: Hallo hier de zedenpolitie!* (The Hague: Daamen N.V., 1960), p. 117.
40 Van Nie, *Recherche zedenpolitie*, p. 131.
41 Groen, *Kamer 13*, p. 117.
42 It is, of course, remarkable that the victims in this sample are very young overall; all except three are under the age of twenty. Additionally, in the period 1960–1969 far fewer cases involving adult victims reached the prosecutor, who, moreover, appears to have been

somewhat quicker to dismiss these cases than the ones involving children. These findings may indicate that older victims were less trusted than children, that older people were less likely to become victims, that they were less likely to report the crime to police, or that evidence gathering was for some reason more problematic when the victim was an adult.
43 Groen, *Kamer 13*, p. 117.
44 Van Nie, *Recherche zedenpolitie*, p. 138.
45 UA, 1234 ARU, 149, 319, 'Processtukken', 1937.
46 This was the case, for example, in UA, 1234 ARU, 549, 1824 'Vonnis', 19 October 1948; UA, 1234 ARU, 555, 1211 'Vonnis', 28 June 1949; UA, 1234 ARU, 559, 2111 'Vonnis', 8 November 1949; UA, 1348 ARU, 1237, 452 'Verdict', 13 March 1959.
47 UA, 1234 ARU, 559, 2111 'Vonnis', 8 November 1949.
48 UA, 1234 ARU, 549, 1824 'Vonnis', 19 October 1948. This points to a problem that is addressed by Sara Serrano Martínez in her contribution to this volume; it may well be the case that some of the suspects in this sample confessed under duress. While I have no indication that corrupt practices were widespread, the court's insouciant handling of retracted confessions does at least seem to be a cause for concern.
49 Bates, 'Forensic Medicine and Female Victimhood'; other researchers have also demonstrated that in England and Scotland medical practitioners were very often involved in rape investigations; Jackson, *Child Sexual Abuse in Victorian England*, pp. 71–89.
50 Wolffram, 'Forensic Psychology in Historical Perspective'; see also Wolffram's contribution to this volume.
51 Patrick P. J. van der Meij, 'De driehoeksverhouding in het strafrechtelijk vooronderzoek: Een onverminderde zoektocht naar evenwicht in de rolverdeling tussen de rechter-commissaris, de officier van justitie en de verdediging' (PhD thesis, Leiden University, 2010), pp. 116–119, 141, 146.
52 Thus, it seems relevant that Pemberton and Burney are specifically concerned with murder cases. Burney and Pemberton, *Murder and the Making of English CSI*.

3

The making of evidence after mass violence: Forensics in the aftermath of the Second World War

Taline Garibian

Introduction

Following the Second World War, the victorious armies deployed a great deal of energy and resources to find and judge those guilty of crimes committed during the conflict. The need for justice, the eagerness of the victors to see the perpetrators of the crimes punished and their difficulties in speaking with one voice undoubtedly explain the disparate nature of the post-war tribunals.[1] Yet all victorious countries took steps to research and collect evidence of the crimes committed during the war. This included gathering testimonies and written material, but also fieldwork on mass graves and corpses. In this context, the use of forensic techniques and tools has been both widespread and discreet; widespread because several armies took action to collect material evidence of crimes in order to identify human remains whenever possible, and discreet because the results of such practices did not receive much exposure, either at the time or subsequently.

The history of these forensic interventions can be placed within the long history of post-conflict corpse management, health and funerary concerns having become increasingly important. Indeed, the bodies of victims resulting from war and violence, and their fate, have attracted growing attention at least since the French Revolution.[2] This echoed a transition in the management of corpses that occurred between the end of the eighteenth and the first half of the nineteenth centuries in the Western world. This shift, which has been studied by many historians and termed the 'funerary transition' by Régis Bertrand,[3] is characterised by a relocation of funerary activity away from the church, the individualisation of graves and a certain secularisation of funerary practices. This development also reflects a growing concern regarding the hygienic problems associated with the dead.[4] After the First World War, the public health challenge posed by the management of the huge number of corpses was evident.[5] Bodies left in conflict zones not only caused logistical and health challenges, but also raised judicial and memorial issues that had political implications.

While the handling of the corpses left by violence has a long history, which has also been investigated by historians of the Second World War, such as Monica Black and Christopher Mauriello,[6] forensic practices have remained relatively unexplored. This omission can partly be explained by the tendency of scholarship to focus on the judiciary institutions created after the war to judge the guilty. In addition to the International Military Tribunal (IMT), led by the four great powers and held in Nuremberg, which has been covered extensively by the historiography, there were the twelve trials conducted by the Americans in the same city between October 1946 and April 1949,[7] as well as numerous other proceedings in Germany and elsewhere, that have received less attention.[8] A milestone in the history of international criminal justice, the IMT of Nuremberg was shaped from the outset by a clear take on the choice of evidence, which left the work of forensic pathologists in the background. The American prosecutor Robert Jackson, who helped to draft the London Charter of the IMT, explained in 1954, 'The prosecution early was confronted with two vital decisions … One was whether chiefly to rely upon living witnesses or upon documents for proof of the case. The decision … was to use and rest on documentary evidence to prove every point possible',[9] a decision that worked well with the bureaucratic structure of the Third Reich.[10] Despite the approach outlined in the London Charter, varying methods prevailed among the nations involved in the establishment of international courts. Several judicial cultures coexisted, and while the American trials tended to rely mostly on documents, British war crimes trials were more inclined to use testimonies.[11] However, both the 'Doctors' Trial', conducted in Nuremberg under the auspices of the United States in the wake of the IMT, and the Hamburg Ravensbrück Trials, held by the British authorities, relied on information gathered by pathologists.[12]

The Nuremberg Tribunal had such an impact on historiography that when the Eichmann trial, another landmark in the history of the Holocaust, which took place almost fifteen years later, took the approach to rely primarily on testimony, many historians saw this as a paradigm shift. Several terms to refer to what was seen as the rise of the figure of the witness have been coined. Shoshana Felman and Dori Laub chose the 'era of testimony', and Annette Wieviorka the 'era of the witness'.[13] These phrases were to characterise the period from the Eichmann trial onwards, during which the testimony of Holocaust survivors became central not only to memory, but also to judicial processes.[14] Until then the paradigm of documentary evidence prevailed in the courts established to judge the crimes of the Third Reich, as the historiography centred on the IMT suggests. Notwithstanding these differing approaches to evidence, however, the IMT and the Eichmann trial shared some common features. Specifically, they both neglected corpses and material evidence.[15] These judicial options have contributed to leaving forensic practices in the shadows, both in the trials and in the historiography.

Recently, forensic practices and the fate of corpses after mass violence events have attracted more attention from scholars of various disciplines, such as anthropology, history and sociology.[16] These scholars have identified a new shift in the handling of mass crime corpses and have noted the extensive use of forensic medicine in mass violence cases since the 1980s, to the point of popularising the expression 'forensic turn'.[17] This has also been used to characterise the use of forensic techniques from the 1980s onwards for much older cases of mass death, such as Robert Jan van Pelt's work on the gas chambers of Auschwitz.[18] The 'forensic turn' that happened in the 1980s is often described as a shift in judicial logics,[19] that followed an 'era of witness' (from the 1960s), which in turn came after a period during which documentary evidence was key, from the late 1940s.

This chronology is intriguing for at least two reasons. Firstly, it took a very long time for forensic techniques to become prevalent in cases of mass violence. As Zuzanna Dziuban has pointed out, although the use of forensic technology for criminal law dates back to the nineteenth century, its pre-eminent role in investigations of mass violence came much later.[20] Secondly, according to Adam Rosenblatt, this growing presence does not necessarily coincide with the development of new techniques or their appropriate use. As he explains, in the 1980s, a form of amateurism still prevailed. When discussing the exhumations carried out in Argentina, he notes, 'These initial exhumations … were haphazard efforts, as the forensic authorities and cemetery workers who conducted them had little knowledge of the appropriate archaeological and anthropological techniques of exhumations. For the most part, they destroyed more evidence than they recovered.'[21]

Thus, the 'forensic turn' that occurred in the 1980s is characterised more by a shift in the evidential paradigm – and the popularisation of specific techniques – in the field of international justice than by scientific advances. However, as Dziuban notes, it profoundly modified the way mass crimes are proven: 'Even if this has not necessarily entailed an overall invalidation of human testimony and its disappearance from the courtrooms and human rights activism, forensically acquired and assessed evidence has assumed critical importance in evincing the existence and nature of the crimes …'[22]

To understand and nuance this timeline, it is worth looking at the origins of forensic interventions in wartime and the context in which they emerged. The emergence of a more 'object oriented juridical culture', as Weizman put it,[23] has a long history. As what follows shows, this history is at least partially linked to the increasing role of scientists and the importance of the expert figure in both the field of justice and that of war and humanitarian practice from the end of the nineteenth century onwards. Indeed, the emergence of an international law of war which provides for the regulation of the use of violence and obligations regarding the treatment of the dead and wounded has led armies in particular to adopt forensic techniques to establish the violations committed by their enemy. In this chapter, I show that a culture of investigation, relying on material evidence, clearly existed among the military command in the aftermath of the Second World War.[24] This culture was sufficiently developed to lead to the creation of units dedicated to this task. This was the result not only of the general use of forensic techniques but also of a reflection on the credibility of different types of sources. Furthermore, the use of forensic tools and the debates surrounding them reveal the issues relating to the broader use of forensic techniques in the field of investigation. In its first section, this chapter traces the origins of forensic practices and highlights their long history. In the following sections, it examines more closely some of the work produced by the British Army War Crimes Investigation Unit in the aftermath of the Second World War.

Tracing the origins of forensic practices

The history of forensic practices relating to war and mass violence is linked to the emergence of an international law of war and the willingness to prosecute those who violated it. The armies were certainly the first to act in this direction. By focusing on the simultaneous establishment of a law of war and the practice of establishing evidence of its violations, this section aims to shed light on the origins of forensic warfare practices. The St Petersburg Declaration, which was signed in 1868 and aimed to monitor violence during conflict, forbade the use of weapons that were deemed to cause 'unnecessary suffering', such as explosive bullets. This formulation undoubtedly helped to provide opportunities for physicians – and military physicians in particular – to study pain, ways to assess it and to define the thresholds of acceptable destructiveness.[25] The Hague Convention, signed in 1899 and 1907, subsequently provided further guidance. Therefore, when the First World War broke out, there were laws that regulated the practice of warfare, the use of weaponry and the handling of corpses. Article 23 of the annex to the Convention (IV) regarding the Laws and Customs of War on Land forbade, among others, the employment of poison or poisoned weapons, the killing or wounding of civilians belonging to the hostile nation or prisoners of war and the employment of arms, projectiles or materiel meant to cause unnecessary suffering.[26] At the same time, the Geneva Convention for the Amelioration of the Condition of the Wounded and Sick in Armies in the Field specified the obligations of the belligerent with regard to the treatment of bodies left on the battlefield.[27] Motivated by the rapid development of weapons technology and the willingness to mitigate war violence, this legislation did not prevent the occurrence of atrocities. However, by making the protection of the integrity of the combatants, the wounded and the dead a legal obligation, these texts created, as I will show, the conditions for the emergence of forensic practices in a war context.

The First World War, the brutality of which has been studied by several historians, was to provide the backdrop to these first interventions. In their book, *German Atrocities*, John Horne and Alan Kramer identify 129 major incidents on the Western Front during Germany's invasion of France and Belgium. During these incidents, a total of 6,147 people were killed.[28] As Annette Becker notes, civilians were not spared violence: 'From the early days of the war, in August 1914, violence was committed against civilians on all fronts that were invaded, particularly crimes against women, many of which were documented by verified testimonies published during the conflict itself.'[29]

To facilitate the documentation of atrocities, governments issued guidelines for the military relating to the collection of evidence. An example of this is provided by an instruction from the French Ministry of War issued in August 1914, which prescribed the recording of acts contrary to the laws of war. It recommended that, 'whenever such an act has been established, a duplicate report should be made, signed by witnesses, military or not, and, if possible, by the perpetrators of the attacks themselves, if they have been captured'.[30] It also suggested questioning prisoners to ascertain whether they acted on their own initiative or whether they followed the orders of their superiors. At the very end of the letter, it was further documented that if prohibited weapons and projectiles were to be used by the enemy, these facts should be accurately recorded, and the ammunition confiscated and sent to the Ministry of War.

Besides these military efforts, several countries set up civil investigation commissions, often composed of lawyers and senior officials. They collected testimonies and gathered medical or forensic data. On 6 November 1914, for example, a medical officer of the French Army testified before the commission of his country and detailed the forensic examination he had carried out a few days earlier on two exhumed corpses.[31] In Eastern Europe, Rodolphe A. Reiss, a criminologist based in Lausanne, took part in a commission, set up by Serbia, to investigate atrocities committed by the invading Central Power. His reports included information on explosive bullets, as well as observations of wounds and bodies found in mass graves.[32] However, what is most striking about these reports is that the boundary between testimony and physical evidence is not as rigid as one might think. Testimony, sworn testimony and physical evidence are obviously not mutually exclusive, but they often work together. As Reiss explained, 'eyewitnesses were examined on the spot and in most cases, they were my guides to the place where the outrages had taken place. Thus, I was afforded the opportunity of verifying the truth of their statements by actual and personal inspection'.[33]

Thus, the establishment of an international law of war and its formulation have greatly facilitated the deployment of forensic techniques in the theatre of war violence. However, it would be wrong to link the development of forensic practices solely to these legal foundations. Indeed, military physicians were – and continue to be – also heavily implicated in researching and improving the effectiveness of weapons.[34] Ballistic expertise, for example, can serve the purposes of attesting breaches of the law of war or improving a weapon's destructiveness. Moreover, the forensic medicine of war/mass crimes cannot be regarded completely independently of military justice. Indeed, if the presence of forensic scientists within the armed forces increased, this was mainly due to the needs of the military court. The First World War prompted the reorganisation of military health services and the development of medico-legal practices to help the military justice department detect malingerers or calculate the pension of disabled veterans.[35] Besides these tasks, certain military physicians also helped establish the first procedures for the identification of bodies and the recording of possible violations of the laws of war.[36] Hence, the First World War was not only a time of formalisation of forensic practices regarding war crimes; a forensic culture in the service of military justice and the draft was also emerging within the armies. Yet, in the aftermath of the First World War, several obstacles prevented the prosecution of crimes committed during the conflict, including disagreements between the victors and the refusal to extradite the Kaiser. Therefore, it would take until after the Second World War for this burgeoning forensic culture to really emerge. At the Nuremberg Trials, the charge included 'crimes against peace', i.e. initiating a war of aggression and war crimes, as provided for in the Nuremberg Charter, which used the terminology of the Hague Convention and added conspiracy and crimes against humanity, which 'seemed specifically created to deliver an idiom of judgment capable of naming, and by extension, condemning the evidence of atrocity so graphically captured in *Nazi Concentration Camps*.[37] After the war, the question of the punishment of crimes took on unprecedented importance, giving rise to significant investigative work.

The British War Crimes Investigation Unit in the aftermath of the Second World War

After the Second World War, investigative practices into war crimes were further formalised within the armed forces. The development of war forensics stemmed not only from the willingness to prosecute war crime, but also from the greater attention paid to the corpses, the challenges they posed and the high demand for identification. In Berlin, as Monica Black explains, 'corpses accumulated in every conceivable place: streets, parks, railway stations, air raid shelters, canals, and cellars'.[38] The large number of unburied or inadequately buried Holocaust victims also provided the US Army with material to punish the German population, forcing them to give these dead a proper burial, often without protective equipment.[39] As Black maintains, 'to control the disposition of the dead is, in any context, a profound gesture of power'.[40] Thus, at the end of the conflict, the bodies were far from being invisible objects or ignored by the authorities. They were present in high numbers and sometimes integrated into the occupation policies of the Allied armies as the example of the US Army shows. The legal obligations of belligerents have also further expanded since the First World War. The Geneva Convention of 1929 stipulates among other things that, if possible, death should be ascertained by medical examination and that the belligerents 'shall organize officially a graves registration service, to render eventual exhumations possible, and to ensure the identification of bodies whatever may be the subsequent site of the grave'.[41] In the interwar period, the identification of bodies – including those of enemies – thus was explicitly mentioned in the legal text. The evolution of these laws reflects the growing demand, often from the public, for the search for, identification and repatriation of soldiers' bodies. But this is obviously only valid for soldiers, whereas the identification of civilians remains unaddressed. Indeed, in the aftermath of the war identification of civilians proved to be often more difficult,[42] although Jean-Marc Dreyfus notes that the French search mission for the corpses of deportees in Germany achieved a high rate of identification.[43]

In 1944, the British created the Missing Research and Enquiry Service within the Royal Air Force, dedicated to the search for overseas casualties. Its work included the tracing of 41,881 missing people and the locations of those who had been buried during the conflict.[44] Japan began repatriation operations in 1953, while the United States and France took similar steps just after the war.[45] The United States relied on physical anthropologists to proceed with the identification of the unknown soldiers.[46]

It is in the context of the implementation of corpse management policies that several investigation teams were set up within the British Army. In 1946, these teams and a war crimes specialist pool were united under the name of the War Crimes Investigation Unit. Based in Bad Oeynhausen, near Bielefeld, the unit took over all the records of cases of the earlier team units.[47] The main tasks of the unit were to exhume the corpses found in mass or isolated graves when a crime was suspected or when there were doubts regarding the identity of the bodies, to identify the corpses and determine the cause of death. The archives of the newly created unit reveal the importance the army command attached to the use of a pathologist for exhumations. When graves were discovered in Bemburg, for example, Colonel A. O. Stott insisted on not proceeding with the exhumations until a pathologist was able to come to the site. He explained, 'When the remains are exposed to the air, it may happen that valuable evidence, which may be detected and noted only by a SPECIALIST, is lost in a few moments.' He then added, 'the function of the graves service is to exhume for identity and to concentrate when necessary; graves service officers are not regarded as competent to report on "evidence of atrocities"'.[48]

The search for the bodies of the missing largely explains the organisation of specific teams dedicated to this mission. Moreover, a form of specialisation was taking place and the establishment of evidence of war crimes was becoming a specific task. Thus, not only did forensic examination take place in the aftermath of the Second World War, but it was also institutionalised with the creation of dedicated teams within the armed forces. This shows that the collection of material evidence was, together with the collection of testimonies and the search for documentary evidence, a means of investigation.

The report on the Ravensbrück concentration camp

The several types of evidence – such as testimonies, documents or material examination – were often used in parallel as the report produced by the War Crimes Investigation Unit on the Ravensbrück concentration camp shows. This camp, situated in the north of Berlin and opened in May 1939, was the largest women's concentration camp of the German Reich. In 1941, a men's camp was added before the Uckermark Jugendschutzlager (youth protection camp) was opened in 1942. According to the *Mahn- und Gedenkstätte Ravensbrück* approximately 120,000 women and children were interned in the camp during the war, in addition to 20,000 men and 1,200 youths. Inmates were subjected to forced labour, medical experiments and executions. Between the end of January 1945 and April 1945, these executions were performed in a gas chamber, where 5,000 to 6,000 prisoners were murdered.[49]

In 1946, Keith A. Mant, one of the pathologists working for the British Army, took part in the investigation of the medical experiments conducted at Ravensbrück.[50] In addition to Mant, seven officers contributed to a report on this issue. Their work is indicative of the prevailing culture of investigation: testimonies were a very important source of information, and the pathologist participated in their collection and analysis.[51] The document details the functioning of the camp and provides general information. The origins of the internees, the structure of the camp and its organisation regarding food, work, punishment, etc., are first described. Then the report details the killing methods, making a distinction between 'the execution of named individuals and [the] extermination of certain categories'.[52] The commission found that in January 1945, the *Jugendschutzlager* (youth camp) was repurposed to execute prisoners. The victims were executed by neck shots from a small-calibre rifle. In March, a gas chamber was built after converting half of one of the barrack stores situated 'conveniently', as the report states, close to the crematorium. According to the report, 'the total number of persons who were burned at the Crematorium was about 6,400 from January until the end of March. [...] The gassing lasted for approximately 5 weeks during which time 2,400 to 2,500 were exterminated. The gas chamber closed shortly after Easter 1945.'[53]

The authors were keen to insist on the application of a certain method. At the very beginning, they state that, 'In order to establish a definite case and determine both which of the accused were to be included in the major case and the direction in which investigations could be most profitably pursued, all witnesses were interrogated prior to examination of any suspect persons',[54] thus revealing an *episteme* of the investigation. This document suggests that witness statements were used in the report in a compilation mode, in which for each accused, the investigators initially presented their own statement and then the other accused's statements regarding their co-accused, before finally presenting the witness testimonies. 'The intention behind their accumulation is simply to serve as a quick reference guide to the most direct a[nd] positive evidence obtained so far against the main accused.'[55] Thus, witness statements were used cautiously and served as peripheral information by comparison with what was considered more solid evidence. Indeed, a certain suspicion of witnesses is apparent, and the report produced by Mant's team is obviously not free from stereotypical assumptions. For instance, in the conclusion, the authors remind their readers that, 'In all, the investigators have attempted to allow for the histrionic exaggerations to be expected from the female sex.'[56] The objectivity and credibility of potential witnesses was a particular concern, especially when they belonged to minority groups, like the Jews who, like women, were suspected of bias.[57]

The medical experiments carried out at Ravensbrück received significant attention and were mainly judged at the Ravensbrück trial, held in Hamburg between 1946 and 1947, although certain defendants were brought before the Nuremberg Doctors' Trial, held at the same time.[58] Mant's findings were used in both trials even if, according to Weindling, tensions related to the evidence gathering process arose with the Americans.[59] Along with the report came a shorter account of the 'Medical Services, Human Experimentation and Other Medical Atrocities Committed in Ravensbrück Concentration Camp', written solely by Mant.[60]

Since the camp was situated in the Soviet Zone, Mant could not access it. Therefore, the report is mainly based on an analysis of the statements made by witnesses, including interned doctors and nurses, patients, persons employed in the administration and the accused. This report proved that Karl Gebhardt, Himmler's surgeon, was personally responsible for all medical experiments.[61] These findings were used in a presentation given by Mant in 1949 and published as an article in the *Medico-Legal Journal*, along with additional elements taken from the transcripts of trials, which took place in Hamburg and Nuremberg, as well as the discussion that followed the presentation. This reflects a form of normalisation of war forensics that was spreading to scientific networks and bodies of criminal law forensics.

Mant's work is interesting for several reasons. Firstly, it confirms the presence of forensic pathologists in the investigation teams and therefore the interest of the military hierarchy in these techniques. Secondly, it shows that they are not only called upon to analyse material evidence but also to produce reports on the basis of testimony. This ultimately reveals a culture of enquiry that relies on scientific expertise and combines different approaches.

Mant's work on exhumed bodies

One of Mant's most important contributions to the field of war forensics is undoubtedly his work on exhumed bodies. This work also constitutes the core material for his doctorate in medicine, submitted in 1950. During this research study, Mant performed more than 150 autopsies and witnessed several hundred exhumations undertaken by the graves service. He explained, 'the time which had elapsed between the original burial and exhumation varied from eight months to five years, and was known accurately, usually to the day, and often hour, of the original burial'.[62] Mant's work was carried out in the context of the investigation of war crimes, as defined by the Royal Warrant, and essentially concerned crimes committed against British or Allied soldiers, excluding those committed in the camps. As he explained, the warrant shapes the investigation: 'The investigations, therefore, were quite different from those undertaken for the trial of the major war criminals at

Nuremberg, where the evidence was for the most part documentary.'[63] This view reflects the various traces left by different crimes; executions committed during combat certainly resulted in less documentation than the organisation of mass extermination policies. As Mant put it: '[the war crimes units] had on many occasions to build up the entire case by investigation in the field'.[64] This also suggests that a different judicial culture prevailed in different spheres, and that supporters of an international tribunal were perhaps, at least initially, less sensitive to forensic evidence than the military, which already had a long history of forensic work and created units dedicated to such practices early on.

As for his work on war crimes committed against British or Allied soldiers, Mant's main task was to exhume the corpses and to perform autopsies, to identify the deceased whenever possible and to determine the cause of death with all the relevant details: the weapon and its calibre, the number of shots and an estimation of the range.[65] This involved at least two types of investigative practices, one on objects surrounding the corpses, which would help with identification, a practice that already had a long history within armies. The other was associated with the bodies themselves and was in the process of being formalised at the time of Mant's work. In addition to marks on clothing (such as name or numbers) and identity discs, Mant used for instance dental charts and tattoo marks. The information was then cross-checked by an estimation of the height, age and build mentioned in the service records.[66] It should be noted that the armies made their own arrangements, which demonstrated different degrees of preparation. American soldiers could often be identified by their fingerprints, for which the army had records, which was not the case for the British Army.[67]

Mass graves involved special precautions, as the bodies had to be treated individually, while allowing for the collection of information regarding the entire grave and the arrangement of the bodies in relation to one another. In his dissertation, Mant also details several cases of shots to the neck. As Mant explains, although they were called neck shots, 'the majority of the victims were actually shot through the base of the skull, the exit hole being situated in the frontal bone'.[68] Interestingly, the work of Mant and his teams involved not only fieldwork, but also laboratory-based practice.

When the bodies were in too bad a condition to be examined, the injured parts were removed and sent to the laboratory.

Mant's thesis is relevant for grasping the issues at stake in the question of testimony versus forensic expertise. Remarkably, Mant was very quickly aware of the changing role of pathologists, whose expertise was increasingly in demand in the years following the war. He writes:

> In the earliest trials of war criminals charged with the murder of members of the Allied Armed Forces, no more than a written report on his findings was usually required of the pathologist. This report, in accordance with the provisions of the Royal Warrant (Paragraph 8), was put into the court and accepted as evidence without his personal appearance. It contained the evidence of identity of the victim, the cause of death and all relevant details concerned with the cause of death, together with the pathologist's remarks on the case.[69]

He viewed this increasing demand for pathologists' expertise as a consequence of a declining reliance on testimony, as he explicitly stated:

> As time progressed, however, more and more was required of the pathologist. This was mainly due to the increasing time-lag between the crime and the trial, and the consequent blunting of the memories of the witnesses, for as the witnesses' statements became more contradictory, so the medical evidence became more important, and was often subjected to searching cross-examination.[70]

However, this opinion must be put into perspective, when we know the precautions taken in relation to the testimonies, which were often used in compilation, and the stereotypical assumptions that surrounded some of them. Mant's analysis must also be understood in light of the quest for recognition and institutionalisation of his discipline, which was far from assured.[71] Before the Coroner's Rule of 1953, any qualified medical practitioner could be asked by the coroner to carry out an autopsy.[72] In the same year, a white paper on mortuaries helped modernise the processes for the management of dead bodies and post-mortem facilities. According to Mant, during the war, bombing raids also led to an improvement of equipment and the building of new mortuaries: 'Where these mortuaries were erected, they replaced the existing parish mortuaries. These wartime mortuaries were spacious ... having both a storage room and a post-mortem room with a standard autopsy table and a gas or electric water heater.'[73] Thus, the increasing reliance on forensic pathologists certainly stemmed from the modernisation and institutionalisation of their discipline.

The work carried out by Mant in post-war Germany influenced forensic medicine, as the exceptional circumstances had provided an unprecedented amount of data. In a paper published in 1987, Mant highlights:

> In Great Britain, exhumations for medico-legal and other purposes other than the removal of bodies from one cemetery to another are of rare occurrence ... The large numbers of exhumations for medico-legal purposes ... which were carried out in Europe after the Second World War provided a unique opportunity for a study of the changes which occur in a cadaver following internment under different conditions. It was not surprising that some of the old traditional teaching was found to be misleading.[74]

At a time when forensic medicine suffered from a lack of recognition as a medical discipline,[75] studies into the deaths of the Second World War were a great opportunity, both in terms of knowledge and acknowledgement.

Conclusion

This chapter has shown that the opposition between testimonies and forensic evidence was thematised very early on by those involved in these investigations. In the aftermath of the Second World War, discussions on the relevance of these different types of sources were already taking place. Forensic investigations did take place, but their use remained limited. Forensic pathologists were crucial for corpse identification and were regularly called to the opening of common graves. However, although their presence in the army was formalised, the options taken in terms of establishing the international tribunals did not leave them much room as documentary evidence and testimonies were the preferred means of evidence.

As the long history of investigation into the Holocaust shows, the culture of evidence not only shaped the judiciary process, but also framed the collective memory of an event. Some are concerned about the death of the last survivors in terms of the transmission of history, others ponder on the means of preserving the material traces, especially former camps.[76] The infatuation with the IMT and subsequently the Eichmann trial has undoubtedly contributed to the scholarship's inclination to focus on documentary evidence, before moving on to the testimonies. However, it would be wrong, in my opinion, to take testimonies and material evidence as fixed entities opposed to one other, the meaning of which has remained unchanged for seventy to one hundred years. I would rather argue that there is a continuum in the making of evidence, a continuum that includes a wide range of techniques and discourses, from oral testimony to forensic reports, from children's drawings to sworn statements. Thus, material evidence never speaks for itself and always needs to be understood in its context, above all in relation to mass violence.

Notes

This research is part of a broader project on forensics and mass violence in the Second World War started at the University of Oxford. It was funded from October 2020 to August 2021 by the British Academy (PF20\100101). I am grateful to this volume's editors, Sébastien Farré and the two anonymous reviewers for their helpful comments and suggestions on earlier drafts.

1 Mark Lewis, *The Birth of the New Justice: The Internationalization of Crime and Punishment, 1919–1950* (Oxford: Oxford University Press, 2014).
2 Erin-Marie Legacey, *Making Space for the Dead: Catacombs, Cemeteries, and the Reimagining of Paris, 1780–1930* (Ithaca: Cornell University Press, 2019).
3 Michel Vovelle and Régis Bertrand, *La ville des morts, essai sur l'imaginaire urbain contemporain d'après les cimetières provençaux* (Paris: Editions du CNRS, 1983); Michel Vovelle, *Mourir autrefois: Attitudes collectives devant la mort aux XVIIe et XVIIIe siècles* (Paris: Gallimard, 1974); Régis Bertrand, *Mort et mémoire: Provence, XVIIIe – XXe siècles: Une approche d'historien* (Marseille: La Thune, 2011).
4 Thomas Laqueur, *The Work of the Dead: A Cultural History of Mortal Remains* (Princeton: Princeton University Press, 2015), p. 222.

5 Adrien Douchet, Taline Garibian and Benoit Pouget, 'Managing the Remains of Citizen Soldiers: France and Its War Dead in 1914 and 1915', *Human Remains and Violence: An Interdisciplinary Journal* 7:1 (2021), pp. 37–51. doi:10.7227/HRV.7.1.4
6 See Christopher E. Mauriello, *Forced Confrontation: The Politics of Dead Bodies in Germany at the End of World War II* (Lanham Lexington Books, 2017) and Monica Black, *Death in Berlin: From Weimar to Divided Germany* (Cambridge and New York: Cambridge University Press, 2010).
7 On the confusion between the IMT and the twelve American trials, see Kim C. Priemel and Alexa Stiller, 'Introduction', in Kim C. Priemel and Alexa Stiller (eds), *Reassessing the Nuremberg Military Tribunals: Transitional Justice, Trial Narratives, and Historiography* (New York and Oxford: Berghahn Books, 2012).
8 See Daniel Bloxham, 'British War Crimes Trial Policy in Germany, 1945–1957: Implementation and Collapse', *Journal of British Studies* 42:1 (2003), pp. 91–118. doi:10.1086/342687 or Frédéric Mégret, 'The Bordeaux Trial: Prosecuting the Oradour-sur-Glane Massacre', in Kevin Jon Heller and Gerry Simpson (eds), *The Hidden Histories of War Crimes Trials* (Oxford: Oxford University Press, 2013), pp. 137–159.
9 Quoted by Shoshana Felman, *The Juridical Unconscious: Trials and Traumas in the Twentieth Century* (Cambridge, Massachusetts and London, England: Harvard University Press, 2002), pp. 132–133.
10 *Ibid.*, p. 133.
11 Paul Weindling, 'Victims, Witnesses, and the Ethical Legacy of the Nuremberg Medical Trial', in Priemel and Stiller, *Reassessing the Nuremberg Military Tribunals*, pp. 74–103, here p. 81.
12 See for example: Ulf Schmidt, ' "The Scars of Ravensbrück": Medical Experiments and British War Crimes Policy, 1945–1950', *German History* 23:1 (2005) pp. 20–49. doi:10.1191/0266355405gh334oa and Paul Weindling, *Nazi Medicine and the Nuremberg Trials: From Medical War Crimes to Informed Consent* (Basingstoke: Palgrave Macmillan, 2004).
13 Shoshana Felman and Dori Laub, *Testimony: Crises of Witnessing in Literature, Psychoanalysis and History* (London: Routledge, 1991); Annette Wieviorka, *The Era of the Witness* (Ithaca: Cornell University Press, 2006, first published in French in 1998).
14 Leora Bilsky, 'The Eichmann Trial: Toward a Jurisprudence of Eyewitness Testimony of Atrocities', *Journal of International Criminal Justice* 12:1 (2014), pp. 27–57. doi:10.1093/jicj/mqt075.

15 See Donald Bloxham, *Genocide on Trial: War Crimes Trials and the Formation of the Holocaust History and Memory* (Oxford: Oxford University Press, 2005); David Cesarani, *After Eichmann: Collective Memory and Holocaust Since 1961* (London: Routledge, 2005).
16 See, for example: Élisabeth Anstett and Jean-Marc Dreyfus (eds), *Destruction and Human Remains. Disposal and Concealment in Genocide and Mass Violence* (Manchester: Manchester University Press, 2014); Élisabeth Anstett and Jean-Marc Dreyfus (eds), *Human Remains and Identification: Mass Violence, Genocide and the 'Forensic Turn'* (Manchester: Manchester University Press, 2015); Francisco Ferrándiz and Antonius C. G. M. Robben (eds), *Necropolitics: Mass Graves and Exhumations in the Age of Human Rights* (Philadelphia: University of Pennsylvania Press, 2015).
17 Élisabeth Anstett and Jean-Marc Dreyfus, 'Introduction. Why Exhume?', in Anstett and Dreyfus, *Human Remains and Identification*, pp. 1–13.
18 Robert Jan van Pelt, *The Case for Auschwitz: Evidence from the Irving Trial* (Bloomington: Indiana University Press, 2016).
19 Zuzanna Dziuban, 'Introduction: Forensics in the Expanded Field', in Zuzanna Dziuban (ed.), *Mapping the 'Forensic Turn'* (Vienna: New Academic Press, 2017), pp. 7–35, here p. 18.
20 *Ibid.*, p. 12.
21 Adam Rosenblatt, *Digging for the Disappeared. Forensic Science After Atrocity* (Stanford: Stanford University Press, 2015), p. 3.
22 Dziuban, 'Introduction: Forensics', p. 19. See also Eyal Weizman, 'Violence at the Threshold of Detectability', in Dziuban, *Mapping the 'Forensic Turn'*, pp. 63–87.
23 Eyal Weizman, *The Least of All Possible Evils. A Short History of Humanitarian Violence* (London: Verso, 2017), p. 114.
24 The example of the International Katyn Commission of Inquiry shows that initiatives were even taken during the war.
25 Taline Garibian, 'Pain, Medicine and the Monitoring of War Violence: the Case of Rifle Bullets (1868–1918)', *Medical History* 66:2 (2022), pp. 155–172, doi.org/10.1017/mdh.2022.4.
26 Annex to the Convention (IV) respecting the Laws and Customs of War on Land, The Hague, 18 October 1907.
27 Convention for the Amelioration of the Condition of the Wounded and Sick in Armies in the Field, 6 July 1906, article 3.
28 John Horne and Alan Kramer, *German Atrocities, 1914: A History of Denial* (New Haven and London: Yale University Press, 2001).
29 Annette Becker, *Les cicatrices rouges, 14–18, France et Belgique occupées* (Paris: Fayard, 2010), p. 23.

30 Service historique de la défense (SHD), GR 16 N 302.
31 *Rapports et procès-verbaux d'enquête de la commission instituée en vue de constater les actes commis par l'ennemi en violation du droit des gens*, vol. 1 (Paris: Imprimerie Nationale, 1915).
32 See Rodolphe Archibald Reiss, 'Les balles explosibles autrichiennes', *Archives d'anthropologie criminelle* 29 (1914), pp. 895–909 and Rodolphe Archibald Reiss, *How Austria-Hungary Waged War in Serbia. Personal Investigation of a Neutral* (Paris: Armand Colin, 1915).
33 Rodolphe Archibald Reiss, *Report Upon the Atrocities Committed by the Austro-Hungarian Army During the First Invasion of Serbia* (London: Simpkin, Marshall, Hamilton, Kent & Co. Ltd, 1916), p. 30.
34 Joanna Bourke, *Wounding the World: How Military Violence and War-Play Invade Our Lives* (London: Virago Press, 2014).
35 Paul Chavigny, 'Le problème de l'organisation du service de la médecine légale aux armées ce qui a été fait à ce sujet dans les diverses armées en campagne pendant la guerre de 1914–1918', *Annales d'hygiène publique et de médecine légale* (1919), pp. 257–267.
36 Paul Chavigny, 'De l'identification des individus particulièrement en temps de guerre', *Annales d'hygiène publique et de médecine légale* (1917), pp. 32–40.
37 Lawrence Douglas, *The Memory of Judgement. Making Law and History in the Trials of the Holocaust* (New Haven and London: Yale University Press, 2001), p. 43; italics in original.
38 Black, *Death in Berlin*, p. 147.
39 Mauriello, *Forced Confrontation*.
40 Black, *Death in Berlin*, p. 148.
41 Convention for the Amelioration of the Condition of the Wounded and Sick in Armies in the Field, Geneva 27 July 1929, article 4.
42 Richard Bessel, 'The Shadow of Death in Germany at the End of the Second World War', in Alon Confino, Paul Betts and Dirk Schumann (eds), *Between Mass Death and Individual Loss. The Place of the Dead in Twentieth-Century Germany* (New York; Oxford: Berghahn Books, 2008), p. 59.
43 Jean-Marc Dreyfus, 'Renationalizing Bodies? The French Search Mission for the Corpses of Deportees in Germany, 1946–1958', in Jean-Marc Dreyfus and Élisabeth Anstett (eds), *Human Remains and Mass Violence. Methodological Approaches* (Manchester: Manchester University Press, 2015), pp. 129–145, here p. 138.
44 Stuart Hadaway, 'Identification Methods of the Royal Air Force Missing Research and Enquiry Service, 1944–52', *Forensic Science International* 318:110487 (2021) [n.p.]. doi: 10.1016/j.forsciint.2020.110487.

45 See Eric Ohtani, Haruyuki Makishima and Kazuhiro Sakaue, 'The Recovery and Repatriation of the Remains of Japanese War Dead and the Roles of Physical Anthropologists', *Forensic Science International* 324:110791 (2021) [n.p.]. doi:10.1016/j.forsciint.2021.110791; Dreyfus, 'Renationalizing Bodies?'; Michael Sledge, *Soldier Dead: How We Recover, Identify, Bury, and Honor Our Military Fallen* (New York, Chichester: Columbia University Press, 2005).
46 Charles E. Snow, 'The Identification of the Unknown War Dead', *American Journal of Physical Anthropology* 6:3 (1948), pp. 223–228.
47 National Archives Kew (hereafter NA), WO 309/372.
48 *Ibid*; emphasis in original.
49 See the *Mahn- und Gedenkstätte* website: www.ravensbrueck-sbg.de/en/history/1939-1945/
50 Born in 1919 in Surrey, Mant studied medicine before serving in the Royal Army Medical Corps from 1944 onwards. In November 1945, he led the War Crimes Investigating Team's pathology division which covered north-western Europe.
51 Paul Weindling, 'Auf der Spur von Medizinverbrechen: Keith Mant (1919–2000) und sein Debüt als forensischer Pathologe', *1999. Zeitschrift für Sozialgeschichte des 20. und 21. Jahrhunderts* 16 (2001), pp. 129–139.
52 Report by War Crimes Investigation Unit, BOAR, on Ravensbrück Concentration Camp, p. 8. NA, RW 2/6.
53 *Ibid.*, p. 10.
54 *Ibid.*, p. 1.
55 *Ibid.*
56 *Ibid.*, p. 14.
57 Donald Bloxham, *Genocide on Trial*, pp. 63–69.
58 Ulf Schmidt, ' "The Scars of Ravensbrück" '.
59 Weindling, 'Auf der Spur von Medizinverbrechen', p. 134.
60 Report by Major Arthur Keith Mant, R.A.M.C. on the Medical Services, Human Experimentation and other Medical Atrocities committed in Ravensbrück Concentration Camp, NA, RW 2/5.
61 Weindling, *Nazi Medicine and the Nuremberg Trials*, p. 63.
62 A. Keith Mant, 'A Study in Exhumation Data' (MD thesis, University of London, 1950).
63 *Ibid.*, p. 2.
64 *Ibid.*, pp. 2–3.
65 *Ibid.*, p. 9.
66 *Ibid.*, p. 47.
67 *Ibid.*, p. 18.
68 *Ibid.*, p. 57.

69 *Ibid.*, p. 5.
70 *Ibid.*, pp. 5–6.
71 A. Keith Mant, 'Forensic Medicine: What is the Future?', *The American Journal of Forensic Medicine and Pathology* 7:1 (1986), pp. 17–22.
72 A. Keith Mant, 'Changes in the Practice of Forensic Pathology, 1950–85', *Medicine, Sciences, and Law* 26:2 (1986), pp. 149–197. The Coroner's Rules of 1953 then stipulate that wherever possible a pathologist with laboratory facilities should be hired.
73 *Ibid.*, p. 152.
74 A. Keith Mant, 'Knowledge Acquired from Post-War Exhumation', in A. Boddington, A. N. Garland and R. C. Janawy (eds), *Death, Decay and Reconstruction. Approaches to Archaeology and Forensic Science* (Manchester: Manchester University Press, 1987), p. 65.
75 A. Keith Mant, 'Forensic Medicine'.
76 This idea was expressed by van Pelt several times in different media. See, for example: Richard Gizbert, 'Save Auschwitz, or Leave it to Rot?', *ABC News*, 6 January 2006, https://abcnews.go.com/Nightline/story?id=128520&page=1 (accessed 23 October 2021).

4

Teaching Grossian criminalistics in Imperial Germany

Heather Wolffram

Introduction

In considering the transition from one forensic culture to another, be that the replacement of an indigenous forensic culture by a colonial one or an older forensic culture by a newer one, historians of the forensic sciences have concentrated on explicating the often lengthy process by which these transformations are achieved.[1] Pointing to moments in which the transmission or teaching of the new culture is evident or cases in which the epistemology and practices that distinguish the new culture are explicit, these historians have illuminated not just the process of cultural change, but the importance of both international and national contexts in determining how forensic cultures are taught, practised and institutionalised in specific countries.[2] Of particular note in this regard is the 2016 book by Ian Burney and Neil Pemberton *Murder and the Making of English CSI*, in which the authors consider the process by which English murder investigation came to be focused on the crime scene and the scientific analysis of the traces found within it. Through their use of 'flash moments', murder cases that highlight the evolution from a body- to trace-centred forensic regime, and their discussions of how English detectives were taught continental or 'Grossian' practices of crime scene investigation (CSI), Burney and Pemberton demonstrate how a peculiarly English form of CSI emerged in the first half of the twentieth century.[3]

While *Murder and the Making of English CSI* goes a long way towards helping us understand how the transition between forensic cultures occurs, it also highlights a number of surprising historiographical gaps. As other historians have done before them and since,

Burney and Pemberton locate the beginnings of CSI in the system of criminalistics developed by the Austrian investigating judge Hans Gross (1847–1915) around the turn of the century.[4] They also point to the frequent comparisons made by English advocates of scientific policing during the interwar period between the well-established systems of criminalistics in Austria, Germany and France and those in England.[5] On this basis, it would be easy to assume both that the transition to and institutionalisation of Grossian criminalistics on the Continent was long complete by the end of the First World War and that the history of this process had been thoroughly canvassed by historians. Closer examination of the extant literature, however, suggests that while Gross's attempt to implement his new system in Austria has attracted some attention, scholars are yet to explore how criminalistics replaced older approaches to crime in other locations, including neighbouring Germany.[6] Perversely, it seems we know more about the process by which the English system of CSI, which built on continental criminalistics, was introduced and replaced older forensic regimes than we do about its adoption among the German practitioners of criminal justice on whom Gross had the most direct influence. In its concentration on the teaching of criminalistics in Imperial Germany (1871–1918), therefore, this chapter seeks to strengthen our understanding of how German criminalists were taught this new forensic culture and the extent to which the processes of transition to and institutionalisation of Grossian criminalistics were complete by 1918. In addition, the chapter sets out to demonstrate, as Burney and Pemberton have done for England, how both national context and international influences shaped German forensic culture.

The use of the term 'forensic culture', rather than another commonly utilised concept, 'forensic regime', is deliberate here. At its most basic level, 'forensic culture' describes all those ideas and values in circulation about the problem of crime and its investigation, not just among investigators, pathologists and scientists, but also among others involved in the criminal justice process as well as the public. 'Forensic regime', by contrast, has been employed by historians as a useful shorthand for the set of assumptions, behaviours and practices associated with death investigation at particular times and places, often with the aim of highlighting the transition between a body-centred forensics and a trace-centred one.[7] A forensic regime is thus an important part of a forensic culture, but not its totality. While discussions of forensic regimes by no means ignore epistemology and popular conceptions of forensic science, they are necessarily focused on the more concrete elements of forensic work and markers of regime change, such as the behaviour of investigators, crime scene procedure and techniques of laboratory analysis. If we are to understand how new forensic ideas are transmitted and accepted among a broader group of people, however, an emphasis solely on these tangible signifiers of cultural change is unlikely to tell us the whole story. As this analysis of the teaching of criminalistics in Imperial Germany, which considers the broader discourse and debate about forensic science at the time, will demonstrate, the acceptance of a new forensic culture among both practitioners and lay people may occur well in advance of any concrete changes to behaviours, practice or institutions.

As the burgeoning historiography of the forensic sciences has demonstrated, the emergence of new forensic cultures, which often result from epistemic and procedural shifts, technological and scientific development and pragmatic need, offer opportunities to understand how forensic culture is transmitted both nationally and internationally and how this process might differ between countries. In England, for instance, the transmission of Grossian criminalistics during the 1930s focused on detectives, who it was hoped would conduct propaganda work for the new system of investigation within their own forces.[8] In Germany by contrast, where circulation of Gross's ideas was already evident at the *fin de siècle*, emphasis was put on the teaching of criminalistics to jurists, who considered themselves best placed to lead the transformation of Germany's forensic culture. This was due to two factors: the holistic view that judges, particularly investigating judges, had of the criminal justice process; and the requirement that higher police officials were trained in law. Tracing the efforts of German jurists to teach criminalistics to their colleagues and other criminal justice practitioners, this chapter will argue that while there was little tangible sign of the institutionalisation of the new forensic culture by 1918, a cultural transformation had nonetheless taken place. This transformation had been facilitated not just by the range of initiatives, beginning early in the twentieth century, to instruct jurists and other investigators in criminalistics, but also through discussion of foreign institutional models and practices, which simultaneously acted as an inspiration and as a source of anxiety about Germany's scientific reputation. German criminalists, this chapter will argue, watched other countries establish apparently robust systems of criminalistics training, service and research during the early twentieth century, leading them to express embarrassment at their nation's slow progress in the field. This prompted a number of vocal advocates of the new culture to practise what might be called 'forensic patriotism'; a largely rhetorical strategy which sought to leverage national pride and concerns about being left behind scientifically to encourage reform. How 'forensic patriotism' was mobilised in the context of the First World War and what impact it had on the understanding of science, in general, and the forensic sciences, in particular, as international pursuits will be examined in the last section of this chapter.

A new forensic culture

In Germany at the *fin de siècle* a modern scientific approach to crime and criminal investigation, embodied most clearly in Hans Gross's system of criminalistics, appears to have been emerging. That contemporaries were engaged in proselytising for this new forensic culture is evident in the range of schools, programmatic statements, handbooks and journals launched by prominent criminalists around 1900. Franz von Liszt's (1851–1919) modern school of criminal law, for instance, signalled not only a shift away from fixed punishments prescribed by the law towards empirically based individualisation of punishment, but the necessity of applying science to all parts of the criminal justice process, including the investigation and prosecution.[9] As Gross stressed, von Liszt's 'modern German school' had firmly integrated criminalistics into its programme of work, introducing a new generation of investigating judges and prosecutors – largely through Gross's own *Handbook for Investigating Judges as a System of Criminalistics* (1893) – to knowledge in the areas of Bertillonage, graphology, forensic photography, witness psychology and the application and evaluation of various expert witnesses as well as to crucial skills such as sketching crime scenes and the preservation of evidence.[10] The birth of this new forensic culture was highlighted further by the foundation of several periodicals in which criminology and criminalistics were key features, including *Archiv für Kriminal-Anthropologie und Kriminalistik* (*Archive for Criminal Anthropology and Criminalistics*) (1898) (hereafter *Archiv*) and *Monatsschrift für Kriminalpsychologie und Strafrechtsreform* (*Monthly Journal for Criminal Psychology and Criminal Law Reform*) (1904) (hereafter *Monatsschrift*).[11] The former had the goal of making criminology and criminalistics practical scientific aids to criminal law, while the latter sought to apply research findings in criminology and criminal psychology to the reform of criminal justice.[12]

This emphasis on the application of science to the criminal justice process was new in the Imperial period, clearly signalling a shift away from a forensic culture in which judicial truth-finding was bound tightly by formal rules of evidence and dependent on confessions and witnesses, to a culture in which the court's free evaluation of evidence fostered the increasing use of expert witnesses and the testimony of those *stumme Zeugen* (mute witnesses), that is, physical evidence, left at crime scenes. The impetus for this transition had been both the procedural changes wrought by the introduction of a new *Strafprozessordnung* (Code of Criminal Procedure) in the late 1870s and empirical psychological research during the late nineteenth century, which threatened to undermine criminal law's reliance on witness testimony for establishing facts. As Christopher Hamlin's work on forensic cultures implies, changes to legal institutions, what he calls 'technologies of judgement' will necessarily impact upon the application of both technologies of witness (forensic techniques) and technologies of testimony (professions recognised to apply and interpret forensic techniques).[13] This was certainly the case in Imperial Germany.

Within the inquisitorial legal systems that had prevailed in the German states prior to the middle of the nineteenth century, the status of the witness, as a means of establishing material truth, had been unsurpassed by documentary evidence, but was dependent on strict rules that excluded certain types of people from testifying as they were deemed unreliable.[14] Expert witnesses, by contrast, played a relatively minor role in proceedings. While the testimony of physicians and midwives was mandatory for some crimes, their role was confined to providing written reports establishing the physical facts of the case, that is, what had happened and whether it was criminal.[15] Changes adopted nationally as part of the 1879 Code of Criminal Procedure, not only introduced public trials, oral testimony and juries for the determination of serious crimes, but also removed the inquisitorial rules of proof, allowing for the free evaluation of evidence (*freie Beweiswürdigung*).[16] This principle left it up to judges and juries to determine the type and volume of evidence that constituted sufficient proof.[17] In terms of witness testimony, this enabled those witnesses, including women and children, who had previously been excluded from testifying, to give evidence, even though suspicion of their credibility had not lessened. It also led to expert testimony, now presented orally and publicly, playing a more significant role in the court's determination of facts and of guilt.[18] In contrast to common law jurisdictions at the same time, where distrust of men of science translated into a need for expert witnesses to prove their value, the willingness of German judges to call experts, particularly medical experts, provides evidence of the growing prestige of science in German society during the late nineteenth and early twentieth centuries.[19]

The procedural changes that altered German courtroom practice following 1871 coincided with psychological research on perception and suggestion that further undermined the value of witness testimony for establishing the facts of a case. Empirical research conducted during the 1880s and 1890s revealed not only that the long-held suspicion of children's testimony was well founded, but that even those witnesses who had been considered reliable under the inquisitorial system were prone to faulty perception, suggestion and falsification of memory.[20] The resulting crisis around the reliability of the witness led to jurists advocating the need for a forensic psychology that would educate them in the sources of witness error, as well as scientific tools, including suitable expert witnesses, which would allow them to establish facts via the physical traces of crime.[21] Jurists' calls for a system of criminalistics that might equip them for this new environment, in which the credibility of all witness testimony was questionable and nearly all evidence was admissible, signalled the transition to a new forensic culture based on empirical science, rather than legal dogma.

Leading proponents of criminalistics in German-speaking Europe, most of whom were legally trained, argued that the implementation of this new culture should be led by jurists. While a few prominent medico-legalists, such as Richard Kockel (1865–1934), maintained that medico-legal institutes might become centres for both forensic services and instruction, warning that these tasks should not be allowed to fall into the hands of jurists or police, the rationale for judges leading the transformation of Germany's forensic culture was compelling.[22] The judges' position, unlike that of any other criminal justice practitioner, including medico-legalists and police investigators, necessitated their involvement in and overview of the entire criminal justice process.[23] While forensic training was naturally required for police and other practitioners involved in criminal investigations, application of their skills would be coordinated and directed by an investigating judge. In this regard, Gross maintained, 'if someone says: that all of this is a matter for the police, not judges, so is this objection as easy as it is incorrect. Above all, the recording of the facts, usually the basis of the entire proceedings, in all important cases are a matter for the investigating judge.'[24]

The education of criminal judges, particularly investigating judges, in criminalistics was, therefore, regarded as the most effective means of ensuring that the whole criminal justice system and all its practitioners adopted the new forensic culture. The requirement that all higher police officials in Germany had a law degree and the fact that many *Kriminalkommissare* (lead detectives), approximately 45 per cent, were legally trained, also suggested efficiencies in concentrating on teaching criminalistics to jurists.[25] This contrasted with the situation in other countries, including Italy, where it was police that were regarded as the most important targets for education in criminalistics. Salvatore Ottolenghi (1861–1934), who founded an Italian school of scientific policing at the turn of the century, noted that he had 'urged the adoption of the new system ... to introduce a scientific method, based on investigation, in all departments of the police' because he wished to 'raise the efficiency of this powerful weapon of social defense'.[26] 'The new pedagogy of scientific police', he stated, was intended to 'teach the officers and the judges how to observe, to reason, and to be absolutely impartial in investigations and reports'.[27] In Italy, as Ottolenghi makes clear, education of the police followed by that of jurists was regarded the surest means of facilitating a change in forensic culture.

As Hamlin has suggested when tracing the changes between early modern forensic culture and that of the eighteenth century, it would be misleading to imagine such changes in terms of abrupt transitions.[28] New cultures must be accepted, transmitted and taught, but impediments, both epistemological and structural, may slow or stall this process. In Germany, the belief that it was jurists, rather than police, who should lead the scientific transformation of criminal justice had unforeseen consequences. The insistence on educating jurists in the new forensic sciences necessitated both an overhaul of legal education and an institutionalisation of forensic services that in the Imperial period, at least, proved difficult to achieve. While those who had embraced the new forensic culture avidly put forward suggestions about curriculum and institutional reform or sought to teach criminalistics through short courses and handbooks, Germany's system of legal training proved difficult to modify and the provision of forensic services hard to either rationalise or institutionalise. In many other countries, or so it appeared to German criminalists, significant progress had been made in systematising and institutionalising the forensic sciences before the First World War, usually in the form of criminalistics institutes or schools of scientific policing. Why were German efforts less successful?

Transmitting criminalistics

The procedural changes introduced towards the end of the nineteenth century altered the role of judges by transferring their accusatory function to the prosecution and, in *Schwurgerichte* (jury courts), their decision-making power to a jury, but their investigative role was largely maintained at the pre-trial stage.[29] In the *Hauptverhandlung* (main trial) also, despite the public and oral presentation of evidence, an inquisitorial core was preserved by making judges responsible for carrying out the hearing of evidence and the passing of judgment (in non-jury trials).[30] While these responsibilities at both the investigative and trial stages arguably put judges in the best position to model the new forensic culture to other criminal justice practitioners, it was clear that the theoretical training offered by German universities ill prepared graduates for the realities of modern judicial practice, which necessitated a sound understanding of criminal and witness psychology as well as the value of expert witnesses for explicating forensic evidence.[31] The question then was how the criminal jurist, particularly the aspiring investigating judge, might acquire this practical knowledge. Gross suggested there were three conceivable ways. First, the individual could acquire such knowledge for themselves through experience and reading. This method, however, Gross warned, was a lengthy process and even the most comprehensive handbook both left things out and was quickly outdated by advances in science and technology.[32] Second, jurists might receive instruction while practising law via courses held at convenient locations such as courthouses. Where adequate numbers of suitable teachers might be found for this purpose, however, was unclear. Third, training in criminalistics might occur in the universities, if professorships in this discipline were created and expertise from other sciences was mobilised to create a programme of instruction.[33] Such a programme, Gross argued, 'must have as its goal the complete criminal-technical training of the investigating judge, because it is he ... that represents the prototype of the criminalist'.[34] But, while Gross initially advocated for the inclusion of criminalistics within the university legal curriculum, imagining that twenty years hence there would be chairs established in this field,[35] he soon concluded that the necessity of continued research in the forensic sciences would require not just space in the universities, but the creation of specific institutes for criminalistics.[36]

By 1912 Gross had established such an institute in Austria, but in Germany little progress had been made towards the incorporation of the forensic sciences within the universities, let alone the foundation of institutes for research and practical instruction in the field. The Berlin-based jurist Albert Hellwig (1880–1950) noted in this regard that, in contrast to other countries, German universities seldom offered lectures on forensic psychology, criminalistics, forensic chemistry and other scientific aids to modern criminal law.[37] This was to some extent a result of the principle of *Lehrfreiheit* (the freedom to teach what one wants). Opportunities for training in criminalistics following university study, however, were limited too, with Hellwig complaining that trainee judges in Berlin, as elsewhere, were dependent on working with a 'good judge', familiar with the works of Hans Gross, if they were to expand their knowledge beyond the dogmatic literature.[38] Similar analyses of the deficiencies of German criminal justice, accompanied by arguments for the necessity of criminalistic knowledge in legal praxis, became common features of criminological congresses and specialist periodicals like the *Archiv* and *Monatsschrift* by the second decade of the century.[39] For instance, at the 11th International Congress of the International Crime Association held in Copenhagen in 1913, the German contingent responded enthusiastically to Professor Josef Heimberger's (1865–1933) suggestions about the specialist training of jurists in scientific aids, including criminalistics, criminology, forensic medicine and penology.[40] But, while there was growing consensus on the importance of the forensic sciences for criminal justice practitioners, there was debate about when and where instruction in it was best supplied.

The desirability of regular courses in criminalistics intended to support the professional development of practising jurists and police investigators was self-evident to proponents of the modern school of criminal law, but the timing and location of basic training in this area was disputed.[41] Professor Heimberger's Copenhagen talk, for example, concluded that, as a rule, such training should occur after university study.[42] This conclusion rested on several factors, including that university study was intended to provide a general legal education, rather than a specialist one, and that the amount of examinable material in the curriculum was already onerous.[43] The counter argument, which was supported by the director of Berlin's Identification Service, Hans Schneickert (1876–1944), stressed that it would be simplest to include the teaching of scientific aids alongside other legal subjects at university. This would ensure both that trainee jurists acquired adequate knowledge of the field and that legal study, which had a well-founded reputation for being dry, was refreshed and enlivened.[44]

While leading figures within the modern school of criminal law remained divided over whether knowledge of criminalistics was best imparted at university or in the latter stages of practical training, they did increasingly agree on the benefits of erecting dedicated institutes for criminalistics, modelled on that of Gross. By the eve of the First World War, jurists and other criminal justice practitioners were presenting plans and petitions for institutes that would provide forensic training, services and research. The Leipzig-based medico-legalist Kockel, for instance, who wished to transform Germany's medico-legal institutes into institutes for forensic medicine and criminalistics, used both Hermann Zangger's institute in Zurich and that established by Gross in Graz as blueprints.[45] The criminal psychologist Hans von Hentig (1887–1974), in contrast, proposed a criminological institute that would facilitate research into criminal sociology and criminal statistics, offer services in psychology and psychopathology and provide laboratories focused on scientific crime detection.[46] Shortly thereafter, the government advisor Heinrich Lindenau, the jurist Franz von Liszt and the forensic pathologist Fritz Strassmann (1858–1940), lobbied the Prussian Ministry of Justice, calling for the erection of a state criminalistics institute, which would run courses for practitioners as well as offer a range of forensic services.[47]

In spite of such proposals, by 1918, Germany was no closer to providing its jurists with systematic instruction in criminalistics or a criminalistics institute than it had been in the first decade of the century. There were several reasons for this. First, a lack of consensus appears to have been a significant hurdle to reform. The discussion of when and where trainee jurists might be taught criminalistics, as we have seen, led to disagreement between those who considered it an important addition to the university legal curriculum and those who saw it as a component of later professional development. Similarly, proposals for the erection of criminalistics institutes created divisions over whether a centralised or decentralised system would work best, providing both sufficient service and the best value for money. Gross, for example, proposed that Germany erect a single Reich Institute for Criminalistics, located at a University in one of the country's larger cities.[48] Figures like Heimberger and Lindenau, however, dismissed this idea, advocating instead for the utmost decentralisation.[49] Without clear agreement on such issues, it proved difficult to make progress towards the institutionalisation of the new culture; a problem that was exacerbated by the resistance to change of existing institutions and systems, including the traditional system of legal training. It was here that the consequences of trusting the transmission of the new forensic culture to jurists becomes most evident.

As leading advocates of the teaching of criminalistics to jurists, such as Lindenau, von Liszt and Strassmann, made clear, the realisation of this ambition hung on the reform of the criminal law curriculum both in the universities and during the period of practical training.[50] Debate on the necessity of reforming legal training had begun shortly after unification, as differences between the curriculum in different states became apparent,[51] and continued into the twentieth century as demands for the inclusion of more socially and scientifically relevant content were suggested to combat claims that German jurists were unworldly.[52] There was a widespread feeling throughout the Imperial period that legal training was inadequate,[53] but, as Silviana Galassi has concluded, there was ultimately little appetite for overhauling legal training in the states and little room for including additional material on topics such as criminology and criminalistics in the curriculum.[54] Furthermore, as Konrad H. Jarausch points out, entrenched bureaucracy and professional organisations had a vested interest in subverting substantial reform of legal training because the existing system enabled trainee jurists to be exploited for their cheap labour and for menial tasks.[55] For these reasons, those advocating the inclusion of criminalistics within the curriculum could make little progress towards an official system for transmitting this knowledge because the broader debate about legal training had stalled.[56] Whereas in other countries, including Austria and Italy, training of jurists and detectives in criminalistics was quite quickly organised and institutionalised, in Germany before 1918 attempts at practical instruction in and theoretical transfer of criminalistic knowledge remained piecemeal and sporadic.

Teaching jurists criminalistics

Gross, in his calls during the 1890s for the complete criminal-technical training of the practical jurist, had not simply been a polemicist.[57] By 1894, he had given two series of lectures to court officials and police instructors in Vienna, which based their programme on the content of his *Handbook*.[58] The course held for police instructors concentrated on transmitting knowledge of practical aids to investigation, including the problem of false perception among witnesses, effective interrogation of suspects, how to proceed at a crime scene, what experts in medicine, chemistry, physics and botany could do and thus what objects were worth protecting, preserving and collecting for later examination.[59] Not long afterward, Gross was establishing a Criminal Museum in Graz and considering the most effective ways of exhibiting and cataloguing objects in order to facilitate the hands-on teaching of criminalistics.[60] By 1912, this museum had been incorporated into Gross's criminalistic institute at the University of Graz, which not only offered forensic services and research facilities, but also instruction in criminal anthropology, criminal psychology, criminalistics and criminal statistics.[61] Students received both theoretical and practical instruction in criminalistics, hearing lectures and working in the institute's laboratories. Practical training courses were also held periodically for court and police officials.[62]

Taking inspiration from Gross's example, German advocates of the teaching of criminalistics experimented with several forms of transmission. As the *Handbook for Investigating Judges* had proved, one means of transferring knowledge to criminal justice practitioners was the publication of guides to the field. Several high-ranking German police officials, pathologists and jurists took this approach. The works of Albert Weingart and Heinrich Lindenau, for instance, sought to provide police officials and other criminal justice practitioners with an overview of the methods of criminal investigation and guidelines for goal-oriented investigative work.[63] Strassmann's *Medizin und Strafrecht: Ein Handbuch für Juristen, Laienrichter und Ärzte* (*Medicine and Criminal Law: A Handbook for Jurists, lay Judges and Doctors*) (1911) built on lectures about forensic medicine given to students of law and sought to provide jurists with an overview of the services legal medicine could offer in the realm of criminal law.[64] Such volumes, which were often well-illustrated, were intended as practical guides to criminalistics that might aid jurists and judges in selecting appropriate expert witnesses, understanding the significance of trace evidence or appreciating the best means of crime scene investigation. Other works had an even wider remit, seeking to inform not just criminal justice practitioners, but also educated lay readers, whose interest in modern criminalistics and concern about judicial competency might help create pressure for more systematic instruction in the forensic sciences. A good example of such a work was Hellwig's 1914 *Moderne Kriminalistik* (*Modern Criminalistics*), which not only introduced readers to the basics of modern crime scene investigation, but argued stridently that the integrity of Germany's criminal justice system was dependent on jurists and other practitioners being well-versed in modern criminalistics. According to Hellwig, this necessitated that the state pursue substantial reform of legal training and invest in the institutionalisation of criminalistics.[65]

Beyond the publication of guides as a means of teaching forensic science and crime scene investigation, German jurists and police also experimented with short training courses reminiscent of those run by Gross in Vienna. The Berlin Police, for example, held advanced training courses in criminalistics from 1906 and repeated these every two years for interested parties.[66] From 1910, the courts in Berlin and Potsdam offered introductions to criminalistics, which initially targeted trainee jurists, but were soon made available to judges and prosecutors.[67] As with similar courses abroad, lectures were provided by experienced detectives, forensic pathologists and chemists, experts in criminal identification and the forensic sciences. Emphasis was placed on practical advice about crime scene protocol and procedure, the significance of trace evidence and an understanding of how particular types of expert might best aid the jurist or detective.[68] Practical demonstrations, photographic illustrations and field trips were all vital components of these courses.[69] According to Hellwig, the richness of such programmes left little to be desired and provided excellent overviews of modern criminalistics, but, he stressed, the criminalist could not become expert in forensic psychiatry or chemistry in a few hours; this required intensive training, which short ad hoc courses could not provide. In the absence of thoroughgoing reform of the legal curriculum, however, Hellwig hoped that such short courses would become standard for court trainees as well as judges and prosecutors in both Prussia and the other German states.[70] Only in this way could German jurists reassure the public that an ignorance of modern investigatory techniques did not contribute to miscarriages of justice.

Forensic patriotism and internationalism

If presenting the issue of training in criminalistics to the broader public as a matter of the competency of criminal justice practitioners was one polemic strategy used to create pressure for reform, another was the mobilisation of anxieties about Germany's backwardness in this field; a strategy that is referred to here as 'forensic patriotism'. International congresses and international networks afforded German jurists a good understanding of how other countries had organised their forensic services during the early twentieth century and provided them with ample ammunition to argue that Germany's systems were inferior.[71] Both prior to and during the First World War, then, 'forensic patriotism' provided further impetus for reform and a compelling argument that financial investment in the teaching of criminalistics was strategically necessary. Armed with information about the detrimental impact of the war on crime rates as well as a range of flexible martial metaphors, campaigning jurists appealed to the authorities' patriotism, seeking ultimately to have the state create and invest in the systems of forensic training required to ensure that the nation's organs of criminal justice were not an international embarrassment.[72] Perhaps surprisingly, given the hostilities between 1914 and 1918, comparisons between Germany's systems of criminalistic training and those of other nations, including enemies, did not lead to jingoism or calls to break off relations with the international scientific community. The idea that science was international, that even enemy nations might have systems worth replicating and that science was necessarily damaged by attempts to confine it to the national level, sat alongside complaints about Germany's comparative failings in criminalistics.

In his 1914 call for an institute for the criminal sciences, Hentig noted that Austria, France and Belgium had all outstripped Germany in this field by establishing modern and exemplary research facilities. He argued that the German preference for theory over practice and belief that books sufficed as a means of transferring knowledge, threatened to undermine any claim by the German police or legal authorities to be operating on a scientific or empirical basis.[73] While this assessment was damning, Hentig remained confident that the thirst for knowledge and drive for professional development among German criminal justice practitioners could soon rectify this situation. Hentig's use of national comparison, scientific anxiety and patriotic pride as a means of pushing for reform, was a common strategy among advocates for the teaching and institutionalisation of criminalistics in Germany during the late Imperial period,[74] but was employed most thoroughly by Hellwig in his 1918 international survey of training opportunities and facilities in the forensic sciences.[75] On the basis of this survey, Hellwig's evaluation of Germany's standing in the field was that, 'For years we have written and spoken more about the absolute necessity of a thoroughgoing criminalistic education, than just about any other civilised nation, but what has been achieved thus far ... is as good as nothing to satisfy even the most frugal requirements.'[76]

The other countries surveyed, as he demonstrated, had done a far better job of implementing systems of forensic training than had Germany. Austria-Hungary, for example, could boast Gross's criminalistic institute at the University of Graz, while nations such as Switzerland and Italy had been running courses or regular lecture series for expert witnesses, students of law and police officials since 1902.[77] Just like Hentig before him, Hellwig was convinced there was no want of enthusiasm among German jurists and police officials for a modern scientific approach to crime, but the transmission and institutionalisation of this new culture, at least in the form of university courses, regular professional development and academic chairs and institutes, was frustratingly slow. He concluded, 'With shame and regret one must opine that in this important cultural issue, in the question of the training of the organs of criminal justice in criminalistics, which is an essential precondition for an actual and effective fight against crime, Germany stands a long way from first position.'[78]

Such patriotic appeals, which relied on a belief that Germany should occupy a leading position in this field, sought to demonstrate to the authorities that their investment in the reform of the legal curriculum and in criminalistic training would pay dividends in combatting crime and in maintaining both the integrity of the justice system and Germany's scientific reputation.[79]

'Forensic patriotism' as a rhetorical strategy was employed by proponents of the new forensic culture from early in the twentieth century, but the First World War saw these calls for reform take on a new urgency. The social, economic and political crises that accompanied the hostilities led to a rise in crime, particularly juvenile crime, which threatened stability on the home front and longer-term economic prosperity. While advocates of the new culture were conscious that the question of the training of criminalists in scientific aids to crime detection had, like thousands of other important social questions, been paused for the duration of the war, they nonetheless argued that those nations that moved quickly to combat the increase in crime would not only avoid a myriad of domestic problems, but would also have the advantage over other states in a post-war world.[80] The most effective means of doing this, they claimed, was to invest in the reform of the legal curriculum and the training of all the organs of criminal justice in modern criminalistics. In this regard, figures like Hellwig argued, it was short-sighted to postpone the urgently required reforms to the training of criminal justice practitioners on the basis of short-term financial or political considerations; indeed, these reforms would ultimately save money, given the impact of crime on the nation's coffers every year.[81] In addition, and perhaps predictably, these patriotic appeals began to more explicitly use martial metaphors and the lessons of warfare in order to make their arguments more persuasive. Rhetorically, polemicists, like Hellwig, wrote of the threat of an 'army of criminals' that, unchecked by improvements to the means of 'fighting' crime, would overrun the state. Furthermore, they pointed to lessons learnt during the war, drawing parallels between what had been discovered at the front and attempts to combat crime. For example, Hellwig declared that the war had taught not only the absolute necessity of choosing the right people for specific tasks and the importance of practical technical and scientific training, but also that money could not be spared if one wanted to achieve something significant.[82]

While the war elicited a more urgent tone and martial language among those who employed 'forensic patriotism' as a means of pushing for reform, it did not lead, as it did in some other sciences, to hostility to foreign scientists or scientific internationalism. Among German physicists, for example, there were calls for scientific autarky and attempts to create a nationalist physics that cited more German than English works and replaced foreign scientific terms with German ones.[83] In contrast, proponents of the new forensic culture rejected scientific autarky and continued to stress the importance of scientific internationalism. The war, Hellwig stated, had naturally shrunk opportunities for international exchange, but a permanent shrinking to the national level would ultimately be detrimental because science and the advance of science were international endeavours.[84] This suggests that advocates of the new forensic culture in Imperial Germany continued to see the transmission of forensic knowledge across national borders as necessary, even in the context of a global war. It also shows that they believed that the best means of achieving the transition from the old forensic culture, which predated 1871, to the new one focused on the use of science to establish legal truth, was to convince the authorities of the necessity of reform through a combination of appeals based on Germany's international scientific reputation and explanations of how the adoption of foreign models of forensic training might ease the nation's financial burden in combatting crime. This is not to suggest that there was no sense of international competition in criminalists' appeals, which argued that those nations that dealt well with rising crime rates caused by the war would have a competitive advantage over others in the post-war era, but that as far as proponents of the new forensic culture were concerned the most patriotic thing they could do was to point to the advantages of other countries' systems, even if those countries were currently enemies.

Conclusion

Clearly, the desire of German criminalists to transmit the new trace-based forensic culture that emerged during the late nineteenth century to all criminal justice practitioners by educating criminal jurists in criminalistics was not fully realised by the end of the Imperial period. Concrete signifiers of cultural change, such as the reform of the legal curriculum and the construction of institutes, were absent, but the polemics, petitions, texts and short courses that promoted a modern scientific approach to the investigation of crime were indications that the basic ideas and values associated with the new culture were in circulation and accepted by leading German criminalists by 1918. The peculiarities of the German context, including its entrenched tradition of legal training and its emphasis on the education of jurists as the best means of transmitting forensic culture, were responsible for the slow institutionalisation of modern criminalistics in Germany. Elsewhere, as this chapter has shown, the teaching of criminalistics focused on police, leading fairly rapidly in places like Italy and Switzerland to the foundation of schools of scientific policing.

This chapter has focused on a moment during the transition between forensic cultures in which epistemology had altered, but systems for fully realising the culture had not. This approach highlights not just how local conditions impact on the transmission of forensic cultures between nations and how new cultures circulated in advance of concrete changes to forensic regimes, but also casts light on the strategies by which contemporaries hoped to rectify this situation. Several strategies were used by proponents of the new forensic culture to encourage reform in Imperial Germany. First were arguments about the financial benefits of embracing modern investigatory procedures and techniques. Second were those pleas based on the human toll of maintaining an incompetent justice system. If criminal justice practitioners were not adequately trained in modern criminalistics, so the argument went, miscarriages of justice could not be prevented. Third were patriotic appeals, which compared the status of German systems of criminalistics to those in other countries in order to argue that Germany would be left behind scientifically if it did not swiftly deal with its inadequate provision of training and service in the forensic sciences.

Analysis of the strategy labelled 'forensic patriotism' in this chapter, underlines further the important role international forensic networks and the example of foreign forensic cultures play in the transition from one forensic culture to another; not least in providing a point of leverage in places where local conditions or traditions militate against change. While in the case examined here, German criminalists mobilised embarrassment over the state of criminalistics in Germany to campaign for reform, claiming the superiority of foreign systems even during the First World War, it is possible to imagine that in other national contexts and at other times, 'forensic patriotism' might have had a range of different purposes, including bids to maintain or increase funding or to insist on or resist restructuring of forensic services. In addition, the internationalism displayed by German criminalists in their use of this strategy is not a given. One can envision a form of 'forensic patriotism' that both boasted of national superiority and rejected foreign models and cooperation. All of this is to suggest that for those historians interested in both shifts in forensic cultures and the interplay of national and international systems of forensic knowledge and expertise, the question of whether the strategy of comparing forensic systems at home and abroad has been employed more broadly and for what purposes, seems worth pursuing.

Notes

1 For a consideration of four different forensic cultures and the transition between them from the sixteenth century to the present day, see Christopher Hamlin, 'Forensic Cultures in Historical Perspective: Technologies of Witness, Testimony, Judgment (and Justice?)', *Studies in History and Philosophy of Biological and Biomedical Sciences* 44 (2013), pp. 4–15. Good examples of the international transfer of forensic knowledge include Ian Burney and Neil Pemberton, *Murder and the Making of English CSI* (Baltimore: Johns Hopkins University Press, 2016), which traces the translation of Hans Gross's manual of criminalistics into English for use in the Indian context, its reception in England and the processes by which continental forms of crime scene investigation were adapted to and put into practice in the English context. Also, Jeffrey Jentzen, 'Death and Empire: Medicolegal Investigations and Practice across the British Empire', in Ian Burney and Christopher Hamlin (eds), *Global Forensic Cultures: Making Fact and Justice in the Modern Era* (Baltimore: Johns Hopkins University Press, 2019), pp. 149–173. On transnational networks, see Heather Wolffram, 'Forensic Knowledge and Forensic Networks in Britain's Empire: The Case of Sydney Smith', in Burney and Hamlin, *Global Forensic Cultures*, pp. 235–256.

2 For examples of works that examine attempts to teach new forensic cultures, see Burney and Pemberton, *Murder and the Making of English CSI*, pp. 103–118; Annette Mülberger, 'Teaching Psychology to Jurists: Initiatives and Reactions Prior to World War I', *History of Psychology* 12:2 (2009), pp. 60–86; Heather Wolffram, 'Teaching Forensic Science to the American Police and Public: The Scientific Crime Detection Laboratory, 1929–1938', *Academic Forensic Pathology* 11:1 (2021), pp. 52–67.

3 Burney and Pemberton, *Murder and the Making of English CSI*, pp. 3, 100–125.
4 Alison Adam, *A History of Forensic Science: British Beginnings in the Twentieth Century* (London: Routledge, 2015), pp. 52–53, 64–67; Christian Bachhiesl, Gernot Kocher, Thomas Mühlbacher (eds), *Hans Gross — ein 'Vater' der Kriminalwissenschaft. Zur 100. Wiederkehr seines Todestages* (Vienna: LIT, 2015); Gal Hertz and Christian Bachhiesl, 'Hans Gross und die Normativität der kriminalistischen Wahrheitsfindung', *Myops* 35 (2019), pp. 34–43; Daniel M. Vyletta, *Crime, Jews and News: Vienna 1895–1914* (New York & Oxford: Berghahn, 2007), pp. 17–27.
5 Burney and Pemberton, *Murder and the Making of English CSI*, p. 115.
6 Christian Bachhiesl, 'Hans Gross und die Anfänge einer naturwissenschaftlich ausgerichteten Kriminologie', *Archiv für Kriminologie* 219 (2007), pp. 46–53; Roland Grassberger, 'Hans Gross (1847–1915)', *The Journal of Criminal Law, Criminology, and Police Science* 47:4 (1956), pp. 397–405; Gernot Kocher, 'Das K.k. Kriminalistische Universitätsinstitut in Graz', in Christian Bachhiesl, Sonja Maria Bachhiesl and Johann Leitner (eds), *Kriminologische Entwicklungslinien. Eine interdisziplinäre Synopsis* (Vienna: LIT, 2014), pp. 21–33.
7 Histories of forensic science that employ this term include Daniel Asen 'Dead Bodies and Forensic Science: Cultures of Expertise in China, 1800–1949' (PhD thesis, Columbia University, 2012); José Ramón Bertomeu-Sánchez, 'Chemistry, Microscopy and Smell: Bloodstains and Nineteenth-Century Legal Medicine', *Annals of Science* 72:4 (2015), pp. 490–516; Burney and Pemberton, *Murder and the Making of English CSI*.
8 Burney and Pemberton, *Murder and the Making of English CSI*, pp. 103–118.
9 Richard F. Wetzell, *Inventing the Criminal: A History of German Criminology, 1880–1945* (Chapel Hill & London: The University of North Carolina Press, 2000), pp. 32–34.
10 Hans Gross, 'Kriminalistik', in *Gesammelte kriminalistische Aufsätze*, vol. 1 (Leipzig: F. C. W. Vogel, 1902), p. 90.
11 Silviana Galassi, *Kriminologie im Deutschen Kaiserreich: Geschichte einer gebrochenen Verwissenschaftlichung* (Stuttgart: Franz Steiner Verlag, 2004), pp. 265–285.
12 Ibid., pp. 265–266, 274.
13 Hamlin, 'Forensic Cultures in Historical Perspective', p. 5.

14 While reforms to procedure began in most German states following 1848 with the adoption of public trials and oral testimony, a uniform national procedure was not achieved until 1879. Mathias Schmoeckel, 'Der Einfluss der Psychologie auf die Entwicklung des Zeugenbeweises im 19. und beginnenden 20. Jahrhundert', in Matthias Schmoeckel (ed.), *Psychologie als Argument in der juristischen Literatur des Kaiserreichs* (Baden-Baden: Nomos, 2009), pp. 57–58; Elisabeth Koch, 'Der Zeugenbeweis in der deutschen Strafprozeßrechtsreform des 19. Jahrhunderts', in Andre Gouron (ed.), *Subjektivierung des justiziellen Beweisverfahrens: Beiträge zum Zeugenbeweis in Europa und den USA (18.-20. Jahrhundert)* (Frankfurt am Main: Vittorio Klostermann, 1994), p. 247.

15 Marcus B. Carrier, 'The Value(s) of Methods: Method Selection in German Forensic Toxicology in the Second Half of the Nineteenth Century', in Burney and Hamlin, *Global Forensic Cultures*, p. 41.

16 Thomas Vormbaum, *A Modern History of German Criminal Law*, trans. Margaret Hiley (Berlin and Heidelberg: Springer, 2014), pp. 87–88, 91–98.

17 Raluca Enescu and Leonie Benker, 'The Birth of Criminalistics and the Transition from Lay to Expert Witnesses in German Courts', *Journal on European History of Law* 9:2 (2018), pp. 59–66, here p. 61. On how the principle of the free evaluation of evidence was developed, see Ronnie Bloemberg, 'The Development of the German Criminal Law of Evidence between 1750 and 1870: From the System of Legal Proofs to the Freie Beweiswürdigung — Part I', *Journal on European History of Law* 9:1 (2018), pp. 2–24.

18 Carrier, 'The Value(s) of Methods', p. 42; Enescu and Benker, 'The Birth of Criminalistics', pp. 59–66.

19 Carol Jones, *Expert Witnesses: Science, Medicine, and the Practice of Law* (Oxford: Clarendon Press, 1994); Richard F. Wetzell, 'Psychiatry and Criminal Justice in Modern Germany, 1880–1933', *Journal of European Studies* 39:3 (2009), pp. 270–289, here p. 273. Enescu and Benker, 'The Birth of Criminalistics', pp. 59–61.

20 Heather Wolffram, *Forensic Psychology in Germany: Witnessing Crime 1880–1939* (Cham: Palgrave Macmillan, 2018), pp. 21–50.

21 Milos Vec, *Die Spur des Täters: Methoden der Identifikation in der Kriminalistik* (Baden-Baden: Nomos, 2002), p. 12.

22 Kockel's bid to have medico-legal institutes claim a monopoly on conducting and teaching criminalistics was connected to the attempt to make forensic medicine an independent discipline, free from social medicine. See Richard Kockel, 'Mitteilungen und Ausblicke',

Vierteljahrsschrift für Medizin und öffentliches Sanitätswesen (3 F.) 45 (1913), pp. 30–31; Friedrich Herber, Gerichtsmedizin unterm Hakenkreuz (Leipzig: Militzke, 2002), pp. 24–27.
23 Gross, 'Kriminalistik', p. 91.
24 Ibid.
25 Raymond B. Fosdick, European Police Systems (New York: The Century Co., 1915), pp. 186–187, 301–302.
26 Salvatore Ottolenghi, 'Scientific Police', Journal of Criminal Law and Criminology 3:6 (1913), pp. 876–877.
27 Ottolenghi, 'Scientific Police', p. 878.
28 Hamlin, 'Forensic Cultures in Historical Perspective', p. 8.
29 Adolf Dochow, Der Reichs-Strafprozess nach der Strafprozessordnung für das deutsche Reich (Berlin: Guttentag, 1879), pp. 156–170; Vormbaum, A Modern History of German Criminal Law, pp. 85–88.
30 Vormbaum, A Modern History of German Criminal Law, p. 88.
31 Hans Gross, 'Die Ausbildung des praktischen Juristen', in Gesammelte kriminalistische Aufsätze, vol. 1 (Leipzig: F. C. W. Vogel, 1902), p. 82.
32 Ibid., p. 84.
33 Ibid., pp. 85–86.
34 Ibid., p. 87.
35 Ibid., p. 89.
36 Gross, 'Kriminalistik', p. 93.
37 Albert Hellwig, 'Kriminalistische Ausbildungskurse', Monatsschrift für Kriminalpsychologie und Strafrechtsreform 7 (April 1910–März 1911), p. 538.
38 Albert Hellwig, 'Einiges über die Ausbildung der Referendare', Archiv für Kriminal-Anthropologie und Kriminalistik 39/40 (1910–1911), p. 303.
39 Hellwig noted that specialist training in forensic psychology and in criminalistics had been called for by the 7th International Congress of Criminal Anthropology in Cologne in 1911, the 31st German Jurists' Conference in Vienna in 1912 and the General Assembly of the International Crime Association in Copenhagen in 1913. Albert Hellwig, 'Zur Frage der Spezialausbildung der Richter', Monatsschrift für Kriminalpsychologie und Strafrechtsreform 11 (April 1914– March 1918), p. 116.
40 Johannes Seidel, 'XII. Internationaler Kongreß der Internationalen Kriminalistischen Vereinigung', Monatsschrift für Kriminalpsychologie und Strafrechtsreform 10 (April 1914–March 1918), pp. 504–505.
41 Hans Schneickert, 'Beiträge zur Frage der kriminalistischen Ausbildung', Monatsschrift für Kriminalpsychologie und Strafrechtsreform 10 (April–März 1914), pp. 221–229.

42 Schneickert, 'Beiträge', pp. 223–224.
43 *Ibid.*
44 *Ibid.*, p. 224.
45 Kockel, 'Mitteilungen und Ausblicke', pp. 30–31. While Kockel pointed to Austrian and Swiss institutes as models for the expansion of Germany's medico-legal institutes into the field of criminalistics, he and other medico-legalists advocating the same thing do not appear to have resorted to the rhetorical strategy of 'forensic patriotism'.
46 Hans von Hentig, 'Institut für Kriminalwissenschaft und angewandtes Strafrecht', *Monatsschrift für Kriminalpsychologie und Strafrechtsreform* 10 (April–März 1914), pp. 216–221.
47 Franz G. Strafella, 'Eine Denkschrift über die Errichtung kriminalistischer Institute', *Archiv für Kriminologie* 66 (1916), pp. 314–323.
48 Hans Gross, 'Kriminalistisches Reichsinstitut für Deutschland. Zur Frage des Unterrichtes in den strafrechtlichen Hilfswissenschaften', *Archiv für Kriminologie* 54 (1913), p. 198.
49 Seidel, 'XII. Internationaler Kongreß', p. 505.
50 Strafella, 'Eine Denkschrift', pp. 314–323.
51 Knut Wolfgang Nörr, 'Rechtsbegriff und Juristenausbildung. Bemerkungen zur Reformdiskussion im Kaiserreich und in der Weimarer Republik am Beispiel Preußens', *Zeitschrift für neuere Rechtsgeschichte* 14: 3/4 (1992), pp. 217–226, here p. 217.
52 Nörr, 'Rechtsbegriff und Juristenausbildung', pp. 219–221.
53 Konrad H. Jarausch, *Students, Society, and Politics in Imperial Germany: The Rise of Academic Illiberalism* (Princeton, New Jersey: Princeton University Press, 1982), p. 142.
54 Galassi, *Kriminologie*, p. 336.
55 Jarausch, *Students, Society, and Politics*, p. 142.
56 Galassi, *Kriminologie*, pp. 290–291, 312.
57 Gross, 'Die Ausbildung', p. 87.
58 Hans Gross, 'Ein Kurs für die Instruktionsoffiziere der k.k. österreichischen Gendarmerie', in *Gesammelte kriminalistische Aufsätze*, vol. 1 (Leipzig: F. C. W. Vogel, 1902), p. 94.
59 *Ibid.*, pp. 94–96.
60 Hans Gross, 'Das Kriminal-Museum in Graz', *Gesammelte kriminalistische Aufsätze*, pp. 112–113.
61 Hans Gross, 'Kriminalistische Institute', *Deutsche Juristen Zeitung* 16 (1911), pp. 320–321.
62 Albert Hellwig, 'Die gegenwärtige Stand der Ausbildung in der Kriminalwissenschaft', *Archiv für Strafrecht und Strafprozeß* 65 (1918), p. 345.

63 Albert Weingart, *Kriminaltaktik: Ein Handbuch für das Untersuchen von Verbrechen* (Leipzig: Duncker & Humblot, 1904), p. v. A. Niceforo and H. Lindenau, *Die Kriminalpolizei und ihre Hilfswissenschaften* (Groß-Lichterfelde-Ost: Dr. P. Langenscheidt, 1908).
64 F. Strassmann (ed.), *Medizin und Strafrecht: Ein Handbuch für Juristen, Laienrichter und Ärzte* (Berlin-Lichterfelde: Dr. P. Langscheidt, 1911).
65 Albert Hellwig, *Moderne Kriminalistik* (Leipzig & Berlin: B. G. Teubner, 1914).
66 Schneickert, 'Beiträge', p. 223.
67 Landgerichtsrate C. Kade, 'Richterfortbildung', *Archiv für Rechts- und Wirtschaftsphilosophie* 4:3 (1911), p. 372; Hellwig, 'Kriminalistische Ausbildungskurse', p. 540; Hellwig, 'Einiges über die Ausbildung', p. 306.
68 Hellwig, 'Einiges über die Ausbildung', p. 306.
69 Hellwig, 'Kriminalistische Ausbildungskurse', pp. 540–542.
70 *Ibid.*
71 Galassi, *Kriminologie*, pp. 288–336.
72 Hellwig, 'Die gegenwärtige Stand', p. 338.
73 Hentig, 'Institut für Kriminalwissenschaft', pp. 220–221.
74 Strafella, 'Eine Denkschrift', p. 316.
75 Hellwig, 'Die gegenwärtige Stand', pp. 337–357.
76 *Ibid.*, p. 337.
77 *Ibid.*, pp. 344–352.
78 *Ibid.*, p. 358.
79 On the belief that economic investment in criminalistics would rapidly be repaid by a decline in criminal statistics, see Hentig, 'Institut für Kriminalwissenschaft', p. 221.
80 Hellwig, 'Die gegenwärtige Stand', pp. 332–333.
81 *Ibid.*, p. 334.
82 *Ibid.*
83 Stefan L. Wolff, 'Physicists in the "Krieg der Geister": Wilhelm Wien's Proclamation', *Historical Studies in the Physical and Biological Sciences* 33:2 (2003), pp. 337–368.
84 *Ibid.*, p. 335.

5

Sober suits, bowler hats and white lab coats: Enclothed impartiality, masculinity and the tailoring of a bourgeois expert persona in British courtrooms, 1920–1960

Pauline Dirven

Introduction

A striking feature of modern forensic culture in England in 1920–1950 was that both the general public and forensic experts showed ample interest in the 'looks' of forensic scientists and doctors. The media – newspapers, crime fiction and popular non-fiction – reported on the personal appearances of forensic experts and advice literature for forensic expert witnesses included instructions on what to wear to court. Interestingly, these texts show that forensic expert witnesses in British courtrooms did not 'dress up' as doctors or scientists, i.e. they did not wear their white coats or the kind of formal clothes that doctors usually wore to distinguish themselves from less highly skilled middle-class men. Instead, they wore a dark-coloured lounge suit, as had become the custom for most British middle-class men. This observation is not trivial: this chapter argues that experts' adoption of such a bourgeois look was a key feature in the performance of forensic expertise because it allowed them to embody one of the crucial virtues of modern forensic culture: impartiality. In making this claim, this chapter defines forensic culture as a set of shared values, beliefs and ideals of what it meant to practise good and trustworthy science and medicine.

In the modern English adversarial justice system, it was far from self-evident that expert witnesses enacted impartiality. Whereas in the Middle Ages and early modern period, experts appeared in court either as jurors or as court advisors, from the eighteenth century onwards expert witnesses had to face the jury as witnesses, for the prosecution or defence party.[1] This put expert witnesses in a difficult position. As scientists, they wanted to embody 'society's preferred model of the cool, objective, correct, impartial man of science'.[2] However, the space that formed the stage for their performance, the modern adversarial courtroom, to the jury suggested their partiality.[3] In 1923 the influential medical journal *The Lancet* described the situation as follows: 'In a popular statement of the degree of untruthfulness the superlative is reserved for the expert witness. When scientific evidence adduced by plaintiff and defendant seems to be mutually contradictory, the layman is puzzled and grows skeptical of scientific values.'[4] In the modern system, expert witnesses, therefore, looked for ways to convince the lay jury that they were not partial 'hired guns' or charlatans, but impartial, objective researchers.

The historiography of forensic science and medicine has shown how forensic experts have attempted to present themselves as trustworthy knowledge-makers by analysing the ways in which they produced forensic evidence. This literature focuses on the question of how the virtue of objectivity was enacted in forensic examination practices, as well as on the technologies, protocols or mathematical models forensic scientists used to create 'objective knowledge'.[5] In this line of thought, historians Ian Burney and Neil Pemberton argue that the English forensic culture around the 1930s was characterised by the development of practices that enacted a sense of objectivity, such as the development of protocols and the emphasis on trace-based evidence.[6] They identify a shift from a regime that was centred around a celebrity, all-round pathologist who personally enjoyed the trust of the public, towards a modern forensic regime that earned credibility through the use of teamwork, protocols for evidence collection and trace-based crime scene investigation practices.

This chapter aims to add to this literature by shifting the focus from examination practices carried out by experts, to the related question of how forensic experts presented themselves as impartial, credible *personae*; how they *embodied* this epistemic virtue. To be specific, I study sartorial performances of forensic experts and reflections on 'the expert look' in newspaper articles, forensic handbooks and autobiographies to answer the question of how they presented themselves as impartial and authoritative knowledge-makers in English forensic culture. Shifting the focus from forensic evidence to advice literature and reflections on the way expert witnesses dressed and presented themselves, illustrates that while between 1920 and 1960 doctors and scientists did not use the notion of 'objectivity', they did refer to the epistemic virtue of impartiality. In this context, impartiality referred to 'their duty to assist in the discovery of truth and the administration of justice, no matter which side may be found to be in the wrong'.[7] It meant being a 'coldly detached person' who does not take sides.[8] This chapter shows that, while a new forensic *regime* – characterised by the enactment of objectivity in protocols, technologies and examination practices – started to develop in the interwar years, popular performances of expert witnesses continued to rely on an older scientific and forensic culture. To be specific, in the courtroom, news media and popular autobiographies, expert witnesses embodied the ideal of impartiality by invoking class-based mechanisms of building trust that had already developed in the nineteenth century.

In the English and Scottish adversarial justice systems, where the choreography of the courtroom suggested to the lay jury an opposition between the parties, expert witnesses had to attain credibility, trust and authority via a performance of impartiality. As I will explain below, this task was particularly difficult as scientists and doctors – both of whom could occupy the position of expert witness – had a long history of negotiating their tenuous social position in British society. To explain why this was the case, I will outline the British history of the gentleman scholar, quackery and the relation of the expert witness with the jury. But first, I will explain the value of studying fashion in a forensic context and illustrate what forensic experts looked like in Britain from 1920 to 1960.

Fashion and forensic virtues

Historians of forensic science and medicine have paid little attention to the embodied performances of forensic experts. That is unfortunate because in judicial cultures based on jury systems, such as England and Scotland, 'lay juries could not usually follow elaborate technical arguments, ... [and expert witnesses were compelled to] let their own credibility be the main support of their testimony'.[9] Thus experts, who struggled to verbally communicate their scientific knowledge-making practices to the jury, could establish their impartiality through a language that their audience did speak: fashion.

Attention to bodily appearance and dress practices can reveal much about the role of forensic experts in British society because the body is 'an instrument that performs socially or culturally constructed sexed or gendered identities', to use the words of Karen Harvey.[10] The study of clothes can help us understand the 'organisation of power and authority' within societies because clothes are active actors in bringing about this order.[11] In this chapter, I use a broad definition of fashion that does not only refer to *haute couture* but also, and primarily, to the look of people in the street. It encompasses the cultural conceptions about what was 'fashionable' to wear and the sartorial language of what specific items of clothing, fabrics and colours meant. This fits the historical context I study. In the twentieth century, being fashionable was no longer reserved for members of the upper classes. As the manufacturing process of clothing became standardised and mass production developed, members of the labouring and lower-middle classes could more actively engage in consumer society.[12] As a consequence, in early and mid-twentieth century Britain, dress culture was an important tool to assess not only a person's social status[13] but also their personality.[14] In other words, fashion became an instrument to communicate the qualities you possessed as a person.

Applied to the context of science and medicine, the 'meaning of dress, and the cultural capital that dress secures, are key to comprehending struggles for authority and trust in medicine', and science.[15] That is because, in the words of Mineke Bosch, 'knowledge cannot be recognised as valuable when it is not performed in a way that the scholar or scientist is seen as a trusted member of the scientific or scholarly community'.[16] An analysis of fashion can reveal much about the way scientists wished to present themselves, the personae they adopted and the gendered and class codes they resorted to in order to enact status and credibility or evoke trust.

A notable exception to the neglect of forensic fashion in the historiography is the work of Kelly Ann Couzens, who has studied the clothes worn by expert witnesses in the nineteenth-century Scottish courtroom.[17] She argues that they wore dark-coloured suits because this signified the formality that was required in the courtroom. She writes

> restraint in physical appearance matched well the atmosphere of solemnity and respect the legal profession wished to inculcate among participants within the courtroom setting. Unlike the judges in their fine robes or the advocates in their wigs and gowns, the dress of the medical expert expressed a suitably inferior sense of respectability and authority that befitted their place within the hierarchy of the court.[18]

According to Couzens, experts' dress emphasised their formal role in the courtroom and enacted a sense of hierarchy between the judiciary and expert witnesses. This argument is compelling. As legal actors could advise expert witnesses on how to dress, it seems fitting that they would have used it to emphasise the hierarchy between the competing professions of medicine and law.[19] However, as I shall argue below, the choice of garment of expert witnesses, the sober lounge suit, did more than emphasise the solemn nature of the trial and establish a hierarchy between these professions. The dress code amongst doctors and scientists had a long social history as it was interwoven with their struggle for status in the British class-based society.

The sober middle-class look

Expert witnesses dressed according to the modern, masculine, middle-class fashion trend of the 1920s to 1950s. They wore sober, dark-coloured, three-piece lounge suits and matching overcoats. Such 'lounge suits' – or business suits, as they are known today – had become the choice of garment for most middle-class and increasingly also working-class men in Britain from the 1920s onwards.[20] They enacted a sense of middle-class professionalism. As an author of *The Lancet* described the situation in 1947, 'correct men's dress today is designed to show that the wearer doesn't work with his hands. Men dress like bankers'.[21] Moreover, the bourgeois ideal enacted by the sober suit was highly gendered and created a shared masculine culture.[22] The practical suit emphasised the increasingly hectic and urban lives of professional men working in public institutions. It was a comfortable garment, suitable for industrial life.[23]

Advice literature for forensic expert witnesses emphasised the importance for forensic scientists and doctors to adopt this neat but sober look. This instruction was part of the general advice in forensic handbooks and journal articles for expert witnesses on how to behave and look in the courtroom. The literature prescribed that experts needed to 'stand up, speak up and dress up' when they were in the witness box and never lose their temper during cross-examination. An author in the *British Medical Journal* explained in 1934 that careful consideration of this 'art of performance' was a vital aspect of the forensic expert's job description because, while 'the professional and private conduct of a doctor in the ordinary course of practice is not obvious to the public eye, … in court, it is open to the inspection of perhaps a hundred people directly and in particularly unlucky cases – to thousands of people through the Press'.[24] Displaying the appropriate behaviour in court was vital if the expert witnesses wanted their testimony to be heard and taken seriously. The authors of the advice literature emphasised that 'the privilege of giving evidence carried with it no small responsibility, and might affect not only the persons involved in the action but *the doctor's own reputation*'.[25] According to some experts, it even impacted the stature of science and medicine as a whole.[26] To explain why this was the case I delve into the question of the social status of doctors and scientists in British society below. However, first I will outline how expert witnesses thought they could win over their audience; in particular, in what kind of costume they thought would make a good impression.

In the early and mid-twentieth century, professional fashion advice was highly gendered as it was only aimed at male experts. They were supposed to wear a simple suit in dark colours. As a professor of forensic medicine, Sir Sydney Smith, explained in his handbook in 1925: 'the witness should pay due regard to his bearing, which should be modest and unassuming, and to his personal appearance, which should be at least clean and tidy; an untidy, unshaved professional witness creates a bad impression on the Court'.[27] Importantly, an expert witness should also not dress up too much. As a columnist in the *British Medical Journal* remarked, forensic experts should avoid appearing 'conceited or vain'.[28] Police surgeon and medical referee Douglas Kerr explained in more detail in 1935:

> Much depends on the impression they [the jury] form of the doctor himself; he should therefore conduct himself as becoming a responsible professional man. He should dress accordingly in a quiet professional manner, and before entering the witness-box should remove his gloves and overcoat. It is not necessary for him to wear a morning coat, but to appear in a sporting-suit, as sometimes happens, is only to leave the jury with the impression that he does not take his profession seriously, and consequently considerably distracts from the value of his evidence.[29]

According to Kerr, dress was a way to enact professionalism and to ensure that the audience, the jury, would take the performing expert seriously. To accomplish this, they should not adopt a casual sporting style nor a too formal look.

In practice, it seems that experts took this advice to heart. Photographs in newspaper articles and portrait pictures of forensic experts, such as Figure 5.1, illustrate that they were clad in sober, middle-class clothes. The first photograph displays Sydney Smith (quoted above), wearing a dark-coloured, three-piece suit of heavy fabric. Pictures of expert witnesses attending the court confirm that in practice experts increasingly chose not to dress distinctively in the period 1920–1960.[30] Figure 5.2, for example, is from 1920 and depicts Home Office analyst John Webster on the left and chemist William Willcox on the right as they arrive or leave at the court. The picture illustrates a change in performance: Webster is still dressed more conservatively in the clothes of the medical trade, wearing a morning suit and top hat. But Willcox has adopted a middle-class look, wearing a lounge suit and bowler hat. This latter trend would set the tone for expert performances during the rest of the century. This is illustrated for example by Figure 5.3, which shows Dr Keith Simpson arriving at the court in a three-piece lounge suit. In general, photos indicate that expert witnesses started to deviate from

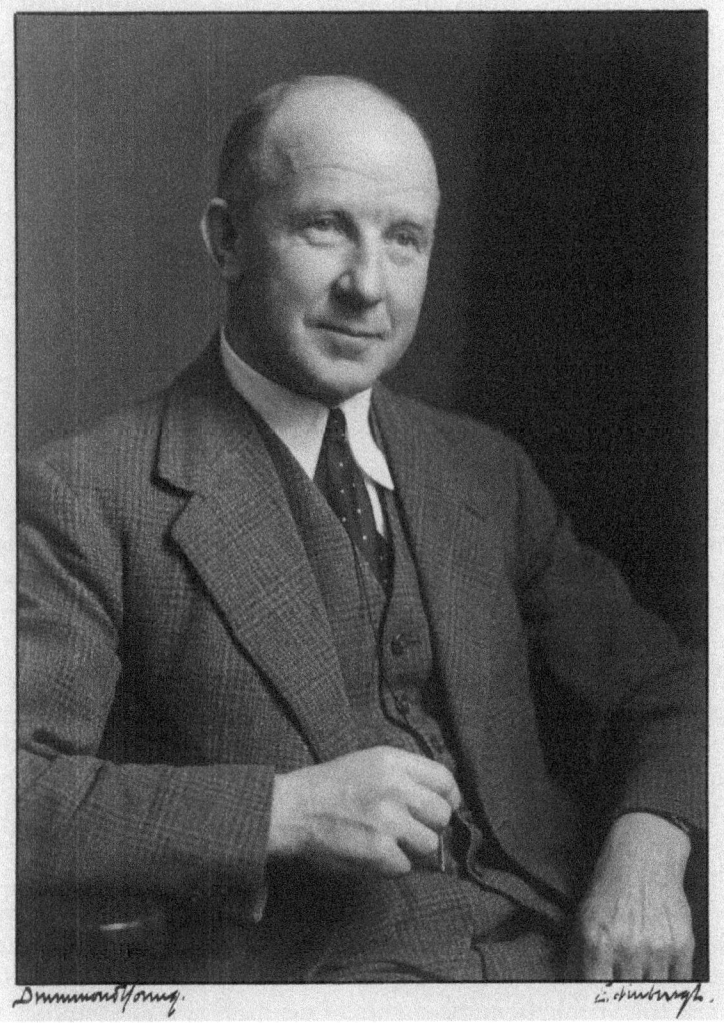

Figure 5.1 Portrait picture of Sir Sydney Alfred Smith (1883–1969), Regius Professor of Forensic Medicine at Edinburgh University from 1928 to 1953. (Photograph by W. & E. Drummond Young, The University of Edinburgh, UA CA1/1 h, 'Sir Sydney Alfred Smith (1883–1969) – Our History', accessed 14 February 2022, http://ourhistory.is.ed.ac.uk/index.php/Sir_Sydney_Alfred_Smith_(1883–1969))

Sober suits, bowler hats and white lab coats 125

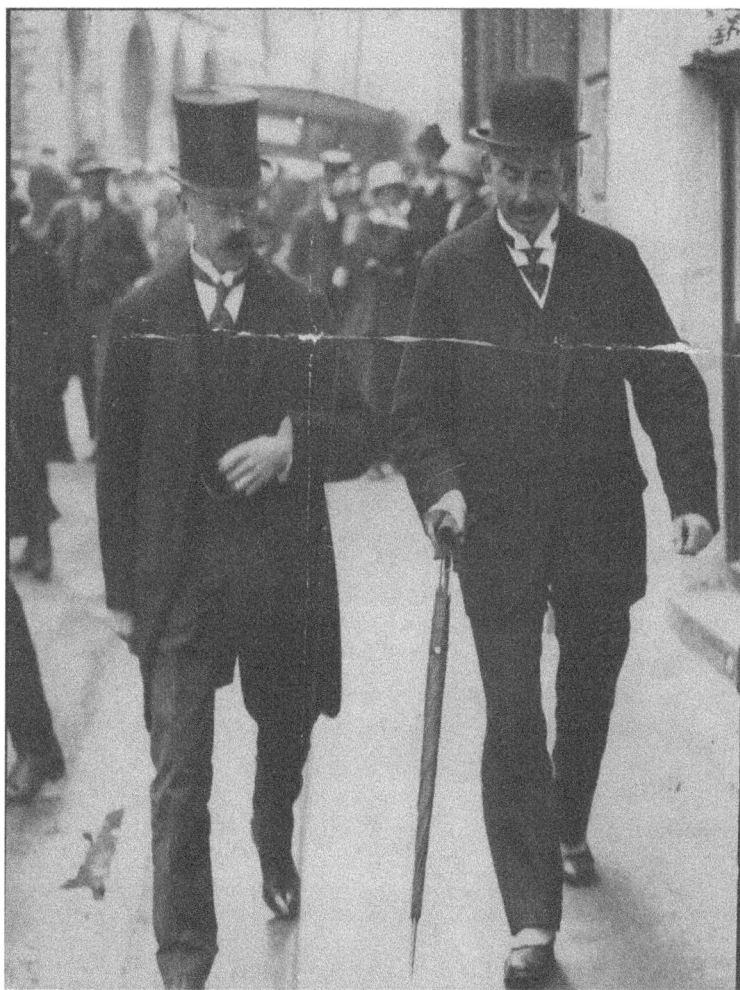

Figure 5.2 Home Office analyst John Webster (left) and chemist William Willcox (right) as they arrive or leave at the court, 1920. (ANL/Shutterstock, accessed 16 December 2021, www.shutterstock.com/nl/editorial/image-editorial/john-webster-l-and-dr-wh-willcox-toxicologists-who-examined-the-body-of-mabel-greenwood-4735558a)

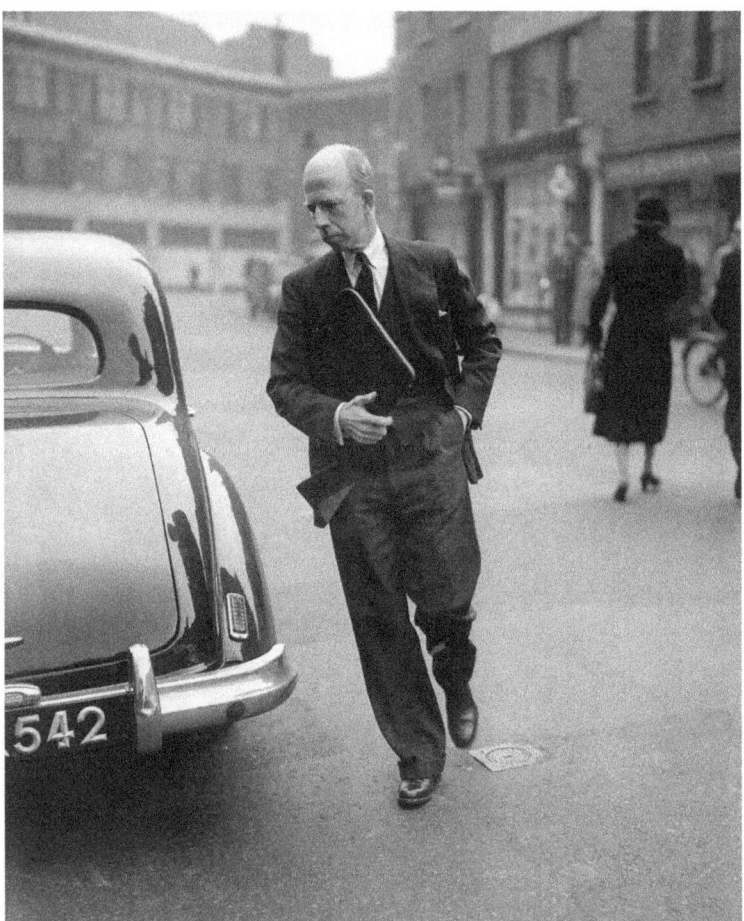

Figure 5.3 Pathologist Keith Simpson arriving at Westminster Coroner Court to give evidence at the inquest of the Ritz Hotel murder and suicide, 13 March 1953. (Trinity Mirror / Mirrorpix/ Alamy Stock Photo, accessed 14 February 2022, www.alamy.com/stock-photo-dr-keith-simpson-the-home-office-pathologist-arriving-at-westminster-83443376.html)

the distinctive enclothed practices of their professions and adopted a sober middle-class look from the 1920s onwards.

Forensic experts' courtroom sartorial presentations were remarkable. In the first half of the twentieth century, it was uncommon for both scientists and doctors to dress like this. As fashion historian Catherine Horwood has argued, doctors were prone to dress more formally than most middle-class men, adorning themselves – depending on the occasion – in morning suits (recognisable by the long, black jacket without tails and striped trousers), evening wear or academic dress.[31] In contrast, scientists and lab assistants enjoyed more freedom than most middle-class men and dressed more casually, for example wearing 'an open-necked shirt, flannels, no socks and sandals'.[32] Despite these customs, forensic experts dressed according to middle-class fashion; doctors dressed down and scientists dressed up when they wore the sober lounge suit in the courtroom.

In general, it was not self-evident that witnesses chose to wear an undistinctive look in the courtroom. By doing so, forensic experts differed from English police officers who could wear their uniform to court to display their professional authority in the witness box.[33] It also set them apart from their Spanish colleagues who emphasised their authority in the courtroom by dressing distinctively, for instance wearing a mortar-board and a symbolic medal.[34]

Newspaper articles and a popular non-fiction book commented on the expert's indistinguishable look, indicating that it was noteworthy or surprising to journalists. In her autobiography in 1940, Molly Lefebure, the secretary of pathologist Keith Simpson, noted that the famous expert witness Sir Bernard Spilsbury

> looked, more than anything else in the world, like a prosperous gentleman farmer. Very tall – though stooping slightly in his later years – powerful, with broad shoulders and a very ruddy, open, earnest face, you would have said he was an expert on dairy herds, or sugar-beet crops, or agricultural fertilizers, but you would not have suspected that he was Sir Bernard Spilsbury.[35]

In a similar vein, the *Dundee Evening Telegraph* claimed in 1938 that a fingerprinting expert 'looks for all the world the successful businessman'.[36] And in 1939 the magazine *John Bull* told its readers that they might mistake poison expert Dr Lynch 'for a lawyer or perhaps an accountant. You would need very unusual penetration to discover in that quiet person one of the greatest investigators of our day.'[37] The article was accompanied by a picture in which Dr Lynch is unremarkable as he looks like an average Englishman in his three-piece lounge suit and Homburg hat.[38]

The fact that forensic experts dressed themselves according to the sober, middle-class fashion trend of the time was not insignificant but a noteworthy occurrence. More to the point, as I shall argue below, it was a performance of judicial impartiality.

The modern courtroom

In the modern courtroom, the sober middle-class look countered the suggestion of partiality that the adversarial legal system had created by moving experts from the jury box to the witness box. It minimised the distance between the jurors and expert witnesses that was implemented in the eighteenth century. That is because the jury, at this time, consisted predominantly of middle-class men. Legal scholar Andrew Watson explains that while it is true that 'after 1919 both men and women could serve as jurors ... the number of females was limited by the need to meet the property qualification'.[39] Moreover, in practice, the jury predominantly consisted of middle-class men due to the ability of the lawyers to challenge specific juror members without having to give a reason for their removal.[40] Because expert witnesses conformed to the bourgeois fashion of the time, wearing sober lounge suits and bowler, Homburg or trilby hats, a familiarity between themselves and the members of the jury was established.

The importance of relating to the jury to win their trust is confirmed by research in legal studies. Watson, for example, has shown that in England barristers altered their performances and adopted a less formal and more 'conversational style' of advocacy when the democratisation of the jury set in with the passing of the Juries Act 1974. He notes that lawyers wanted to appeal to the more diverse group of jurors but at the same time were 'anxious to avoid appearing patronizing to jurors or of under-estimating their intelligence'.[41] Legal scholar William McMahon has made a similar claim concerning the way American lawyers dressed. He argues that an attorney's use of clothing could have an impact on the outcome of a case because of the performative nature of their jobs. He explains that the clothes or 'costumes' they wear have an impact on their audience, the jurors, to whom they want to relate by not dressing as if they are different or better than them, but as if they were one of them.[42]

While McMahon's observations are of a different context, his general point helps to explain the fashion choices of expert witnesses in England during the 1920s to 1960s. Like these lawyers, expert witnesses were performing for an audience that would respond to their appearance. By putting on the common suit forensic experts masked personal or social differences amongst themselves and between themselves and the jury. This is illustrated by Figures 5.4 and 5.5, depicting

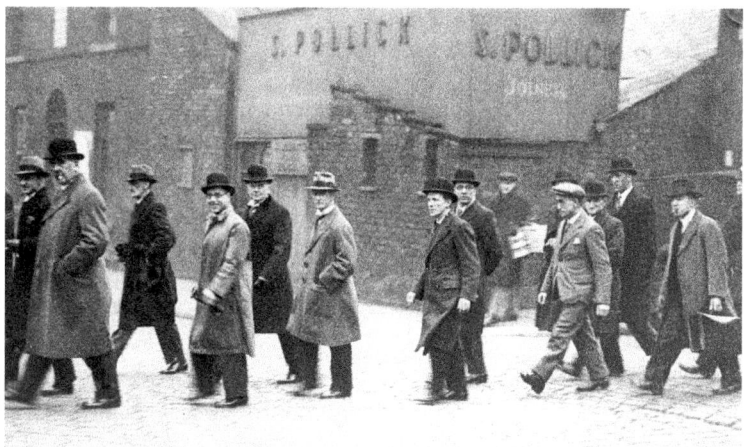

Figure 5.4 The jurors in the Dr Ruxton murder trial as they return to court to return their verdict of guilty, 1935. (Photo by Mirrorpix/Mirrorpix via Getty Images, accessed 14 February 2022, www.gettyimages.nl/detail/nieuwsfoto%27s/dr-ruxton-murder-case-members-of-the-jury-at-he-trial-who-nieuwsfotos/591974956)

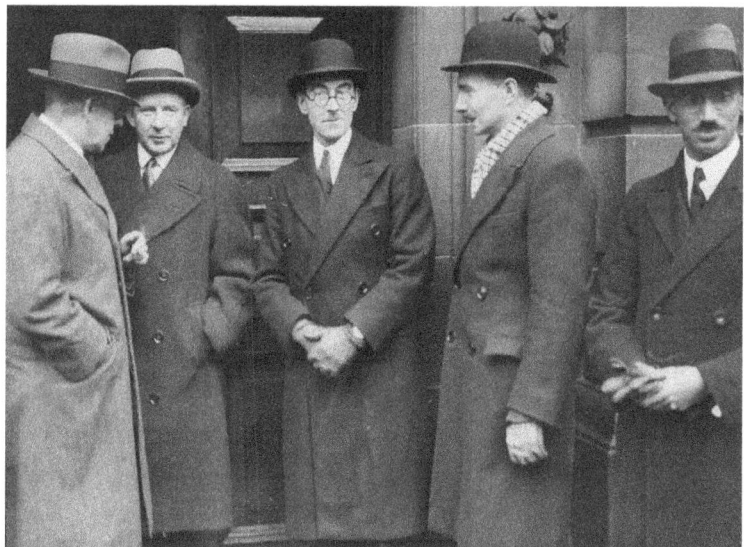

Figure 5.5 Team of expert witnesses who worked on the *Ruxton* case. (ANL/Shutterstock, accessed 14 February 2022, www.shutterstock.com/editorial/image-editorial/forensic-experts-working-on-the-ravine-murders-lr-prof-js-brash-prof-sydney-smith-prof-john-glaister-dr-wg-millar-and-dr-cl-godfrey-box-651-2407121527-ajpg-5727859a)

respectively the jury members and the expert witnesses involved in the infamous Ruxton murder case. Figure 5.4 shows that jurors were dressed in overcoats and lounge suits and wore bowler and trilby hats, with the exception of only one jury member wearing a cap. Figure 5.5 displays the expert witnesses, dressed similarly in overcoats, bowler and trilby hats. Thus, by adhering to the dominant middle-class fashion, forensic experts bridged the gap between themselves and the jury and suggested that they were not so different from them; i.e. they had not become theatrical showmen or 'hired guns' but like the jury were still impartial, 'humble servants' to the court.

The white lab coat

The choice of expert witnesses to wear indistinctive middle-class clothes is remarkable if we take into account that at this time a specific sartorial symbol for science came into being: the white lab coat. This garment became popular in the nineteenth and early twentieth century; not just in science, but also in the field of medicine, where physicians and surgeons started to trade in their gentleman's frockcoat for white lab coats.[43] According to fashion historians Susan Hardy and Anthony Corones this make-over signified a change in 'professional identity replete with new forms of credibility and new forms of trust'.[44] More specifically, it points to a significant development within medicine as it symbolised 'scientificisation': the growing impact of bacteriology and a new emphasis placed on hygiene within the field.[45]

Following this new trend, forensic experts started to wear special work clothes when they carried out examinations. Scientists, and increasingly doctors, would wear a white lab coat, and pathologists clad themselves in a post-mortem gown, rubber apron and rubber gloves (Figure 5.6).

According to pathologist Keith Simpson, this was a positive development. He exclaimed in 1947:

> I have entered a mortuary unexpectedly, to find a doctor fully dressed, bowler hat on head, umbrella over arm, leaning against a wall smoking a pipe and making jotted notes in a book while the mortuary assistant pulled out and cut up organs for a Coroner's autopsy. Such scandalous days are fast receding into the dark Middle Ages of forensic pathology.[46]

Sober suits, bowler hats and white lab coats 131

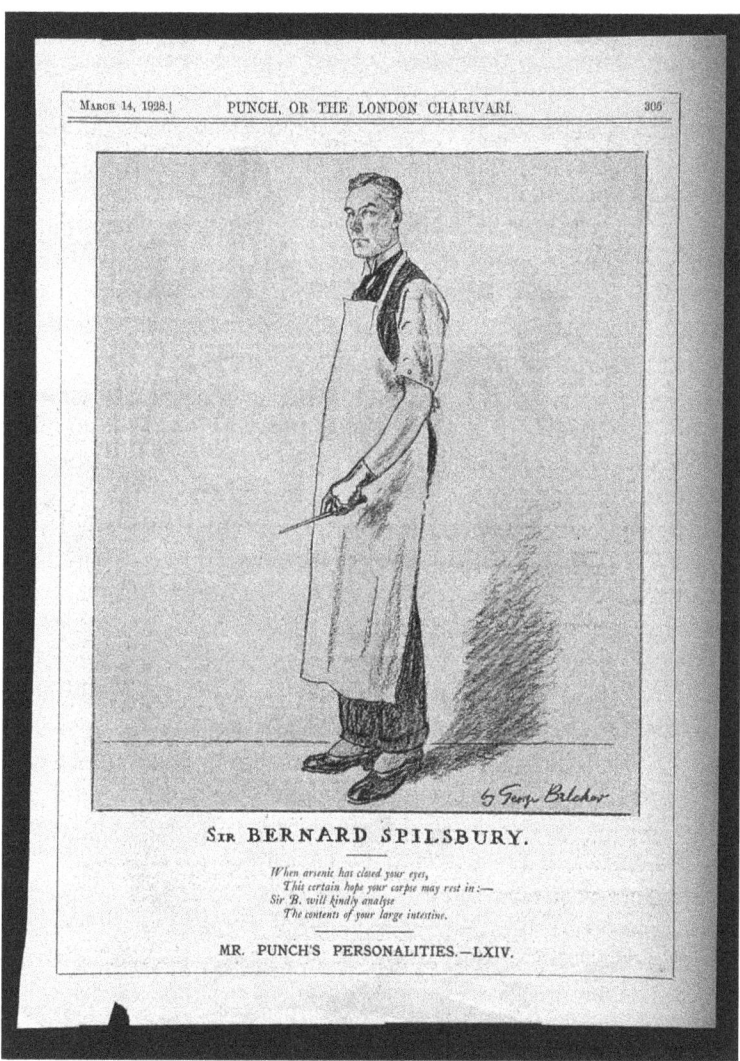

Figure 5.6 Bernard Spilsbury in post-mortem garment. (Wellcome Images / Wikimedia, CC BY-SA 4.0: Library reference: ICV No 11802, Photo number: V0011537, accessed 14 October 2022, https://commons.wikimedia.org/wiki/File:Sir_Bernard_Spilsbury,_a_famous_pathologist._Reproduction_of_Wellcome_V0011537.jpg)

Whether Simpson's account of this encounter is truthful or simply a rhetorical strategy does not matter, the point of the anecdote is clear. The way the pathologist is dressed is scandalous and old-fashioned to Simpson because it exemplifies his passive attitude; adorned in the male uniform of the time he is unable to get his hands dirty and apply his manual skills. Whereas in the courtroom this outfit would have been appropriate and suggested impartiality, in the examination space the same look depicted a 'backward' and 'outdated' practice. In the investigative space, the modern expert was characterised by his skills and ability to engage with his object of study, as symbolised by his special work garb.

It seems that this new performance of expertise was context-bound, as it continued to be limited to the space of laboratory and morgue, at least until the 1960s. In the courtroom experts did not use their white lab coats or working outfits to perform the ideal of trained judgment and specialised skills. Nor were they prone to use this new symbol of science in the media. An exception is Sir Bernard Spilsbury, who did have his pictures taken dressed in a white lab coat or post-mortem garb (Figure 5.7).

However, seeing that Spilsbury was a unique figure in the history of forensic medicine who enjoyed celebrity status, his public performances do not represent a general trend in the performance of forensic expertise. I only found one other example of a public performance displaying forensic experts dressed in lab coats: a 1946 newsreel called *Science Fights Crime*.[47] This Pathé clip responded to the post-war social fear of a 'crime wave'. In this promotional film, forensic scientists are depicted in white lab coats doing tests. In other visual material of the time, experts are not portrayed as such but appear plain-clothed. Images issued by experts themselves, for example, do not show them wearing lab coats or other symbols of science. Nor do newspapers use pictures of experts dressed in examination garb. Usually, these experts are shown either sitting in a neutral setting or rushing to or from a crime scene or courtroom. In all these pictures they are wearing a simple lounge suit.

This changed around 1960 when forensic experts who used to conform to this sober self-representation started to present themselves in lab coats and in the context of the laboratory in popular media outlets, such as on the cover of their autobiographies.

Sober suits, bowler hats and white lab coats 133

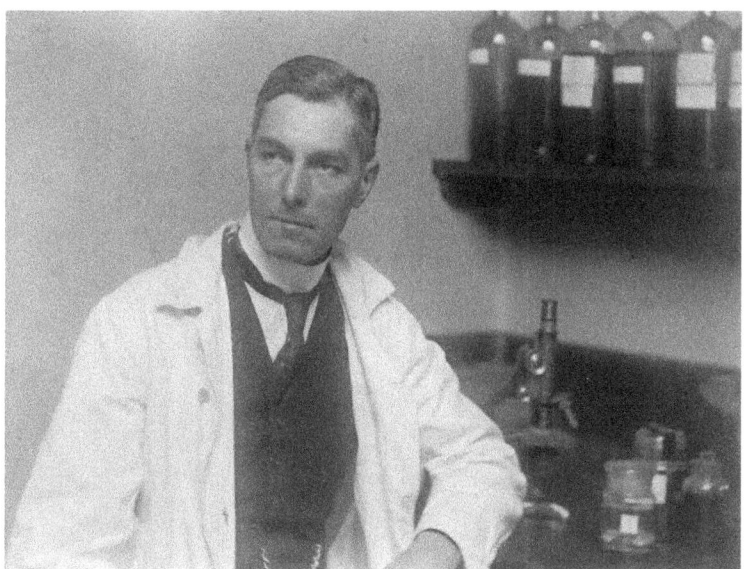

Figure 5.7 Photograph of Sir Bernard Spilsbury posing in the laboratory wearing a white lab coat, 1920s. (Photograph by Edward Cahen, National Portrait Gallery, London, accessed 16 December 2021, www.npg.org.uk/collections/search/use-this-image/?mkey=mw189943)

Figure 5.8 shows the photograph pathologist Sydney Smith used on the cover of his autobiography published in 1959; in it he is posing as a scientist wearing a white lab coat and holding a test tube. John Glaister Jr appeared in a similar manner on the cover of his autobiography in 1964: in the laboratory wearing a white coat.[48] As did specialist in spectrography Hamish Walls on the book jacket of his memoirs in 1972.[49] Keith Simpson never swapped his middle-class suit for a lab coat but he did follow the trend of posing with instruments of the trade, such as a skull, a knife and flask in a picture taken in 1978 (see Figure 5.9). In general, the period after the 1960s is characterised by a shift in popular media representations of forensic experts. In forensic books written for a lay audience, as well as in films and television programmes, experts were depicted as anonymous scientists, immediately recognisable by their white coats and handling of instruments, such as microscopes, beakers or test tubes.[50] Examples of this include the book *The Modern Sherlock*

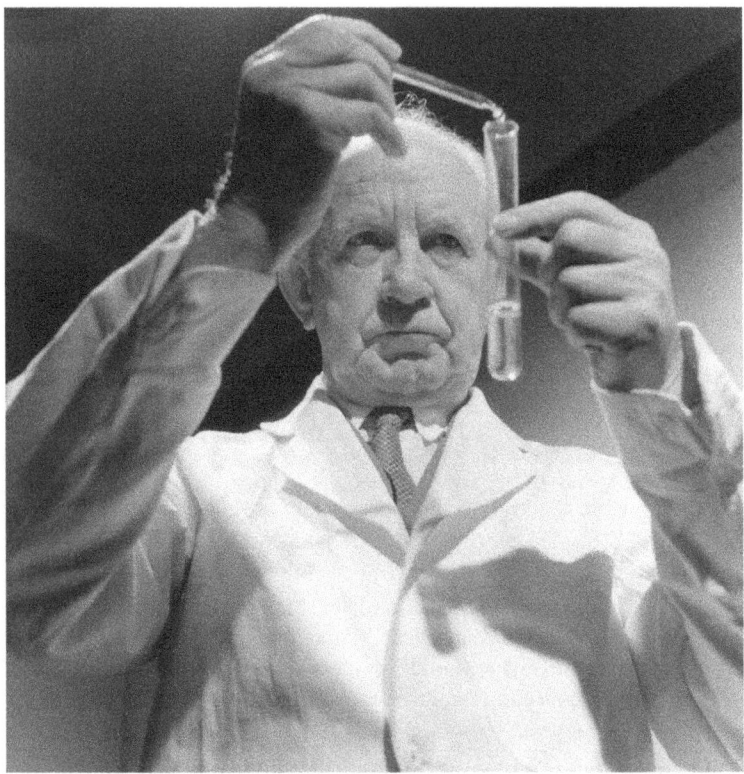

Figure 5.8 Photograph of Sydney Smith in white lab coat posing as a scientist, used on the cover of his autobiography *Mostly Murder*. (Accessed through Royal College of Physicians of Edinburgh)

Holmes intended to inform laypeople about forensic science and the true-crime book *Great Cases of Scotland Yard*.[51] During the second half of the twentieth century, it seems that performances of forensic expertise were more lab-based, and relied on images of technologies and specific institutions to assert authority or trust.

Before the 1960s, however, this look was not part of a public performance of forensic expertise. Public appearances were instead based on the performance of a bourgeois persona as expert witnesses appeared in the courtroom and media in their dark-coloured lounge suits. To understand why experts continued to rely on this

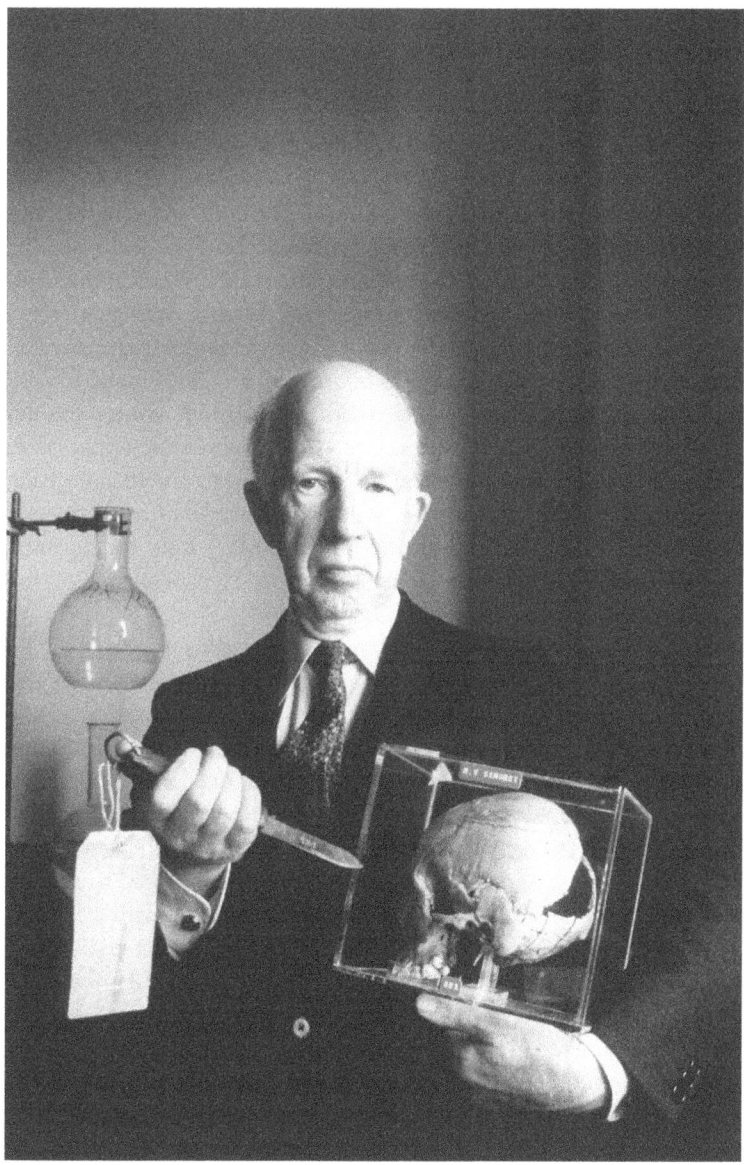

Figure 5.9 (Cedric) Keith Simpson posing with murder weapon, skull and flask in 1978. (Photograph by Judith Aronson, 1978, National Portrait Gallery, London, accessed 19 August 2022, www.npg.org.uk/collections/search/portrait/mw62365/Cedric-Keith-Simpson?LinkID=mp61813&role=sit&rNo=6)

middle-class look for public performances, I turn to the history of British intellectual, medical and scientific culture.

Impartiality and middle-class modesty

The reliance on the gentleman-look should be understood in the light of the long history of class struggles in the medical and scientific community. Already since the seventeenth century, medical men had wanted to secure social status by displaying themselves as gentlemen. They did so because they aimed to counter the popular comparison between surgeons and manual labourers, especially butchers.[52] To shake off the association of their work with 'crude' manual labour, surgeons chose to present themselves as members of the upper class, depicted hosting dinner parties, or conforming to the image of the man of letters, the philosopher, who was considered a gentleman, surrounded by books and sitting at his desk.[53] Like the forensic experts prior to 1960, they were seldom depicted in their working space or with the instruments of their trade.[54]

In their performance, physicians and surgeons needed to find a balance between 'dressing up' and not appearing flamboyant. It was important for them not to appear pompous because of the long history of competition between qualified and unqualified doctors in Britain. 'Quacks' were never outlawed in Britain, and therefore registered practitioners looked for ways to visibly distance themselves from these 'charlatans'.[55] In the nineteenth century, 'the quacks, or unqualified practitioners, continued to rely on eighteenth-century flamboyance, extravagance, exoticism and a bit of showmanship as the time-honoured way to attract patients'.[56] Qualified practitioners attempted to contrast this flamboyance by adopting a sober and simple gentlemanly appearance. At the end of the nineteenth century, 'there was a return, as in so many respects, to the moral aesthetics of Tudor and Stuart times', in the sense that doctors 'were invariably depicted as soberly respectable, clad in greys and blacks'.[57] This performance of sobriety continued to impact the sartorial display of doctors in the twentieth century, as the fear of quacks continued to exist.[58] This anxiety influenced expert witnesses especially, since their reputations could be hurt by the comparison with quacks, due to the performative nature of their courtroom appearances and the fact that they received fees to appear in the witness box. The sober suit-wearing of the expert witnesses must therefore be understood in the medical sartorial tradition of warding off suggestions of quackery or 'bought' evidence.

Forensic experts did not exclusively have backgrounds in medicine; scientists, and especially chemists, were also increasingly asked to contribute to criminal investigations. They too had a history of class struggle. Especially in the seventeenth and eighteenth centuries, the amateur gentleman-scientist was an idealised knowledge-maker because his moral code of behaviour and financial independence was considered to ensure impartiality.[59] A similar ideal existed in the popular imagination of the detective, who was represented as a financially independent gentleman-detective who solved crimes as a hobby, to prove intellectual superiority or out of public service.[60] However, in the nineteenth century 'new men of science', skilled artisans or tradesmen, started to emerge on the stage. They were becoming more influential because they developed the scientific technologies that aided the modernisation project of the manufacturing and industrialised classes. However, these scientists were in an ambiguous position; as contributors to the industrial society they obtained a position of influence but because of their bourgeois background the elite, especially the judiciary, did not trust them upon their word, as they would trust their gentlemanly counterparts.[61] In the words of Carol Jones, 'in England, there was a prevailing cultural snobbery which determined that men of letters could look down upon men of science'.[62] This distrust also stemmed from the professionalisation of science. As Tal Golan explains:

> The scientific gentleman was supposed to labor for the love of knowledge, not for money, and his heart was supposed to be in his researches, oriented toward communal interests rather than toward individual self-interest. No matter how useful the professionals were, if their object in life was to obtain money, they were morally tainted. And among these professionals, none was more repugnant than the so-called scientific expert who had made his living from his appearances in court, tailoring his opinions to the wants of his clients.[63]

To sum up, scientists, and expert witnesses especially, were initially disadvantaged by the professionalisation of the trade.

The historiography is ambivalent as to how the situation developed. Some historians of science have pointed out that the professionalisation of science changed the culture of trust and authority in science: around the turn of the century, gentlemanly codes of behaviour were traded for the modern ideology of professionalism, institutionalisation and technological advancement.[64] This line of thought complements the argument of Burney and Pemberton that in the early twentieth century a modern forensic regime developed that was characterised by the institutionalisation and professionalisation of forensic services.

However, other scholars have argued that a degree of continuity existed because these new men of science adopted and appropriated the gentlemanly ideal. They explain that with the emergence of 'new men of science' the gentlemanly ideal did not disappear but changed. While historians do not agree on the exact moment of this shift, the literature on the British middle class shows that at some point during the nineteenth or early twentieth century the conception of the gentleman altered. It no longer referred to someone's noble birth but became 'a repository of cultural value to which anyone could aspire'.[65] Based on this reconceptualisation of the gentleman, new men of science turned the tables on the aristocracy. They argued that they were not less reliable because they were professionals but rather more so. Unlike members of the upper class, they argued, they were not driven by impulse or extravagant lifestyles.[66] Moreover, they emphasised that in bourgeois society, legitimate knowledge was warranted by objectivity, not by any feudal claims to privileged, personal authority.[67] From this perspective, they fashioned a new scientific persona, that of the bourgeois gentleman-scientist, who was humble, disciplined and impartial, and who served society by contributing to its technological and industrious development.[68] Presenting themselves as sober middle-class professionals, these scientists sought to win the trust of the public by enacting a sense of impartiality that went hand in hand with a display of disciplined devotion and civil service. The impact of this updated understanding of who a scientist ought to be is illustrated by the course taken by scientists appearing as expert witnesses in court: it was 'the sober, middle-class scientist' who was believed to earn the trust of the lay jury and expert witnesses modelled their performance on this image. This increased importance of the bourgeois scientist persona, as distinguished from the upper-class gentleman scholar, helps explain why the middle-class look was successful in the courtroom and the media. The middle-class lounge suit enacted a sense of sobriety that contrasted with connotations of arrogance, vanity or extravagance. This was important to forensic experts who were warned 'not to appear conceited or vain, [but] to look simple while being wise' when entering the witness box.[69] Arrogance was a vice that would 'irritate the court and damn the witness'.[70] The secretary of pathologist Keith Simpson, Molly Lefebure, emphasised Sir Bernard Spilsbury's modesty and love for science to counter the common perception of him as an arrogant and flamboyant man. She writes,

> He was reserved, modest and courteous in manner, very serious, very intent on his work. Indeed, he appeared to exist for nothing but his work. And above everything was his complete integrity [...] Despite these adulations Sir Bernard was a deeply modest man; a quiet, withheld man, withheld not in pride but in natural reticence.[71]

The modest, simple, bourgeois look became important for the performance of forensic expertise at a time when forensic culture revolved around the fear of partiality. Humility connoted integrity, a love for science and civil service. It was a middle-class virtue that enacted a sense of servitude, a virtue that was of pivotal importance in the British culture of trust in science. As STS scholar Sheila Jasanoff has argued, in Great Britain the public's trust in experts depended less on professional standing (as it did in the United States) or institutional affiliation (as it did in Germany) and more on 'the embodied virtue of its individual members' of research councils and their 'demonstrated record of service to society'.[72] Therefore, in the British context, it did not make sense for experts to rely on enclothed markers of professionalism or institutional affiliation. Instead, expert witnesses enclothed themselves familiarly, in an outfit that denoted middle-class virtuousness and professionalism. In the medical tradition and according to the new ideals in science, their outfits illustrated that they eschewed personal gain and served justice, not themselves.[73]

Conclusion

The sober suit that forensic experts wore in the courtroom was an important actor in the enactment of impartiality in the modern English and Scottish jury systems. The middle-class lounge suit conjured up a sense of familiarity between the experts and the jury, consisting predominantly of middle-class men. It demonstrated that these experts, like the jurors, were neutral servants of the court. The relation between the sober suit and impartiality derived from a history of class struggle experienced both by physicians and new men of science. In the medical context, a sober suit enabled physicians and surgeons to distinguish themselves from both quacks, who were characterised by their flamboyance, and manual labour. In the scientific world, the simple professional look signified the development of a new bourgeois scientific persona whose impartiality was safeguarded by his sobriety and servitude.

The literature on forensic science and medicine in the UK suggests that a modern forensic regime developed around the 1930s. Ian Burney and Neil Pemberton have argued that this modern regime developed with the establishment of the metropolitan police laboratory, team-based investigative practices and the new protocols for the collection of trace-based evidence. In line with this finding, the analysis of experts' dress practices has illustrated that in the mid-twentieth century forensic pathologists started to value hands-on skills and the collection of evidence in the mortuary. However, my analysis also shows that in different forensic spaces – the courtroom and news media – other expert performances were in place. In the public domain specifically, experts continued to rely on the performance of a bourgeois scientist persona to win trust and credibility. It was only around the 1960s that they started to rely on self-representations in white lab coats, symbolising the team-based, anonymised, technology-driven research practices and institutional affiliations.

The occurrence of this change in forensic culture reflected a general shift in British medical and scientific life. Historian Steven Shapin argues that in the 1960s and 1970s 'heroically self-denying bodies and especially virtuous persons are being replaced as guarantees of truth in our culture, and in their stead we now have notions of "expertise" and of the "rigorous policing" exerted on members by the institutions in which expertise lives'.[74] In this line of thought, it was no longer the person of the expert who ensured impartiality but the forensic institutes, their protocols and training programmes that endorsed objectivity and won the trust of the British population.

Notes

This project has received funding from the European Research Council (ERC) under the European Union's Horizon 2020 research and innovation programme (grant agreement No 770402).

1 Tal Golan, *Laws of Men and Laws of Nature: The History of Scientific Expert Testimony in England and America* (Cambridge, MA: Harvard University Press, 2004), pp. 6–20.
2 Carol A. G. Jones, *Expert Witnesses: Science, Medicine and the Practice of Law* (Oxford: Clarendon Press, 1994), p. 14.
3 Jones, *Expert Witnesses*, p. 14.
4 'The Expert Witness', *The Lancet*, 3 November 1923, p. 991.
5 Alison Adam, *Crime and the Construction of Forensic Objectivity from 1850* (London: Palgrave, 2020); Willemijn Ruberg and Nathanje Dijkstra, 'De forensische wetenschap in Nederland (1800–1930): een terreinverkenning', *Studium* 3:9 (2016), pp. 121–143.
6 Ian Burney and Neil Pemberton, *Murder and the Making of English CSI* (Baltimore, MD: Johns Hopkins University Press, 2016).
7 'The Duties of the Medical Witness III', *British Medical Journal*, Medico-Legal, 31 March 1934, p. 600.
8 H. A. Burridge, *An Introduction to Forensic Medicine for Medical Students and Practitioners* (London: H. K. Lewis & Co, 1924), p. 23; Keith Simpson, *Forensic Medicine* (London: Edward Arnold & Co, 1947), p. 211.
9 Golan, *Laws of Men*, p. 58.
10 Karen Harvey, 'Craftsmen in Common: Skills, Objects and Masculinity in the Eighteenth and Nineteenth Centuries', in Jane Hamlett, Leonie Hannan and Hannah Grieg (eds), *Gender and Material Culture c.1750–1950* (London: Palgrave Macmillan, 2015), pp. 68–89, here p. 83.
11 Laura Ugolini, *Men and Menswear: Sartorial Consumption in Britain 1880–1939* (Aldershot: Ashgate, 2007); Brent Shannon, *The Cut of His Coat: Men, Dress, and Consumer Culture in Britain, 1860–1914*

(Athens, OH: Ohio University Press, 2006); David Kuchta, *The Three-Piece Suit and Modern Masculinity: England, 1550–1850* (Berkeley, Los Angeles, London: University of California Press, 2002); Catherine F. Horwood, *Keeping Up Appearances: Fashion and Class Between the Wars* (The Mill, Brimcombe Port: The History Press, 2005); Jane Tynan, 'Military Dress and Men's Outdoor Leisurewear: Burberry's Trench Coat in First World War Britain', *Journal of Design History* 24:2 (2011), pp. 139–156; Quintin Colville, 'Jack Tar and the Gentleman Officer: The Role of Uniform in Shaping the Class and Gender-Related Identities of British Naval Personal, 1930–1939', *Transactions of the RHS* 13 (2003), pp. 105–129; Hajo Adam and Adam D. Galinsky, 'Enclothed Cognition', *Journal of Experimental Social Psychology* (February 2012), pp. 1–28, here pp. 5–6.

12 Katerina Honeyman, 'Following Suit: Men, Masculinity and Gendered Practices in the Clothing Trade in Leeds, England, 1890–1940', *Gender and History* 14:3 (2002), pp. 428–429; Frank Mort, *Cultures of Consumption* (London and New York: Routledge, 1996), p. 137.

13 *Ibid.*; Simon Szreter and Kate Fisher, *Sex Before the Sexual Revolution: Intimate Life in England 1918–1963* (Cambridge, New York: Cambridge University Press, 2010), p. 295.

14 Szreter and Fisher, *Sex Before the Sexual Revolution*, pp. 295–296.

15 Susan Hardey and Anthoney Corones, 'Dressed to Heal: The Changing Semiotics of Surgical Dress', *Fashion Theory* 20:1 (2015), pp. 27–49, here p. 28.

16 Mineke Bosch, 'Scholarly Personae and Twentieth-Century Historians: Explorations of a Concept', *BMGN – Low Countries Historical Review* 131:4 (2016), pp. 33–54, here pp. 53–54.

17 Kelly-Ann Couzens, '"Upon My Word, I Do Not See the Use of Medical Evidence Here": Persuasion, Authority and Medical Expertise in the Edinburgh High Court of Justiciary', *History* 104: 359 (2019), pp. 42–62. For literature on clothes of victims and perpetrators see: Alison Matthews David and Serah-Marie McMahon, *Killer Style: How Fashion Has Injured, Maimed, and Murdered Through History* (Berkeley: Owlkids Books, 2019); Alison Matthews David, *Fashion Victims: The Dangers of Dress Past and Present* (London and New York: Bloomsbury, 2015).

18 Couzens, '"Upon My Word", p. 51.

19 Jones, *Expert Witnesses*, p. 148.

20 Elizabeth Wilson, *Adorned in Dreams: Fashion and Modernity* (New York: Rutgers University Press, 2003), p. 33; Ann Hollander, *Sex and Suits: The Evolution of Modern Dress* (New York, Bloomsbury,

1994), p. 109; Brent Shannon, *The Cut of His Coat: Men, Dress, and Consumer Culture in Britain, 1860–1914* (Ohio: Cambridge University Press, 2006).
21 'Clothes and Psychic Health', *The Lancet*, 8 October 1949, p. 679.
22 Mort, *Cultures of Consumption*, p. 137; Kuchta, *The Three-Piece Suit and Modern Masculinity*, p. 178; Beth Jenkins, 'Gender, Embodiment and Professional Identity in Britain, c.1890–1930', *Cultural and Social History* 17:4 (2020), pp. 499–514, here p. 501; Honeyman, 'Following Suit', p. 334.
23 Fred Miller Robinson, *The Man in the Bowler Hat: His History and Iconography* (Chapel Hill, 1993), p. 27.
24 'The Duties of the Medical Witness I', *The British Medical Journal*, Medico-Legal, 3 March 1934, p. 407.
25 'The Doctor in the Law Courts', *The British Medical Journal*, 22 March 1930, p. 549; emphasis added.
26 Richard Ellis, 'Initiation', *The Lancet*, 27 August 1955, pp. 403–404; Ordway Hilton, 'The Essence of Good Testimony', *Medicine, Science and the Law* 8:2 (April 1968), pp. 85–87; A. L. Wells, 'The Expert Witness', *The Lancet*, Letters to the Editor, 30 May 1953, pp. 1103–1104; Melitta Schmideberg, 'Point of View of the Psychiatrist', in *The Court and the Expert: Writing Reports*, Essays in Comparative Forensic Psychiatry (*International Journal of Offender Therapy*, 1971); Michael Cleary, 'Personal View', *British Medical Journal*, 1 June 1974, p. 498; Gerald Pearce, *The Medical Report and Testimony* (London, George Allen & Unwin LTD, 1979).
27 Sydney Smith, *Forensic Medicine: A Textbook for Students and Practitioners* (London: J.A. Churchill, 1925), p. 5.
28 'The Doctor in the Law Courts', *The British Medical Journal*, 22 March 1930, p. 550.
29 Douglas J. A. Kerr, *Forensic Medicine: A Textbook for Students and a Guide for the Practitioner* (London: A&C Black LTD, 1935), p. 29.
30 See for example: 'Dramatic Scenes at Gloucester Assizes', *Gloucestershire Chronicle*, 8 November 1924, p. 13.
31 Horwood, *Keeping Up Appearances*, p. 47. And see the dress codes and description of dress in: 'The Harvey Tercentenary: Celebration by the Royal College of Physicians of London', *The Lancet*, 24 March 1928, pp. 621–622; 'Scotland: Medical Women's International Association', *The Lancet*, 27 July 1937, pp. 212–213. For Keith Simpson's description of his teacher in 1923 see: Keith Simpson, *Forty Years of Murder: An Autobiography* (London, 1980), p. 23.
32 Horwood, *Keeping Up Appearances*, p. 45.

33 For information on the impact the police uniform could have on the jury, see: London, National Archives, J 82/1371, Mr Justice Ashworth, Summing Up, 30 January 1969, p. 17.
34 According to this ideal that pictured forensic physicians as a stable element of Francoist courts, in 1947 and 1949 forensic physicians were allowed the use of a corporative medal, a lawyer's cap (*birrete*), they were granted to report in court located spatially as prosecutors and lawyers, instead of as witnesses, and they were legally considered as authorities while in service: BOE, 199, 18 July 1947, 'Ley de 17 de julio de 1947 orgánica del Cuerpo Nacional de Médicos Forenses', 4018; BOE, 1, 1 January 1949, 'Orden de 9 de diciembre de 1948 por la que se aprueban las normas descriptivas a que deberán ajustarse en su forma y características la Medalla y Placa que usarán los Médicos forenses', p. 10; Ricardo Royo-Vilanova Morales, Blas Aznar and Bonifacio Piga, *Lecciones de Medicina Legal* (Madrid: Benzal, 1952), p. 25.
35 Molly Lefebure, *Evidence for the Crown: Experiences of a Pathologist's Secretary* (London, Melbourne, Toronto: Lippincott, 1955), p. 10.
36 ' "FINGERPRINT EXPERT WAS 'IDEAL WITNESS' 'Darkie of the Yard' Retiring" ', *Dundee Evening Telegraph*, 12 November 1938.
37 'The Amazing Dr. Lynch', *John Bull*, 29 July 1939, p. 34.
38 Kuchta described this look as iconic for British men: Kuchta, *The Three-Piece Suit and Modern Masculinity*, p. 178.
39 Andrew Watson, *Speaking in Court: Developments in Court Advocacy from the Seventeenth to the Twenty-First Century* (New York: Palgrave Macmillan, 2019), p. 209.
40 Watson, *Speaking in Court*, p. 217.
41 *Ibid.*, p. 210.
42 McMahon, 'Declining Professionalism in Court', p. 849.
43 Hardey and Corones, 'Dressed to Heal'.
44 *Ibid.*, p. 44.
45 *Ibid.*; Mark Hochberg, 'The Doctor's White Coat: An Historical Perspective', *AMA Journal of Ethics* 9:4 (2007), pp. 310–314.
46 Simpson, *Forensic Medicine*, p. 203.
47 *Science Fights Crime (1946)*, 2014, www.youtube.com/watch?v=2MAjELT0WEc&t=238s.
48 John Glaister, *Final Diagnosis* (London, Sydney, Toronto and New York: Hutchinson & Co Ltd, 1964) cover image.
49 H. J. Walls, *Expert Witness: My Thirty Years in Forensic Science*, 1st ed. (London: Random House UK, 1972).

50 See for example: Christopher Menaul, 'Prime Suspect', mini-series, 7 April 1991.
51 Judy Williams, *The Modern Sherlock Holmes: An Introduction to Forensic Science Today* (Glasgow: Eagle Colourbooks, 1991); Reader's Digest Association, *Great Cases of Scotland Yard* (Pleasantville, NY: Reader's Digest Association, 1978), http://archive.org/details/greatcasesofscot00read.
52 Christopher Lawrence, 'Medical Minds, Surgical Bodies: Corporeality and the Doctors', in Christopher Lawrence and Steven Shapin (eds), *Science Incarnate: Historical Embodiments of Natural Knowledge* (Chicago and London: University of Chicago Press, 1998); Keren Rosa Hammerschlag, 'The Gentleman Artist-Surgeon in Late Victorian Group Portraiture', *Visual Culture in Britain* 14:2 (2013), pp. 154–178; Hardey and Corones, 'Dressed to Heal'.
53 Hammerschlag, 'The Gentleman Artist-Surgeon in Late Victorian Group Portraiture'.
54 Lawrence, 'Medical Minds, Surgical Bodies: Corporeality and the Doctors', p. 118; Hammerschlag, 'The Gentleman Artist-Surgeon in Late Victorian Group Portraiture', p. 158; L. J. Jordanova, *Defining Features: Scientific and Medical Portraits, 1660–2000* (London: Reaktion, 2000) p. 163, http://archive.org/details/definingfeatures0000jord.
55 Anne Digby, *The Evolution of British General Practice: 1850–1948* (Oxford and New York: Oxford University Press, 1999), p. 38; Roy Porter, *Bodies Politic: Disease, Death and Doctors in Britain, 1650–1900* (London: The University of Chicago Press, 2014), p. 255.
56 Hardey and Corones, 'Dressed to Heal', p. 31.
57 Porter, *Bodies Politic*, p. 260.
58 See examples in: Rebecca Crites, 'Husbands' Violence against Wives in England and Wales, 1914–1939: A Review of Contemporary Understandings of and Responses to Men's Marital Violence' (PhD thesis, University of Warwick, 2016), p. 180; Jane Custance Baker, 'Fear and Clothing: Dress in English Detective Fiction Between the First and Second World Wars' (PhD thesis, University of London, 2019), p. 118; See also contemporary remarks in: L. W. Harrison, 'Some Disadvantages of Medical Evidence on Venereal Diseases, to the Public Health and to the Administration of Justice', *Transactions of the Medico-Legal Society* 26:154 (1932–1931), p. 155.
59 Jones, *Expert Witnesses*, p. 95.
60 Haia Shpayer-Makov, *The Ascent of the Detective: Police Sleuths in Victorian and Edwardian England* (Oxford: Oxford University Press, 2011), p. 248.

61 Jordanova, *Defining Features*, p. 74; Jones, *Expert Witnesses*, p. 59; Golan, *Laws of Men*, p. 51.
62 Jones, *Expert Witnesses*, p. 72.
63 Golan, *Laws of Men*, p. 125.
64 *Ibid.*, p. 123.
65 Andrew Miles and Mike Savage, 'The Strange Survival Story of the English Gentleman, 1945–2010', *Cultural and Social History* 9:4 (2012), pp. 595–612, here p. 598.
66 Kuchta, *The Three-Piece Suit and Modern Masculinity*, p. 142.
67 Jones, *Expert Witnesses*, p. 65.
68 Heather Ellis, *Masculinity and Science in Britain, 1831–1918* (London: Palgrave MacMillan, 2017).
69 'The Doctor in the Law Courts', p. 550.
70 A. L. Wells, 'The Expert Witness', *The Lancet*, Letters to the Editor, 30 May 1953, p. 190.
71 Lefebure, *Evidence for the Crown*, pp. 10–11.
72 Sheila Jasanoff, *Designs on Nature: Democracy in Europe and the United States* (Princeton: Princeton University Press, 2005), pp. 187, 262, 266, 268.
73 Jordanova, *Defining Features*, p. 95.
74 Steven Shapin, *Never Pure: Historical Studies of Science as if it Was Produced, by People with Bodies, Situated in Time, Space, Culture, and Society, and Struggling for Credibility and Authority* (Baltimore: Johns Hopkins University Press, 2010), p. 257.

6

Reassessing the legacy of Cesare Lombroso: Criminal anthropology in the expert testimony of Mario Carrara, 1910–1930

Franco Orlandi

Introduction

The legacy of Cesare Lombroso (1835–1909) and the impact of his criminological theories in Liberal and Fascist Italy are still controversial among historians. There are at least two points of debate in the scholarship concerning Lombroso. First, there is the question of whether Lombroso's death in 1909 marked the end of his school of criminal anthropology. A number of scholars have argued that the Lombrosian school had already entered a period of irreversible decline and scientific marginalisation by the late nineteenth century and that its influence on Italian legal culture in the Liberal and Fascist eras was completely marginal.[1] A second strand of scholarship, however, suggests that the impact of Lombrosian criminal anthropology on the Italian criminal justice system was extremely significant throughout the first half of the twentieth century and that Lombroso's theories continued to shape criminal law and policing practices long after his death.[2]

The second area of contention concerns the relationship between Lombrosian criminal anthropology and the Fascist regime. According to Mary Gibson, not only did the Lombrosian school contribute to the repression of juvenile delinquency and prostitution in Fascist Italy, but it also 'created an intellectual environment conducive to the dictatorship' and undergirded Mussolini's project of imperial conquest in Africa.[3] These conclusions, however, are not shared by other studies, which have pointed out that rather than finding its way into the criminal policy of Mussolini's regime, Lombroso's ideas were distorted by the Fascist government for its own political ends to the point of unrecognisability.[4]

This chapter seeks to contribute to this ongoing debate on Cesare Lombroso's controversial legacy by assessing the influence of Lombrosian forensic psychiatrists in Italian court cases of murder in the first decades of the twentieth century, an aspect which has been totally neglected in previous research. In so doing, it attempts to shed light on the fate of criminal anthropology after Lombroso's death and the relationship of the Lombrosian school with the Fascist regime. Did Lombrosian criminal anthropology die with Lombroso, as some scholars have claimed, or were his theories still influential in the 1930s? What was the attitude of the Fascist judiciary towards Lombrosian criminal anthropology? Did it reject Lombroso's theories or did it employ them for repressive purposes, as it has been argued in previous studies?

This research is based on the quantitative analysis of seventy-three murder trials and on the qualitative analysis of one murder trial held at the Court of Assize of Turin between 1907 and 1932 in which the criminal anthropologist Mario Carrara (1866–1937), Cesare Lombroso's son-in-law and his successor to the Chair of Forensic Medicine at the University of Turin, was invited as an expert witness to determine the liability of the defendant to punishment. The Court of Assize was (and still is) the body responsible for judging the most serious crimes in Italy.

My key research questions are: To what extent did Carrara make use of Lombroso's theories to carry out his psychiatric evaluations? How often did his expert testimony influence the jury's final verdict in murder trials? Why were his conclusions accepted or rejected by the court? As for the last question, it should be noted that until 1931 the verdicts issued by the Italian Courts of Assize contained only the defendant's sentence and did not explicitly state the reasons for the judgment. This makes it impossible to reconstruct the reasons why the court came up with its judgments in the 1910s and 1920s. After the 1931 jury reform, however, the presidents of the Courts of Assize had to explain why they had reached their verdict and, if an expert testimony had been required during the preliminary investigation or the trial, why they had accepted or rejected the expert's conclusions. Criminal trial verdicts issued after 1931 are therefore extremely valuable sources for assessing the influence of medical witnesses in Fascist Italy and, in this specific case, that of Lombrosian forensic psychiatrists.

Mario Carrara started his academic career as Lombroso's assistant at the University of Turin in 1893, where he became professor of Forensic Medicine ten years later, holding the chair once occupied by his maestro. After the death of Lombroso in 1909, he succeeded him as the head of the Lombrosian school. Carrara took over the editorship of the *Archivio di antropologia criminale* (the journal founded by Lombroso in 1880), the directorship of the Lombroso Museum and he was appointed as a lecturer in Criminal Anthropology, all positions formerly held by Lombroso. During his career, he became one of the most influential Italian criminal anthropologists of his time and was widely regarded as Lombroso's true scientific heir. While it might be misleading to consider post-Lombroso Italian criminal anthropology as exclusively dominated by Carrara, his importance within the Lombrosian school can hardly be overstated. For this reason, an analysis of Carrara's activity as a forensic expert can help to shed light on the legacy of Lombroso in Liberal and Fascist Italy.

The focus of this study on Carrara is further justified by more practical reasons. Firstly, as far as we know, Carrara is the only Lombrosian forensic expert who testified regularly in the court of Turin in the Liberal and Fascist eras and one of the few remaining Lombrosian experts in Italy in the 1930s. Secondly, he is the only Lombrosian forensic expert we know of whose documents and psychiatric evaluations are preserved in a private archive accessible to scholars, which was donated to the University of Turin by Carrara's heirs in 2009. While prominent Lombrosians like Salvatore Ottolenghi (1861–1934) and his pupil Benigno di Tullio (1896–1979) probably also gave expert testimony in the court of Rome in the same years of Carrara, the lack of documentation makes it especially hard to identify and study the court cases in which they participated as forensic experts.

I have decided to focus on murder trials for two reasons: firstly, most of the Assize court records for this period survive in the State archives. This makes it possible to compare Carrara's forensic conclusions with the verdicts reached by the jury. Secondly, criminal anthropologists believed that the most serious and violent crimes were generally committed by the most biologically deviant individuals, who were thought to exhibit a higher number of physical and mental anomalies than non-criminals. An analysis of the psychiatric evaluations carried out by Carrara on subjects charged with murder allows establishing the extent to which the criminological theories of Lombroso, notably the assumption that the physical body could mirror moral perversion and a special criminal predisposition, were actually put into practice by his followers to assess the degree of legal responsibility and dangerousness of the defendants.

The originality of this work lies in its focus on criminal anthropology as practice rather than as scientific discourse. While scholarship on the Lombrosian school has mostly centred on the evolution and circulation of its theories, little attention has been paid to the ways in which the latter were put into practice in specific locations such as the courtroom. I believe that in order to study the history and assess the influence of a forensic culture, one should look not only at how its main ideas were expressed and discussed in books, medical journals or conferences, but also at how they were practically applied to real forensic cases. Forensic practices are embedded in legal systems, cultural contexts and political regimes that may shape the way they are performed. This embeddedness also interacts with the production of scholarly knowledge. For this reason, in my opinion, a good way to analyse a forensic culture is to compare its theory with its practice, trying to understand whether the approach to forensic cases advocated in textbooks finds correspondence in the daily practice of forensic experts. In this specific case, I will analyse how a leading Lombrosian forensic expert like Carrara translated Lombroso's theories into practice when carrying out his psychiatric assessment reports.

Before discussing my findings, I will briefly outline how the role of the forensic expert was regulated by the Italian Code of Criminal Procedure (CCP), how Italian forensic culture compared to other European countries and how Lombrosian criminal anthropologists were instructed to perform their examinations when called to testify.

Criminal law, medical expert witness testimony and forensic culture in Liberal and Fascist Italy

According to the Italian Criminal Code of 1889, a person could not be held criminally responsible for a criminal offence 'if, at the moment in which he committed the crime, he was in such a state of infirmity of mind as to deprive him of the awareness or the freedom of his actions' (art. 46). The penalty could also be reduced in case of diminished mental capacity (art. 47). In a similar vein, the Criminal Code of 1930, which was introduced under the Fascist regime, provided that 'a person who, at the moment in which he committed the crime, was, by reason of infirmity, in such a state of mind as to exclude his capacity to intend or will' could not be held legally accountable (art. 88). The penalty could be reduced in case of partial mental infirmity (art. 89).

According to the CCP of 1930, the judge could request an expert testimony whenever the investigation required 'special knowledge of certain sciences or arts', such as psychiatry, traumatology or toxicology.[5] The expert could be called to testify during both the preliminary investigation (*fase istruttoria*) and the trial. While in theory anyone deemed 'suitable' by the judge could be called to act as an expert witness, in practice only those with a specialist qualification were designated for this role. The title of specialist was attributed by the Ministry of Education to well-educated and experienced professionals working in the field of psychiatry or forensic medicine, such as university professors or directors of mental hospitals.[6] These vague selection criteria and the lack of a professional register for forensic experts were criticised by the Lombrosian school, which called for stricter selections, as in France and Germany.[7]

In case a psychiatric evaluation was requested, the judge would ask the expert to state in his report what the defendant's state of mind was at the moment in which he committed the crime and at the moment the evaluation had been carried out, and whether he was a socially dangerous person, that is, whether he was likely to commit other crimes in the future. The 1930 CCP specified that expert reports could not establish 'the habitual or professional nature of the crime, the tendency toward criminality, the character and personality of the defendant, and in general the psychological features of the defendant which do not depend on mental pathologies' (art. 134).[8] With this provision, which was the expression of profound scepticism towards the human sciences, particularly criminal anthropology, criminology and psychology, the legislator aimed to keep 'sciences that relied on uncertain data' out of criminal trials.[9] The judge, and not the medical witness, was thus the only authority responsible for the evaluation of the defendant's personality. That this provision stood in the way of criminal anthropologists was clear to Carrara, who demanded corrective provisions in this regard.[10] Not all Lombrosians, however, admitted their defeat.[11]

During the trial, the findings of the expert would be read aloud before the court. Afterwards, with the permission of the judge, the public prosecutor and the defence could call the officially designated expert to give oral explanations on his written report. The same privilege was not granted to the defence expert. Any public discussion between the official and the defence experts was absolutely prohibited during the trial, so as to avoid debates that would confuse and negatively impress the jury and the public.[12] Italy was quite unique in this respect. In France and Germany, countries that like Italy had adopted an inquisitorial system of criminal procedure, battles between experts were allowed in the courtroom.[13]

In Italy, the expert's conclusions were by no means binding for the jurors' final verdict. Before 1931, the Italian Court of Assize was composed of ten lay judges and a president 'chosen from among the ranks of superior judges'.[14] At the end of the trial, the jurors did not have to render a 'guilty' or 'non-guilty' verdict, but they had to answer 'yes' or 'no' to a series of questions posed by the president of the court (for example, if the defendant was sound of mind at the moment of the crime). After the jury's decision, the judge pronounced the sentence. Until 1951, the decision of the Court of Assize was final and subject to appeal only on procedural grounds. Lombrosians opposed trials by jury, as they argued that the final verdict on the mental state of the defendant should be left to men of science trained in criminal anthropology and not to incompetent laymen. From the point of view of criminal anthropology, the fact that the judge could demand a medical expertise and then disregard the expert's conclusions was also dismissed. Lombroso lamented that not only were judges and jury members not scientists, but they were also for the most part 'adverse to science' and 'disgusted' by the subtleties of forensic experts' scientific analysis.[15]

In 1931 the Court of Assize was reformed. Jury trials were abolished and replaced by mixed courts made up of two judges and five laymen called 'assessors'. The judges were appointed every year by the Ministry of Justice, while the assessors had to meet a series of eligibility requirements, such as being 'morally and politically above reproach'.[16] The Court was thus entirely selected by the Fascist government and the judiciary was a direct expression of the Regime. The procedure to reach the final verdict changed. Judges and assessors deliberated and established the punishment together, on the basis of the majority principle.[17] After the deliberation, the president of the court drafted the sentence, which did not necessarily represent his personal opinion.

Lombrosian criminal anthropologists and expert testimony

In 1905 Cesare Lombroso published his famous manual for the expert witness, *La perizia psichiatrico-legale*. Consistent with his theory of the 'born criminal', which explained criminal behaviour and moral insanity as the result of a biological predisposition that left visible traces on the body, Lombroso advised his colleagues to:

> gather the results of tests on height, weight, and urine, of the examination of general anthropological characteristics, of the skin and cutaneous processes, of the skull, limbs, etc., then the data on sensitivity to weather, to touch, to pain, to drugs, on affectivity and emotionality, on feelings, [and] on the association of ideas ... so that, in the end, based on all these characteristics, you can offer a synthesis that will illuminate the judge.[18]

In *The Criminal Man*, Lombroso provided examples of how criminal anthropology could help solve criminal cases. He bragged that, as an expert witness, he had been able to identify the culprit among a group of suspects based on his physical appearance on several occasions.[19] According to Lombrosian criminologists, anthropological examinations could not only help to categorise criminals and identify the authors of a crime, but also save innocents from wrongful convictions.[20] The spread of Lombroso's ideas across the country is demonstrated by the number of other guides for the expert witness that were written by adherents of the Lombrosian school in those years.[21]

Many years later Mario Carrara, in his *Handbook of Forensic Medicine*, which was published after his death in 1940 and became a reference book for generations of students, also stressed the importance of physical examination in the assessment and diagnosis of mental illness, claiming that accumulation of somatic anomalies in one individual could be a sign of psychiatric disease. For this reason, he recommended his readers to:

> note the height of the subject, his weight, his skeletal conformation, with particular regard to that of the skull (which will be examined in its shape, its volume and its diameter), and of the face; to examine the state of the skin, particularly of the face, in relation to the existence of wrinkles, the characters of the skin appendages; the shape of the ear, the shape of the nose, the shape of the hand, that of the foot and so on.[22]

Other forensic cultures that had emerged in Italy in the meantime, however, opposed Lombroso's claim that cranial and physical traits could provide valuable evidence of criminality and mental illness. The most important proponent of this alternative scientific paradigm was Eugenio Tanzi (1856–1934), a major figure in the history of twentieth-century Italian psychiatry and neurology. A professor of Psychiatry at the University of Florence, director of the local asylum of San Salvi, co-founder of the *Journal of Nervous and Mental Pathology* and Honorary Fellow of the Royal Medico-Psychological Association, Tanzi had become an authority in the field after the publication of his *Textbook of Mental Diseases*, which went through three editions between 1904 and 1923 and was translated into English in 1909. The treatise soon became the Italian standard textbook in psychiatry. In his works, which were reviewed with disdain by Lombroso,[23] Tanzi distanced himself from orthodox Lombrosian criminal anthropology. Deeply influenced by the work of the German psychiatrist Emil Kraepelin, he downplayed the importance of physical examinations for establishing a psychiatric diagnosis and denied the existence of a close link between epilepsy and criminality. 'The physical signs of degeneration', he wrote in his guide for the expert witness, 'are of no value in determining the presence of a mental disorder or even a simple predisposition to it'.[24] For Tanzi, the vast majority of criminals showed no stigmata of degeneration and only a very small part of them were epileptics. Furthermore, most of their physical defects were not the product of atavism or hereditary degeneration, as Lombroso had argued, but were due to pathological causes, in particular cerebral palsy contracted during childhood.[25] Unlike Lombroso, Tanzi maintained that criminal behaviour mostly resulted from social rather than biological causes. In his view, this was proved by the fact that women committed remarkably fewer crimes than men. If, as Lombroso had maintained, hereditary degeneration played such an important role in the aetiology of crime, both sexes should have been equally affected and therefore there should have been no gender gap in offending. The difference between male and female crime rates, Tanzi argued, was a product of patriarchal society and not of biology, as women mostly lived in the seclusion of their families, which reduced opportunities and temptations to break the law:

> As crime is almost always a reaction to a social anomaly, injustice, or prejudice, the male sex, which stands in the vanguard in the struggle for life and happiness, is guilty of law-breaking much more frequently than the female sex; women, who are the slaves and parasites of man, are in much less degree exposed to dangers and to temptations to crime.[26]

This does not mean, however, that Tanzi did not believe in the existence of the born criminal. What he opposed, though, was Lombroso's assumption that the born criminal bore a cluster of physical anomalies. Most of the born criminals, Tanzi contended, did not exhibit any physical sign of degeneration nor epilepsy. The only feature that distinguished this category of criminals from others was their appalling moral insensitivity. Like Kraepelin in Germany, Tanzi 'stripped Lombroso's notion of the born criminal of its anthropological characteristics and redefined the born criminal in purely psychiatric terms as someone with a "moral defect"'.[27] Tanzi rejected Lombroso's concept of 'moral insanity' and replaced it with that of 'constitutional immorality', which he defined as 'a constitutional and mostly congenital affective anomaly consisting in the deficiency of moral feelings in individuals of sound and complete intelligence'.[28] Since the born criminal's moral insensitivity did not affect his intellectual faculties, Tanzi maintained, unlike the Lombrosian school, that he be held fully responsible for his misdeeds and punished by the law. For Tanzi, the diagnosis of constitutional immorality was 'always subordinate to a judgment of an ethical nature'[29] and not to an anthropometric examination as Lombrosian forensic experts believed.

As we have seen, more than forty years after the publication of the last edition of *The Criminal Man*, Mario Carrara was still faithfully following the theories of Lombroso that correlated physical anomalies with moral insensitivity, at least on paper. But to what extent was this criminological approach appreciated in the courtroom? Which forensic culture most appealed to the jury, Lombrosian criminal anthropology as interpreted by Carrara or Kraepelin's psychiatry as advocated by Eugenio Tanzi?

Mario Carrara in the courtroom

Over the course of his career, Carrara carried out over 300 psychiatric evaluations for the court of Turin, which demonstrates he enjoyed a considerable reputation in the city as a forensic expert. About a third of his forensic reports concerned homicide cases. I was able to reconstruct the outcome of seventy-three murder cases in which Carrara was summoned as a medical witness to the Court of Assize and I have compared his forensic conclusions with the final verdicts reached by the court. From 1907 to 1932, out of seventy-three trials, Carrara argued the liability of the defendant to punishment in thirty cases (41 per cent), a conclusion that was shared by the jury twenty-three times (77 per cent); he argued the partial infirmity of mind in thirty cases (41 per cent), a conclusion shared by the jury seventeen times (57 per cent). It should be noted, however, that this figure varies considerably depending on the period under consideration: from 1910 to 1916, out of nine trials, the conclusion of partial infirmity of mind was always rejected by the court, whereas from 1919 to 1933, out of twenty-one trials, it was accepted seventeen times (81 per cent). This may indicate that over the years, the nosographic category of partial insanity had become increasingly accepted by the general public. Finally, Carrara argued the infirmity of mind in thirteen cases (18 per cent), a conclusion accepted only five times (38 per cent). The defendant's gender was male in sixty-eight cases (93 per cent), and female in five (7 per cent). These figures seem to demonstrate that jurors tended to agree with medical witnesses when they concluded that the defendant was sound of mind, but that they were much more reluctant to accept a diagnosis of mental infirmity. Considering the esteem that Carrara enjoyed in Turin, the jury's reluctance in accepting insanity pleas probably reflects a wider trend within Italian forensic culture rather than distrust towards his expertise. Carrara was without any doubt a very respected professional and one of the most consulted psychiatric experts in town. In 1932, in a defensive memoire submitted to the investigating judge on the case, a defendant's lawyer wrote that in his career he had never met a better medical witness than Carrara, which explained why 'the judiciary of Turin has been daily relying on his scientific expertise for many years now'.[30]

Why, then, did the jury dismiss most of the psychiatric evaluations that proclaimed the defendant's unaccountability? A possible explanation is that jurors did not want insane convicts to escape imprisonment, as they believed that their acquittal might pose a significant threat to the security of society. The 1904 national law on mental asylums prescribed that 'criminals acquitted on the grounds of insanity could be interned only in civil asylums'.[31] The consequence of this provision was that potentially dangerous individuals were sent to mental hospitals intended for non-criminal patients, which were therefore often ill-equipped for their treatment and surveillance. The inadequate facilities of civil asylums offered acquitted criminals more opportunities to escape and harm staff and inmates than did prison. The dangers of riots, mass breakouts and attacks on staff prompted directors of civil asylums to get rid of the criminally insane by handing them back to their families.[32] Once released back onto the streets, however, they would often end up committing other crimes. Aware of this problematic situation and concerned with the security of law-abiding citizens, jurors and judges tended to sentence the criminally insane to life imprisonment or at least to reduced punishment by reason of partial insanity for fear that they might escape or be released from civil asylums.[33] Moreover, the memory of the riot that had broken out at the mental hospital of Turin (based in the nearby village of Collegno) in 1912, then directed by Lombroso's collaborator Antonio Marro, in which a group of armed criminally insane had taken four nurses hostage to denounce their poor conditions of detention (a protest that ended without casualties),[34] was certainly still vivid in town, which might also explain this tendency to reject insanity pleas.

The rise of the Fascist dictatorship in the 1920s does not seem to have affected the reception of criminal anthropology in the courtroom, as the agreement/disagreement ratio between Carrara and the jury members remained constant over the years, as did the number of psychiatric evaluations he carried out per year. This conclusion is not contradicted by the aforementioned finding that from the 1920s onwards the jury tended to agree with Carrara in cases of partial mental infirmity, since this trend can be observed from 1919, while the fascistisation of the Italian judiciary was not completed until 1926.[35] The fact that Carrara (who was known for being a socialist and an anti-fascist)[36] continued to be invited as an expert witness after 1931 – the year he was expelled from the university of Turin for refusing to take the loyalty oath imposed by the Fascist dictatorship upon all Italian university professors – seems to demonstrate that he continued to enjoy the esteem of the Fascist judiciary despite his political position. In 1934, however, he was forced to leave the post of medical witness since it became mandatory to be a member of the Fascist Party in order to exercise the profession.

Carrara in action: The case of Francesco Monticone

In order to understand how Carrara made use of the theories of Lombroso in his assessments and to what extent the latter were accepted by the judiciary, I will now focus on the paradigmatic case of Francesco Monticone, a 28-year-old labourer who murdered and robbed a merchant in 1931. This case stands out from the sample collected for this study for two reasons. Firstly, this is the only case where the subject of Carrara's expertise exhibits a cluster of physical and functional anomalies that bear a striking resemblance to those Lombroso attributed to the 'criminal type' and the 'born criminal'. Secondly, this is the only case where the president of the Court of Assize makes explicit use of a scientific authority to uphold his final decision and undermine the forensic conclusions reached by Carrara.

Monticone's psychiatric evaluation was carried out by Carrara together with Francesco Agosti, the expert appointed by the defence. A lecturer in Nervous and Mental Diseases at the University of Turin and a doctor at the local mental asylum, Agosti had undertaken studies in criminal anthropology in the past.[37] The report pointed out that Monticone bore a 'profoundly degenerative' appearance. He exhibited unusually long arms, overdeveloped sinuses, prominent cheekbones, prognathism, thick eyebrows, a flattened nose, deformed ears and brachycephaly.[38] Monticone also showed abnormal reflexes, dullness of touch and low sensitivity to pain. The psychiatric examination revealed that he suffered from a 'mental deficiency' (*deficienza psichica*), the most evident sign of which was a speech disorder. This conclusion was based upon the results of the interrogation conducted by the two medical experts, during which Monticone had repeatedly given proof of his limited intelligence. Even the way in which he had behaved after committing the crime, thoughtlessly hiding the murder weapon and the stolen goods in his own house, served as evidence for establishing the diagnosis. According to Carrara and Agosti, Monticone's mental deficiency was associated with moral defectiveness. This was proved by the fact that Monticone had a criminal record of thefts, had used violence on his wife and had always felt revulsion for work, which is why he had a reputation for being lazy and violent in his village. This lack of moral sense was also reflected in the formal and unconvincing way in which Monticone had expressed regret for his crime during the interrogation. While no clinical evidence was found that he descended from a family of madmen, the police reported that almost all his family members were 'immoral'[39]. For all these reasons, Carrara and Agosti concluded that Monticone's deficiency was a condition inherited from his family and therefore 'constitutional' in nature.[40] It followed that Monticone had to be considered a dangerous individual, since his psychopathic moral alteration would have lasted for all his life, even after he had served out his sentence. However, the two medical experts maintained that Monticone had to be held partially accountable for the murder since he was not completely unsound of mind. This was evidenced by the fact that he had been able to marry and to live in society until then.

What makes Monticone's case so interesting? To begin with, it shows that more than twenty years after the death of Lombroso criminal anthropologists like Carrara and Agosti were still performing anthropometric measurements and sensitivity tests to reach a clinical diagnosis. A comparison between Carrara's early and later psychiatric reports reveals that from the 1910s to the 1930s little had changed in the way he performed his anthropological examinations. Each of his evaluations included body and craniometrical measures of the defendant, as well as the results of sensory and functional tests. This proves that throughout his career Carrara remained faithful to the biocriminological theories of Lombroso, which he put into practice to carry out his psychiatric assessments.

What is striking, however, is that Carrara was reluctant to adopt a 'Lombrosian' language in his reports and to make explicit use of anthropometric findings to support his forensic conclusions. This case study is particularly revealing in this regard. The physical abnormalities that Carrara found in Monticone corresponded to the marks of degeneration typical of the born criminal. Insensitivity to pain was another feature that he shared with this category of offenders, a condition that criminal anthropologists believed to reflect an inner lack of emotion and morality. From the fourth edition of *The Criminal Man* on, Lombroso had equated congenital criminality with the psychiatric phenomenon of moral insanity and the disorder of epilepsy, although he never clearly defined the differences between these three pathologies.[41] In his *Handbook*, Carrara reaffirmed that the morally insane shared the same anthropological stigmata and functional anomalies of the born criminal, as well as some of his psychological characteristics, such as impulsiveness, egoism and a lack of a sense of justice.[42] He also pointed out that from a biological point of view it was not easy to draw a clear-cut distinction between the criminal and the insane man, since these two categories were often overlapping.[43] Carrara's description of the physical and psychological traits of the 'criminally insane' as provided in his *Handbook* matched perfectly with Monticone's profile. Yet, the fact that the latter belonged to this category of criminals – which is something that must have been plainly evident to Carrara – was never explicitly mentioned in the forensic report nor was it used as an argument for the psychiatric assessment. While it is true that the two medical witnesses wrote that even a layman would have realised that Monticone was feeble-minded (*deficiente*) judging by his 'physical appearance' and his 'behaviour', they used intellectual and cognitive assessments rather than anthropological arguments to justify their conclusion: the fact, for example, that the defendant struggled to pronounce words in a comprehensible way or that he was not able to understand the content of a text.

This reluctance to make use of 'anthropological evidence' is even clearer if one considers the way in which the two experts defended the diagnosis of a congenital moral alteration. Instead of highlighting that Monticone exhibited all the physical and psychological features of the 'criminally insane', which is what one would expect from a Lombrosian criminal anthropologist, Carrara simply recalled his history of petty thefts and domestic violence. Particularly telling is also the fact that in the report Carrara never used the expression 'moral insanity' (*pazzia morale*) to refer to Monticone's condition, contrary to his commenting on similar criminal cases in his scientific publications.[44]

How should we interpret this discrepancy between theory and practice? Why was Carrara so cautious in openly using the tools and findings of criminal anthropology to assess the mental state of the defendants he was to examine? I believe that the answer is that he feared his forensic conclusions would not be accepted by the court if he presented them in a 'Lombrosian' fashion. To put it another way, since criminal anthropology was generally held in disrepute by judges and members of the jury, Carrara adopted the strategy of dissimulating his scientific *modus operandi* and the way in which he reached his forensic conclusions. At this point one question arises: why did Carrara include anthropometric measurements in his reports in the first place? As his *Handbook of Forensic Medicine* demonstrates, Carrara fully believed in the diagnostic value of cranial and skeletal malformations. For this case, he had relied almost exclusively on the results of the physical examination and sensitivity tests to conclude that Monticone was morally insane. The latter's criminal record or the fact that he was violent with his wife did not seem to justify per se Carrara's diagnosis. It was the extreme resemblance between Monticone and the 'born criminal' (marks of degeneration, insensitivity to pain, etc.) that led Carrara to this conclusion, although he did not openly admit it in the report. This silence can be interpreted as an attempt to conceal his scientific ideas in a more or less hostile context, as they would probably be met with resistance from the jury members. Affirming his belief in Lombroso's doctrine would thus be counterproductive, and in addition, Carrara must also have been aware that for the judge and the jurors any form of biological determinism, which entails the denial of free will, would be seen as a direct challenge to their authority. Carrara had little choice but to translate and adapt his conclusions into a language that would resonate well with the various courtroom actors, making it clear that his medical opinion was subordinated to that of the jury.

The court rejected Carrara and Agosti's conclusions, holding that their arguments were not based on concrete evidence. None of Monticone's family members had suffered from nervous or mental disease and none of the witnesses interviewed during the trial had maintained that he was unsound of mind. Commenting on the psychiatric report, the judge wrote:

> The physical signs of degeneration that professors Carrara and Agosti claim to have found on the subject of the expertise are not worth attention, since somatic anomalies are found in every part of the body and in every kind of people. Many of the physiognomic features that are considered as degenerative in nature are merely unesthetic traits that make a physiognomy ugly, unpleasant and suspicious. These features are caused by many different factors that are not easy to identify.[45]

The judge quoted almost verbatim a passage from *Forensic Psychiatry*, the guide for the expert witness that Eugenio Tanzi had written in 1911. As we have seen in the previous section, Tanzi denied the existence of any close link between criminal behaviour and physical characteristics and claimed that the born criminal, whom he labelled 'constitutionally immoral' (*immorale costituzionale*), was morally defective but without any intellectual defect. This assumption was fully supported by the president of the court, who went on to uphold the verdict by relying on Tanzi's scientific authority:

> Apart from the circumstance that all the witnesses heard today excluded in the most absolute way that in [the village of] Caramagna Monticone was considered an abnormal individual, it is clear that alterations of the personality in the ethical sphere can only be

labelled as moral insanity. Moral aberrations, when they do not have a pathological origin, cannot be a reason for diminished criminal responsibility ... Therefore, those who commit crimes because of a constitutional moral defect must be punished in the same way as normal individuals. Mental capacity, a key requirement for holding a person accountable, refers to intellectual ability, not to moral awareness. Therefore, when the ability to understand the consequences of one's acts is intact, it is clear that the requirements to hold the person accountable are fulfilled as much in constitutionally immoral as in normal individuals. Moreover, the treatment of congenital, constitutionally immoral individuals has always been the most debated issue between the criminalists of the classical school and those of the positive school. But given the principles of current criminal legislation ... constitutional immorality is not ground for any sentence reduction and even less for acquittal.[46]

This passage seems to confirm Mary Gibson's claim that Italian judges remained mostly faithful to the classical school of criminal law, which argued against Lombroso's deterministic explanations of crime and understood criminal behaviour as a product of free will.[47] Furthermore, Monticone's verdict shows that in Turin, the cradle and stronghold of the Lombrosian school, judges dismissed Lombroso's theory of the born criminal in favour of Tanzi's theory of constitutional immorality. Monticone was sentenced to life imprisonment. According to the press, he received the news with 'complete indifference'.[48]

Conclusion

What does the analysis conducted so far tell us about the controversial legacy of Cesare Lombroso? First of all, that his school did not die with him. Criminal anthropologists like Mario Carrara continued to defend the validity of his theories and to put his teachings into practice for many more years. Secondly, this research reveals that the establishment of the Fascist dictatorship in the 1920s did not affect the reception of criminal anthropology in the courtroom and that the Fascist judiciary was not necessarily benevolent towards Lombrosian medical witnesses. This finding partially challenges the claim that criminal anthropology provided the Fascist regime with theoretical and practical tools to repress deviance. While it is true that Carrara was called to testify by the Court of Assize of Turin fairly frequently despite his reputation for being anti-Fascist, which might be interpreted as evidence of the judiciary's attraction towards Lombroso's theories, one should bear in mind that in the eyes of the judge (and those of the Code of Criminal Procedure) Carrara's scientific authority derived from his being a professor of Forensic Medicine at the local university and a specialist in forensic psychiatry, rather than a lecturer in Criminal Anthropology.

Thirdly, the case of Monticone seems to suggest that, at least by the 1930s, but probably much earlier, the Lombrosian school of criminal anthropology had entered a period of decline and scientific marginalisation. While Carrara, Lombroso's scientific heir and one of the most influential criminal anthropologists of his time, could reaffirm in his publications the existence of the 'born criminal' and urge his colleagues to perform anthropometric measurements and sensitivity tests on the defendant to reach a diagnosis, he was aware that in the courtroom the criminological theories of his master were held in disrepute. The fact that the judge dismissed the psychiatric evaluation due to his recognition of Lombrosianism in the listing of Monticone's physical abnormalities, despite Carrara's attempt to hide his faith in biological determinism, shows that Carrara had no choice but to conceal his Lombrosian beliefs if he hoped his forensic conclusions might be taken into account by the court. Although Monticone exhibited all the features of the 'born criminal', Carrara did not explicitly state so in his report, to sound more convincing to the jury. Carrara remained an esteemed medical expert both in the Liberal age and under the Fascist dictatorship, although this research has demonstrated that, at least in Turin, it was Emil Kraepelin's psychiatry as advocated by Eugenio Tanzi and not Lombrosian criminal anthropology that was the dominant scientific paradigm in the courtroom.

What can we conclude from reading this case study through the prism of the notion of 'forensic culture'? First of all, that it can take many years for a forensic culture to change. This is apparent if we compare Lombroso's 1905 guide for the expert witness with Carrara's 1940 *Handbook of Forensic Medicine*. Following his master's theories, Carrara continued to stress the importance of physical examination to reach a clinical diagnosis, claiming the existence of a link between body and behaviour. However, the way in which Lombrosian forensic culture was embedded in textbooks and guides for the expert witness differed a great deal from how it came to the fore in other locations. Indeed, the case of Monticone is paradigmatic in showing that the theory of a forensic culture can stand in contrast with its practice. While Lombrosian criminal anthropologists defended the concept of the born criminal in their scientific publications, they were more reluctant to do so in the courtroom. Legal procedures, the marginal influence of Lombroso's theories on Italian legal culture, and the adherence of the majority of judges and jurists to the classical tradition of criminal law did not prevent Lombrosian forensic experts from defending the validity of Lombroso's theories in their publications or using them in their psychiatric assessment reports, but they did limit the ways in which the latter could be voiced. As we have seen, Carrara was reluctant to employ a 'Lombrosian' language in his psychiatric evaluations and to make explicit use of anthropometric measurements to support his conclusions. This, I believe, testifies to the scientific disrepute into which Lombrosian criminal anthropology had fallen in the interwar period.

Notes

1 Renzo Villa, 'Lombroso and his School: From Anthropology to Medicine and Law', in P. Knepper and P.J. Ystehede (eds), *The Cesare Lombroso Handbook* (Abingdon: Routledge, 2013), pp. 8–29; Silvano Montaldo, *Donne delinquenti: Il genere e la nascita della criminologia* (Rome: Carocci, 2019); Paul Garfinkel, *Criminal Law in Liberal and Fascist Italy* (New York: Cambridge University Press, 2016); Pierpaolo Martucci, 'Un'eredità senza eredi: L'Antropologia criminale in Italia dopo la morte di Lombroso', in S. Montaldo and P. Tappero (eds), *Cesare Lombroso cento anni dopo* (Torino: Utet, 2009), pp. 291–300.

2 Mary Gibson, *Born to Crime: Cesare Lombroso and the Origins of Biological Criminology* (Westport: Praeger, 2002); Liliosa Azara and Luca Tedesco (eds), *La donna delinquente e la prostituta: L'eredità di Lombroso nella cultura e nelle società italiane* (Rome: Viella, 2019); Sandro Bellassai, *La legge del desiderio: Il progetto Merlin e l'Italia degli anni Cinquanta* (Rome: Carocci, 2006); Jonathan Dunnage,

'The Legacy of Cesare Lombroso and Criminal Anthropology in the Post-war Italian Police: a Study of the Culture, Narrative and Memory of a Post-Fascist Institution', *Journal of Modern Italian Studies* 22:3 (2017), pp. 365–384. doi: 10.1080/1354571X.2017.1321934; Emilia Musumeci, 'Against the Rising Tide of Crime: Cesare Lombroso and Control of the "Dangerous Classes" in Italy, 1861–1940, *Crime, History & Society* 22:2 (2018), pp. 83–106. doi: 10.4000/chs.2313.
3 Gibson, *Born to Crime*.
4 Musumeci, 'Against the Rising Tide of Crime'; Renzo Villa, *Il deviante e i suoi segni. Lombroso e la nascita dell'antropologia criminale* (Milan: Franco Angeli, 1985); Delia Frigessi, *Cesare Lombroso* (Turin: Einaudi, 2003).
5 *Codice penale e di procedura italiana con relazioni a S. M. il Re* (Rome: Istituto Poligrafico dello Stato, 1931) art. 314, p. 305.
6 Morris Ploscowe, 'The Expert Witness in Criminal Cases in France, Germany and Italy', *Law and Contemporary Problems* 2:4 (1935), p. 505.
7 *Ibid.*
8 *Codice penale e di procedura italiana*, art. 314, p. 305.
9 Adelmo Borrettini, *La perizia nel processo penale italiano* (Padova: Cedam, 1940), p. 139.
10 Mario Carrara, 'L'anthropologie criminelle et la procédure pénale', *Revue de Droit pénale et de Criminologie et Archives Internationales de Médicine légale* 13:11 (1933), pp. 921–935.
11 Giuseppe Falco, 'Salvatore Ottolenghi', *Bollettino della Scuola superiore di Polizia e dei servizi tecnici annessi*, 22–23 (1932–1933), pp. 3–16.
12 Francesco Rotondo, 'Un dibattito per l'egemonia: La perizia medico-legale nel processo penale italiano di fine Ottocento', *Rechtsgeschichte* 12 (2008), pp. 139–173.
13 Ploscowe, 'The Expert Witness'.
14 Morris Ploscowe, 'Jury Reform in Italy', *Journal of Criminal Law and Criminology* 25:4 (1934), p. 577.
15 Cesare Lombroso, *La perizia psichiatrico-legale, coi metodi per eseguirla e la casuistica penale classificata antropologicamente* (Turin: Bocca, 1905), p. 487.
16 *Ibid.*, p. 580.
17 Claudia Passarella, 'From Scandalous Verdicts to "Suicidal Sentences": The Reform of the Court of Assize under the Fascist Regime', *Studia Iuridica* 80 (2019), pp. 251–264, here p. 254.
18 Passage quoted from Mary Gibson, 'Forensic Psychiatry and the Birth of the Criminal Insane Asylum in Modern Italy', *International*

Journal of Law and Psychiatry 37:1 (2014), pp. 117–126, here p. 119. doi: https://doi.org/10.1016/j.ijlp.2013.09.011

19 Cesare Lombroso, *The Criminal Man* (Durham: Duke University Press, 2006), p. 351.
20 Gina Lombroso, *Criminal Man According to the Classification of Cesare Lombroso* (New York: Putnam, 1911), p. 265.
21 Gaetano Angiolella, *Manuale di antropologia criminale ad uso dei medici e degli studenti di giurisprudenza* (Milan: Vallardi, 1906); Giuseppe Antonini, *I principi fondamentali della Antropologia criminale: Guida per i giudizi medico-forensi nelle questioni di imputabilità* (Milan, Hoepli: 1906); Attilio Ascarelli, *Compendio di Medicina legale. Guida alle perizie medico-forensi, ad uso dei medici esercenti* (Rome: G. Bertero, 1912).
22 Mario Carrara, *Manuale di Medicina Legale* (Turin: Utet, 1937–1940) vol. 2:2, p. 167.
23 Cesare Lombroso, 'Il problema del genio e del delitto risolto dall'on. prof. Tanzi', *Archivio di Antropologia criminale* 25 (1904), pp. 428–429.
24 Eugenio Tanzi, *Psichiatria Forense* (Milan: Vallardi, 1911), p. 505.
25 Eugenio Tanzi, *Trattato delle malattie mentali*, 3rd ed. (Milan: Società Editrice Libraria: 1923), vol. 2:1, p. 736.
26 Eugenio Tanzi, *A Textbook of Mental Diseases* (London: Rebman, 1909), p. 59.
27 Richard Wetzell, *Inventing the Criminal. A History of German Criminology, 1880–1945* (Chapel Hill: The University of North Carolina Press, 2000), p. 297.
28 Eugenio Tanzi and Ernesto Lugaro, 'Immoralità Costituzionale', in *Enciclopedia Italiana* (Rome: Istituto Giovanni Treccani, 1933), www.treccani.it/enciclopedia/immoralita-costituzionale_%28Enciclopedia-Italiana%29/
29 Tanzi, *A Textbook of Mental Diseases*, p. 687.
30 Archivio di Stato di Torino (ASTO), Corte d'Assise di Torino (CATO), Sentenze penali 1932–1933, vol. 22, 'Martellozzo Giuseppe', Memoria difensiva al giudice istruttore, p. 7.
31 Gibson, 'Forensic Psychiatry', p. 125.
32 Giuseppe Antonini, 'La moderna biologia e il Progetto di Codice Penale Italiano', *La Scuola Positiva* 32:1–3 (1923), pp. 163–170.
33 *Ibid.*; Augusto Tamburini, Giulio Cesare Ferrari and Giuseppe Antonini, *L'assistenza degli alienati in Italia e nelle varie nazioni* (Turin: Utet, 1918).
34 Alessia Anna Bortolomai, 'Il Regio Manicomio di Collegno: la rivolta dei "pazzi criminali" nel 1912', *Studi Piemontesi* 49:1 (2020), pp. 135–147.

35 Mimmo Franzinelli, *L'amnistia Togliatti: 1946. Colpo di spugna sui crimini fascisti* (Milan: Mondadori, 2006) p. 11.
36 Franco Orlandi, 'In the Name of Lombroso: Mario Carrara and the Refusal of the 1931 Fascist Loyalty Oath', *Annali di Storia delle università italiane* 26:1 (2022), pp. 205–225. Doi: https://doi.org/10.17396/104330.
37 Francesco Agosti, 'La delinquenza nei giovani. Studi e ricerche fatte su 40 ricoverati dell'Istituto di educazione e correzione dei minorenni discoli del Piemonte', *Archivio di Antropologia criminale* 29 (1908), pp. 1–23.
38 ASTO, CATO, Sentenze penali 1930–1931, vol. 24, 'Francesco Monticone', Perizia psichiatrica, pp. 14–16.
39 *Ibid.*, p. 13.
40 *Ibid.*, p. 31.
41 Lombroso, *The Criminal Man*, p. 11.
42 Carrara, *Manuale di Medicina Legale*, p. 324.
43 *Ibid.*, p. 323.
44 See, for example, Mario Carrara, 'Tipo completo di pazzia morale a base epilettica', *Archivio di Antropologia criminale* 16 (1895), pp. 247–251.
45 ASTO, CATO, 1930–1931, vol. 24., 'Francesco Monticone', Sentenza.
46 *Ibid.*
47 Gibson, 'Forensic Psychiatry'.
48 *La Stampa* (16 December 1931) p. 4.

7

Expert evidence and uncertainty in English infanticide trials, c. 1725–1945

Rachel Dixon and Tony Ward

Introduction

Not only forensic scientists but any scientist whose expertise forms the basis for public decision-making must confront the problem of how to convey uncertainty about their conclusions in a way that will maintain public trust.[1] From the early days of forensic medicine this problem has confronted medical witnesses in criminal trials. Landsman has argued that the courts 'pressed medical witnesses for ever more certain opinions that might help satisfy the increasing demanding burdens of proof',[2] and that expert witnesses, in infanticide trials among others, displayed 'rectitude' in resisting this process. Such 'rectitude' contrasts with the examples of overstated certainty that have been highlighted by historians and sociologists of science and legal medicine.[3] According to Adam, mid-twentieth-century English judges reinforced experts' reluctance to explain areas of doubt in their disciplines, with their demands for 'facts, not probabilities'.[4]

While it is true that medical witnesses in infanticide trials faced some pressure to give unequivocal evidence, it is also apparent that the uncertainty they created was not entirely unwelcome. Indeed, one could argue that lawyers, judges, medical men and juries all worked together to produce a situation in which fewer than 10 per cent of charges of murdering newborn babies (in Katherine Watson's study) resulted in conviction between 1700 and 1914.[5] Infanticide cases were different from many other instances of scientific uncertainty in two crucial respects. Firstly, the uncertainty was not the result of disagreement between different experts testifying in the same cases – almost invariably, there was either a single expert or two or more experts were in broad agreement. Secondly, frustrating the conviction of the guilty was a result that was widely accepted, and in particular did not appear to trouble many judges.[6]

In discussing expert evidence in English and Welsh criminal justice it is important to keep in mind the procedural context in which it was given. Serious criminal cases were (and are) tried by juries, although their interpretation of the evidence could be guided to a considerable extent by the judge. From the mid-eighteenth century these trials were increasingly dominated by lawyers.[7] There was no appeal in criminal cases before 1907, although there was a procedure by which disputed points of law could be 'reserved' to a meeting of all twelve common-law judges, or after 1848 to the Court for Crown Cases Reserved.[8] In capital cases, the sentence would be reviewed by officials of the Home Office to decide whether the Royal prerogative of mercy should be exercised to commute the sentence. In practice it was, by the second half of the nineteenth century, very unlikely that a woman would be executed for infanticide; the last execution of a woman for killing her infant child occurred in 1849.[9]

A common theme in the historiography of expert evidence is that lawyers expected science to deliver objective, certain truths, and that when the science turned out to be uncertain and disputable, as it often did, expert witnesses were portrayed as falling short of true scientific standards.[10] The word 'objectivity' was not much used in nineteenth-century medico-legal literature but it sums up a quality that medical men were often criticised for lacking, as when Mary Anne Baines, a writer on infant welfare, observed in 1866 that the duty of medical men in infanticide cases is 'not to assist in the escape of a criminal, but to further the ends of justice by a conscientious interpretation of the facts submitted to them'.[11] The simplest everyday meaning of 'objective' is 'that an objective judgment is free from prejudice and bias',[12] and is therefore trustworthy.[13] Courts have tended to assume that experts who were objective in this sense would agree in their findings, and that disputes between experts were therefore indications of partisanship on the part of one or both protagonists.[14] By 'certain' evidence we do not mean evidence that purports to be infallible, but rather evidence that is couched in such terms that if fully accepted by the jury it would be sufficient to prove a legally material fact 'beyond reasonable doubt'. A perceived lack of objectivity on the expert's part will undermine certainty because it gives the jury a reason to withhold full acceptance of the expert's testimony. A lack of certainty on the expert's part does not, however, undermine their claim to objectivity: on the contrary, it could be taken as a sign of fair-mindedness, which is one meaning of objectivity.[15] This was particularly the case in nineteenth- and twentieth-century trials where only the prosecution called expert evidence, and that evidence to some extent assisted the defence, as in some cases where the defendant's sanity was in doubt,[16] and many trials for the murder of newborn children.

In these cases, the most important form of uncertainty was over whether the infant who had died was born alive. Between 1624 and 1803 the law avoided the difficulty of proving this point by a statutory presumption that the death of a bastard child whose birth the mother had concealed was murder. In 1803 this presumption was abolished by Lord Ellenborough's Act and the meaning of a child's being 'born alive', and how it could be proved, became crucial issues. In 1922 the Infanticide Act avoided the difficulty of obtaining murder convictions in cases of neonaticide by introducing the lesser offence of infanticide to cover those mothers who killed their newly born child in a 'disturbed' mental state.[17] The uncertainty over live birth in trials for infant murder between 1803 and 1922 is discussed at length both in Katherine Watson's study of eighteenth- and nineteenth-century forensic medicine[18] and in Rachel Dixon's monograph, which argues not only that medical uncertainty was an important factor in securing acquittals, but that it was positively valued by the courts.[19] In this chapter we add two new points to this argument. Firstly, we show that the requirement that a child be 'wholly born alive' became firmly established in legal precedent *in response* to medical testimony about the difficulty of demonstrating this very point, which strongly suggests that uncertainty on this point was welcome, or at least not so unwelcome as to lead to a less defendant-friendly interpretation of the law. Secondly, we show that even after the Infanticide Act of 1922 created a simpler way to avoid a capital conviction – by pleading guilty to the lesser offence of infanticide – uncertainty about live birth and the mother's mental state continued to figure both in trials and in the coroner's inquest, a form of judicial inquiry (with a jury) into sudden deaths, which in the period under discussion had the power to commit people suspected of homicide to trial.[20] It was not, therefore, simply abhorrence at passing a death sentence (unlikely as it was to be carried out) on an infanticidal mother that led lawyers and juries to make use of the uncertainty over live birth to avoid finding that an infant had been unlawfully killed.

The remainder of this chapter falls into three sections. The first deals with medical and legal aspects of proving that a baby was born alive in the eighteenth and early nineteenth centuries. Passing swiftly over the later nineteenth century, which has been amply discussed elsewhere, we then move on to consider the developments leading up to the passing of the Infanticide Act 1922, where the relevant medical uncertainties concerned not live birth but the mother's mental state. We then discuss the continuing uncertainty over live birth in the aftermath of the 1922 Act. Together these discussions of two different periods refine and reinforce Dixon's earlier argument about the courts' receptivity to medical uncertainty, within a legal culture that gave scope to juries to take account of a range of social and moral concerns beyond those formally recognised in law.[21] A brief concluding section relates this point to contemporary debates over forensic science.

Being born alive, c. 1720–1840

Forensic medicine in England was slow to evolve, lagging 'centuries behind the rise of this science on the continent',[22] with medical witnesses making only occasional appearances in court from the eighteenth century.[23] At the trials where expert witnesses did present medical findings, Landsman has argued that experts faced a gradually increasing 'demand ... for greater certainty and detail in opinions'.[24] By the early nineteenth century, 'it became routine for the court and counsel to press medical witnesses on the question of certainty and listen carefully to the precise wording of their answers'.[25] Where the expert testified for the prosecution this pressure might well, as in the example Landsman cites from an infanticide trial in 1802, come from defence counsel anxious to establish a sufficient degree of *un*certainty to justify an acquittal.[26]

By resisting the temptation to make stronger statements than they considered justified, experts established their impartiality and 'rectitude' and, by raising an element of doubt over the defendant's culpability, created space for a sympathetic jury to deliver a 'not guilty' verdict in many child murder cases.

During the eighteenth century, a forensic culture developed in England, and the desire to use the body as a source of evidence in murder cases increased, as it was generally believed that the body could provide 'medical knowledge in a legal context' to determine cause of death.[27] This in turn created a correlative demand for increasing knowledge of pathology and developing skills of anatomical dissection, as surgeons became eager to showcase their knowledge and skills, by demonstrating and sharing them in the presence of public gatherings.[28] Such high-profile public demonstrations of scientific techniques with the potential for forensic application arguably triggered an increasing demand for a public performance in the courtroom, with judges testing the strength of the science and pressing medical witnesses for definitive answers. Landsman has argued that 'the growing demand for certainty is documented in the changing behaviour of the judges towards medical witnesses, the increasing use of experimental and symptoms-based evidence, and the special treatment afforded particularly doubtful cases', where the certainty potentially afforded by scientific evidence took on particular importance.[29] In response to this demand, and the increasing pressure medical men faced from the court to provide definitive answers to anatomical questions in infanticide cases, scientific experimentation became widely used, and the desire for autopsy during trials and coroners' inquests became increasingly evident.

Clayton has noted the rising number of requests made by coroners for surgeons to perform autopsies on the infant's body, the aim being to determine 'whether the child had lived or was stillborn; whether it was full term; whether the child had any injuries and, if so, whether they could have been caused during the birth or by the mother after the birth'.[30] Medical men were expected to provide definitive answers relating to live birth and cause of death, and the lung test aimed to establish that a child had inspired (taken a breath) and had therefore been born alive. The lungs were removed from the cadaver and placed into water: if the lungs floated to the surface, it was an indication that the child had breathed, whereas if the lungs sank, it could be a sign that the child had not taken a breath and was therefore stillborn.[31] For example, at the trial of Sarah Perry in 1817 at the Old Bailey, for the wilful murder of her newly born female infant, the surgeon, Edward Leese testified that:

> there was a redness about its neck and head as if arising from strangulation – supposing the child to have been alive, it was quite sufficient to strangle it – it could not breathe. The child appeared to me to be perfect, and I have no doubt but that it was born alive.[32]

Leese was cross-examined by the defence barrister Thomas Andrews, 'a man of "athletic proportions" and a "John Bull-ish" expression, possessed [of] a "fine strong sonorous voice" and "great fluency and readiness of expression"'.[33] As usual, we have no record of what Andrews said; but it seems to have been effective, as Leese now conceded that 'it is difficult to tell whether a child is born alive or not – I will not swear it' and that 'if the child had fallen on the stones at its birth, it would have caused its death'.[34] In spite of these concessions, however, Sarah was convicted and hanged.

Leese's readiness to endanger a woman's life by expressing greater certainty than he could justify recalls the anatomist and obstetrician William Hunter's complaint, in his famous posthumous paper of 1783, that 'some of us [medical men] are a little disposed to grasp at authority in a public examination, when it should have been guarded with doubt'.[35] In Hunter's paper scientific doubts (such as whether the putrefaction might cause the lungs to float although the infant had never breathed)[36] are closely interwoven with the humanitarian sentiments highlighted in Mark Jackson's analysis of changing attitudes to infanticide.[37] To the extent that medical witnesses followed Hunter's lead, it is reasonable to suppose that they were intentionally reducing the likelihood of a capital conviction for women.

The use of the lung test became increasingly controversial, with courts questioning its reliability and accuracy. Its unreliability was partly a product of the legal requirement that the child must have lived entirely outside the mother's body: something the lung test could not determine, as the child might inhale while only partly out of the womb.[38] This was the most important form of medical uncertainty accounting for the high acquittal rate on charges of newborn child murder, as Watson's recent study confirms.[39] The definition of 'live birth' does not appear to have been authoritatively settled before 1830,[40] and crystallised in a series of judicial rulings in response to the uncertainty of medical evidence. The earliest reported case in this series was that of Maria (or Ann) Poulton, where three medical witnesses agreed that it could not be determined by the lung test whether an infant had been fully born alive.[41] Poulton, a cook in a London tavern, was represented by a prominent barrister, Thomas Clarkson, while the prosecution had no counsel; the parish[42] where the baby died had withdrawn funding on the ground that it would be 'acting with great illiberality and injustice to employ Counsel against a defenceless woman, charged with an awful crime'.[43] Mr Justice Littledale summed up in a way that steered the jury strongly towards acquittal:

> With respect to the birth, the being born *must mean that the whole body is brought into the world*; and it is not sufficient that the child respires in the progress of the birth. Whether the child was born alive or not depends mainly upon the evidence of the medical men. None of them say that the child was born alive; they only say that it had breathed: and if there is all this uncertainty among these medical men, perhaps you would think it too much for you to say that you are satisfied that the child was born alive.[44]

This was certainly not a new idea in 1832. For example, in the trial of Hannah Connolly in 1806, the judge put it to the medical witness that 'The lungs might be inflated before it was born. It might have died in the act of delivery, therefore you cannot at all say whether the child was born alive or no', and the witness agreed.[45] Nevertheless, the phrase we have italicised in Littledale's direction, for which he cited no authority, was considered sufficiently novel and important to warrant publication in Carrington and Payne's law reports, which provided a record of judicial rulings which could be cited as precedents in future cases, as *Poulton* was in two further cases which were also included in the same reports.[46]

In one of those cases, in 1837, Mr Justice Parke did express some doubt as to whether proof of complete birth should be required where the medical evidence positively indicated that the child had been strangled while partially born; but he found that the way the indictment against Ann Crutchley was drafted made her acquittal of murder inevitable.[47] In the case of *R v Elizabeth Sellis*, where the defendant confessed that she had cut off her baby's head after it was fully born, the medical witness was able to say 'decidedly that the child had breathed' but he also underlined that it was possible for a child to die after breathing but 'before the entire body was born' as a result of 'contraction of the muscles and the uterus'.[48] Mr Justice Coltman told the jury they must be satisfied that the child both was 'wholly born into the world in a living state'[49] and was still alive when decapitated; the jury 'almost immediately found the prisoner Not Guilty of murder, but Guilty of concealing the birth'.[50]

The limit of judicial generosity was reached in *R v Milborough Trilloe*,[51] where Mr Justice Erskine ruled that a baby was born alive when it was fully outside the mother's body and had, according to the surgeon, an 'independent circulation', but the umbilical cord had not been cut.[52] He reserved the point for the consideration of all the judges, and they upheld his ruling. The decisions of meetings of the judges were treated as binding precedents, laying down legal rules that trial judges were obliged to follow.[53]

What these cases show is that the inability of medical evidence to establish live birth in many cases of neonaticide was not the result of the experts trying and failing to meet an already firmly established legal test; it was, rather, the judges who firmly defined the criterion of live birth in such a way as to ensure that the limits of medical knowledge would usually result in acquittals. Any ruling on a point of common law is likely to reflect the sometimes-conflicting pressures of how the judge 'want[s] to come out' and the constraints of precedent.[54] The *Crutchley* case in 1837[55] shows that at that point it would have been possible to rule that stabbing or strangling a baby who was not yet fully born was murder. But this would only have placed the judges more often in the invidious position of sentencing to death women for whom there was often considerable public sympathy, before working behind the scenes to ensure the sentence would not be carried out.[56]

As Watson observes, 'by the 1840s trials for newborn child murder followed a familiar script in which everyone from the judge to the jury knew their role'.[57] In leaving the court uncertain whether the child had been fully born alive, the medical witnesses were playing their role, not failing in it. As Watson further observes, counsel for the defence were often commended by the judges for their 'powerful pleading', thereby enhancing their professional reputations.[58] The judges, on the other hand, could justify acquittal for murder (usually coupled with conviction of the lesser offence of concealment of birth) on the basis of the strict application of a legal rule. This was consistent with what Atiyah and Summers have characterised as a deeply engrained characteristic of the English judiciary, their 'anxiety lest the effect of legal prohibitions should be weakened by equitable modifications designed to show mercy or compassion (or even justice) to those who committed prohibited acts in situations of stress or ignorance or lack of cognitive understanding'.[59] The jury, meanwhile, could introduce just such an equitable modification without departing from the judge's instructions.

The uncertainty of expert knowledge was harnessed in a way that reflected the structure of the common-law trial and parallels the development of the insanity defence which also crystallised in the 1840s.[60] It was for judges, not medical men, to define through case law the legal meaning of birth and insanity, and it was for juries to determine whether the legal criteria were met in a particular case. In the cases of both insanity and live birth, the judges laid down definitions which, in many cases, made it very difficult for medical witnesses to say with certainty whether the criteria were met, and the oral evidence and cross-examination of the witness enabled these uncertainties to be probed in open court. The construction of medical uncertainty gave expert witnesses an important role while ensuring their epistemic subordination to the judge and jury, and it allowed a merciful exercise of discretion by juries to be combined with strictly delimited rules of criminal law.[61]

From murder to infanticide, 1840–1922

The judges' reluctance to recognise formally that the typical case of infanticide – where a poor, unmarried mother gave birth in secret and killed the child shortly afterwards – should not constitute murder which attracted an automatic death sentence, was reflected in judicial and legislative resistance to attempts to reform the law, despite mounting criticism of the low conviction rate after 1860.[62] Lord Redesdale, an important figure in the upper house of Parliament,[63] put the point dramatically when he declared that it would be 'far better that all the murderesses in the country should be acquitted' than to have Parliament declare 'that the wilful or the malicious killing of a child was not murder'.[64]

As Hilary Marland has observed, the medical profession played an ambiguous role in debates about infanticide at this time.[65] Medical coroners like Thomas Wakley and Edwin Lankester, and medical writers like William Burke Ryan, played a prominent role in raising alarm about the numbers of infants who were murdered, but medical men were also instrumental in securing lenient verdicts, whether on the basis of insanity (the focus of Marland's work), of the mother's mental state reducing the offence from murder to manslaughter, or of uncertainty over the question of live birth. These two roles were not entirely contradictory, because a lenient verdict was at least a conviction, or in the case of the verdict of 'not guilty by reason of insanity' before 1883 (when the form of words changed to 'guilty but insane') a technical acquittal followed by indefinite detention in a secure asylum.

The cultural context of the sympathy extended to many infanticidal mothers has been explored by scholars including Anne Higginbotham, Christine Krueger and Josephine McDonough.[66] As Krueger argues, works of fiction afford insights into these attitudes because they articulate views that were criticised by writers like Ryan, but were not often explicitly defended. Although the heroine of Frances Trollope's 1843 novel *Jessie Phillips: A Tale of the Present Day* was innocent of infanticide, the novel effectively portrays the harshness of the 1834 Poor Law towards unmarried mothers and their children and the callousness of Jessie's seducer. In George Eliot's *Adam Bede*, the mother (Hetty Sorrel) is guilty and the seducer (Arthur Donnithorne) is weak rather than wicked, but in Adam Bede's words, 'if there's been any crime, it is at his door'.[67] This view of the 'seducer's' guilt and the unfairness of the mother's position is often alluded to in debates of the 1860s and, as we have shown elsewhere, remained a theme in infanticide trials well into the twentieth century.[68]

The leniency demonstrated towards infanticidal women by the courts was reflected in other European countries. In France for example, the 1791 Penal Code, Article 300, defined infanticide as 'premeditated murder of the new-born', and Article 302 'introduced the death penalty'.[69] The penal code under Article 319, during the nineteenth century allowed for non-premeditated murder, punishable either with fines or prison sentence.[70] Similarly with German law, French judges made allowances for mitigating circumstances for infanticidal women during the nineteenth century, but any leniency demonstrated towards the woman did not extend to any accomplices.[71] The incidence of infanticide remained high amongst unmarried women in rural areas of France, and Donovan has observed that courts showed leniency to many of these women, a fact that is reflected in the high number of acquittals during the later years of the nineteenth century and into the twentieth century.[72]

In England, while the defence of insanity had a strict and narrow legal definition, it was often stretched in practice and mothers diagnosed with puerperal insanity, as well as some fathers who killed young children, could benefit from this flexibility.[73] The *mens rea* of murder, on the other hand, was broad and vague, and juries in effect had a discretion whether to convict of murder or manslaughter when the killer's intention was unclear. Even in cases where medical men felt able to express a high degree of certainty about the cause of death, they could raise doubts about the mother's mental state.

A typical example is the testimony of the pathologist Ludwig Freyberger at the trial of Louisa Lunn, at the Old Bailey in 1904, for the wilful murder of her newborn female infant.[74] He testified that:

> the cause of death was suffocation by strangulation by some soft material being tightly wound round the neck; my reasons for that opinion are the width to the encircling mark, which was from 1 in. to 1½ in., and the absence of haemorrhages in the skin – I formed the opinion that the child had been completely born, and I do not think there can be any doubt about it; my reasons are the absence of any foreign substance in the air passages, the complete inflation of the lungs, and the presence of air in the stomach, which shows that breathing had been going on for some time.[75]

Having clearly provided the jury with possible grounds for a conviction, he stated on cross-examination that:

> a woman having her first child may, in a way, be affected mentally; there would be pain during the birth, which would be accentuated by depression – child birth is very often followed by a period of partial or total unconsciousness – a woman might not know what was going on around her, or what she was doing herself.[76]

The jury's verdict that Louisa Lunn was not guilty of murder, but guilty of manslaughter, indicates their acceptance both of Freyberger's expressed certainty over the cause of death, and the doubt he acknowledged about her *mens rea*, the mental element of criminal liability. She was 'discharged on her own recognisances as she was willing to go into a home for two years'.[77]

The difficulty with this kind of evidence was not that it led to 'battles of the experts' – which hardly occurred in infanticide cases – or that it threatened the authority of the court. Rather, the problem was that by leaving it to the court to decide whether to give the benefit of whatever doubt the expert left open, it left scope for verdicts that appeared unpredictable and harsh. This problem came to a head with the trial of Edith Roberts in 1921.[78] The expert evidence in this case was similar to that in Louisa Lunn's case: the baby had been born alive and had been suffocated, but 'it was perfectly possible the girl was unconscious through the pain she suffered and that she might not realise what she was doing'. In these circumstances it would have been 'perfectly possible' to return a manslaughter verdict but Mr Justice Avory – a judge with a formidable reputation for coldness and severity[79] – told the jury 'to steel their hearts against being led away by sympathy for a woman'.[80] This admonition must have been effective as the all-male jury – defence counsel having challenged all of the newly eligible women jurors who were summonsed – convicted her of murder in fifteen minutes, albeit with a strong recommendation to mercy. The distressing scenes as Avory passed a sentence of death which he knew would never be carried out led to a campaign of which the ultimate result was the passage of the Infanticide Act 1922. The Act provided that where a woman killed her 'newly-born child' in circumstances that would otherwise amount to murder, but she had not recovered from the effects of giving birth and 'the balance of her mind was disturbed' as a result, she would be guilty not of murder but of the newly created offence of infanticide.

Uncertainty remains, 1922–1945

It might be thought that the 1922 Act would have removed the significance of medical uncertainty in infanticide cases. It was no longer necessary to raise the degree of doubt about the intentional nature of a mother's actions that would persuade a jury to convict of manslaughter rather than murder. The distinction between these offences was not clearly or consistently defined in the case law of the period, and we rarely have any detailed record of how the judge explained it to the jury, but by speculating that the defendant might have suffered some kind of partial unconsciousness, doctors probably did enough in the eyes of most judges to displace the legal presumption that she intended the natural and probable consequence of her actions.[81] Under the 1922 Act, all that was necessary was evidence that the mother's pain and distress would have disturbed 'the balance of her mind', a phrase with no strictly defined meaning[82] but one which judges and jurors appear to have had no difficulty in applying to typical cases of neonaticide. A conviction for infanticide, however, required proof of a 'wilful act or omission', which implied some degree of consciousness and intentionality on the mother's part. Even when there was no risk of a death sentence, doubts about whether the mother's deliberate act had caused the death of a living child remained significant, not only at the trial but at the inquest held to establish the cause of the child's death. A verdict of wilful murder or infanticide at the inquest would result in the mother being sent to trial.

Uncertainty over live birth was a decisive factor in the trial of Caroline Bingham of Brigg, Lincolnshire, in 1931. She was charged with infanticide rather than murder, as the prosecution accepted that 'the balance of her mind was disturbed'. At the Lincoln Assizes, Dr Lambert of Lincoln described how a towel had been tied around the child's neck, covering his head: 'It had evidently been tied by a person who had shown great determination, a post-mortem examination showed that the child had breathed and had had a separate existence, he could only come to the conclusion that death had been caused by strangulation.'[83] Had the charge been murder, this reference to 'great determination' would have been damning. On cross-examination, Dr Lambert denied that the child might have breathed and yet not have had a separate existence. Mr Sandlands, the defence lawyer, said that as Dr Lambert was unable to 'assure the court beyond reasonable doubt that the towel had not been tied after the child had died, he submitted that there was no case for him to answer'.[84] Without leaving the jury box, the jury returned a verdict of not guilty of infanticide, as there was insufficient evidence.[85]

Similarly, in the case of Dora Whiter, who was charged with the murder of her newly born child in November 1937 after the body of her infant was discovered wrapped in paper in the River Witham in Lincolnshire, the medical evidence at the inquest revealed that 'the child had been dead for some 10 or 14 days, but apparently it had only been in the water for a few hours'. According to the prosecutor, 'The doctor was definitely of the opinion that the child had had a separate existence'.[86] Dr Lakes, who carried out the post-mortem, stated that the child had:

> breathed and cried, its lungs were fully expanded, very well preserved and were pink and mottled. There was no evidence of decomposition. The body was that of a full time male child weighing 7lb 5oz. Externally there was considerable decomposition. On the right side of the skull was a bruise, the size of a 5s piece, which in itself was not sufficient to cause death.[87]

Dr Lakes continued by stating:

> there was no evidence to show how the child had died. He could not go further than to say that had any determined effort been made to keep the child alive, it would have been alive. It might have died through violence or it might have died through neglect. If the child had been wrapped up and placed in a cupboard for two or three weeks he would expect to find conditions similar to those he had found in this case.[88]

Despite the certainty he portrays regarding the child having taken a breath and having a separate existence prior to death, the evidence given by Dr Lakes is notable for the precision with which he conveys the degree of uncertainty over the cause of death. The jury found Dora guilty of the lesser offence of concealment of birth, and she was sentenced to three months' imprisonment.

In the case of Edith Marjery Cobner in 1931, the issue of live birth arose at both the inquest and the trial, with opposite results. Edith's newly born child was discovered in a shoebox under her bed. At the inquest Dr Ashwin, the local doctor called by Edith's employer, explained how a sleeve from a blouse had been 'tied around the child's neck and a portion of cloth was in the child's mouth, the knot was sufficient to cause death. Death could have been caused by any form of suffocation, which was always a great danger at unattended births.'[89] However, Edith's solicitor argued that it was possible that the blouse had been placed over the child's head in an attempt to dress the infant, as the sleeve was not tied very tightly. The jury found that the 'child had been born alive and was suffocated by the mother, by tying a piece of cloth round its neck, but that Cobner had not fully recovered and her mind was disturbed. A verdict of infanticide was returned.'[90] At the York Assizes Dr Ashwin stated:

> the blouse was tied sufficiently tight to cause death. The child had had a separate existence. In his opinion, death was due to strangulation. He stated that the girl's condition was consistent with a collapse immediately after birth. The jury found the prisoner not guilty and she was discharged.[91]

Ashwin's evidence, which resulted in an acquittal, seems on the face of it less helpful to the defence than what he said at the inquest, but this may be simply because the part where he left open the possibility of strangulation during birth was not reported in the newspaper.

Similarly, at the inquest into the death of the infant of Elsie Lilley, in September 1944, Dr Philip Science, police surgeon, carried out an autopsy. He stated that:

> the child had had a separate existence and had lived about one day. The body was so much burned that it was impossible to detect any signs of violence. It was also impossible to say whether the child was dead or alive when it was taken from the fire. In his opinion, the cause of death was shock following extensive burns. 'That is providing the child was alive when it was put on the fire', observed the coroner. 'Yes,' Dr Science replied.[92]

Elsie had a relationship with another man and was expecting his baby, in her husband's absence. Her husband was away serving in the armed forces, and they had two children. Elsie had informed her neighbours that she was planning to have this child adopted, however, this was not the case.[93] Elsie was convicted under the Infanticide Act 1938, which extended the offence of infanticide to cover not only 'newly born' children but those under the age of one year.[94] The judge at the York Assizes postponed sentencing, while he asked the authorities to find an establishment for her, for not less than twelve months.[95]

The East Riding and Lincolnshire cases collectively demonstrate how medical evidence remained crucial throughout the inquest stage between 1922 and 1945. The focus on the body, and the 'scientifically satisfying procedure for inquiring into unexplained deaths'[96] emphasises the significance of the part which the medical witness continued to play in the twentieth-century infanticide inquest. It is possible that 'the jury's tendency to an alarmist empathy with the deceased precluded its normal capacity for rational judgement',[97] but medical uncertainty was sufficient to provide a rational basis for avoiding verdicts of murder in most cases.

Conclusion

The pressures on scientific witnesses to deliver certainty have often been commented on in the historical and sociological literature. Some branches of forensic science have been criticised for succumbing to these pressures and cultivating an unjustified image of near-infallible objectivity; others have been lauded for their 'rectitude' in resisting such pressures and carefully communicating the uncertainties of their sciences to the courts.[98] The history of medical evidence in infanticide cases illustrates how uncertainty as well as certainty can be a valuable resource for lawyers and the courts. Particularly in the context of the adversarial, jury trial, it created lines of defence for defendants whose position would otherwise be legally hopeless and gave a sympathetic jury an opportunity to acquit those with whose predicaments they sympathised.

As Watson has shown, the difficulties of proving infanticide formed an important part of training in forensic medicine in the nineteenth and early twentieth centuries.[99] Medical witnesses were careful to acknowledge the limits of their knowledge, and this left the result of prosecutions dependent on how their evidence was interpreted by judges and juries. This was both the strength and the weakness of the legal approach to infanticide before 1922. The law could be mercifully applied but it was criticised both for being too lenient and for being arbitrarily punitive in cases like Edith Roberts's where the judge and jury were less indulgent than usual. Despite the parallels we have noted with the insanity defence, the cautious forensic culture of the medical profession in these cases was very different from that of experts who, as in many insanity cases, produced uncertainty by publicly airing their differences in an adversarial trial. Although the reasons for this caution were specific to infanticide, a culture of forensic 'rectitude' and careful explanation of the limits of knowledge is one that has much to commend it today.[100]

Notes

1 See for example Robert O. Keohane, Melissa Lane and Michael Oppenheimer, 'The Ethics of Scientific Communication under Uncertainty', *Politics, Philosophy & Economics* 13:4 (2014), pp. 343–368; Maya J. Goldenberg, *Vaccine Hesitancy: Public Trust, Expertise and the War on Science* (Pittsburgh, PA: University of Pittsburgh Press, 2021), esp. pp. 170–172.
2 Stephan Landsman, 'One Hundred Years of Rectitude: Medical Witnesses at the Old Bailey, 1717–1817', *Law and History Review* 16:3 (1998), pp. 445–494, here p. 482.
3 E.g. Carol Jones, *Expert Witnesses, Science, Medicine and the Practice of Law* (Oxford: Clarendon Press, 1994); Simon A. Cole, *Suspect Identities: A History of Fingerprinting and Criminal Identification* (Cambridge, MA: Harvard University Press 2002); Andrew Rose, *Lethal Witness: Sir Bernard Spilsbury, Honorary Pathologist* (Kent, OH: Kent State University Press, 2009); Alison Adam, *A History of Forensic Science* (Abingdon: Routledge, 2016), pp. 35–40.
4 *Ibid.*, p. 39.
5 Katherine D. Watson, *Medicine and Justice: Medico-Legal Practice in England and Wales, 1700–1914* (Abingdon: Routledge, 2020) table 4.6, p. 152.
6 One judge who did protest against it was Mr Justice Willes, in a charge to a grand jury in 1865; but he very fairly placed the blame on the state of the law, rather than medicine.
7 John H. Langbein, *The Origins of Adversary Criminal Trial* (Oxford: Oxford University Press, 2003).
8 As in the case of *R v Trilloe* (1842) Car. & M. 650.
9 Katherine D. Watson, 'Religion, Community and The Infanticidal Mother: Evidence From 1840s Rural Wiltshire', *Family & Community History* 11:2 (2008), pp. 116–133.
10 See e.g. Roger Smith, 'Forensic Pathology, Scientific Expertise and the Criminal Law', in Roger Smith and Brian Wynne (eds), *Expert*

Evidence: Interpreting Science in the Law (London: Routledge, 1989); Jones, Expert Witnesses; Brian Wynne, Rationality and Ritual: Participation and Exclusion in Nuclear Decision-Making (2nd edn, London: Routledge, 2011).
11. Mrs Baines, 'A Few Thoughts Concerning Infanticide', Journal of Social Science 10 (1866), pp. 535–540, here p. 536.
12. Stephen Gaukroger, Objectivity: A Very Short Introduction (Oxford: Oxford University Press, 2012), p. 4.
13. Heather Douglas argues that the implication of trustworthiness is what connects the many meanings of 'objectivity': 'The Irreducible Complexity of Objectivity', Synthese 138:3 (2004), pp. 453–473, here p. 453.
14. See for example Wynne, Rationality and Ritual; Jones, Expert Witnesses, pp. 97–102.
15. Gaukroger, Objectivity, p. 4.
16. Tony Ward, 'Law, Common Sense and the Authority of Science: Expert Witnesses and Criminal Insanity in England, ca. 1840–1940, Social & Legal Studies 6:3 (1997), pp. 343–362.
17. See e.g. George K. Behlmer, 'Deadly Motherhood: Infanticide and Medical Opinion in Mid-Victorian England', Journal of the History of Medicine and Allied Sciences 34:4 (1979), pp. 403–427.
18. Watson, Medicine and Justice.
19. Rachel Dixon, Infanticide: Expert Evidence and Testimony in Child Murder Cases, 1688–1955 (Abingdon: Routledge, 2022).
20. This point is touched on in Dixon, Infanticide, pp. 181–184, but we present additional evidence for it below.
21. See Robert P. Burns, A Theory of the Trial (Princeton: Princeton University Press, 1999).
22. Thomas Forbes, 'Early Forensic Medicine in England: The Angus Murder Trial', Journal of the History of Medicine 36:3 (1981), pp. 296–309.
23. Landsman, 'One Hundred Years'.
24. Ibid., p. 456.
25. Ibid., p. 458.
26. Ibid., pp. 458–459; Old Bailey Proceedings (available at: www.oldbaileyonline.org, version 8.0, March 2018) (hereafter OBP), Joanna M'Carthy, September 1802, t18020918-134.
27. Katherine Watson, Forensic Medicine in Western Society: A History (Abingdon: Routledge, 2011), p. 26.
28. Peter Linebaugh, 'The Tyburn Riot Against the Surgeons', in Douglas Hay et al. (eds), Albion's Fatal Tree: Crime and Society in Eighteenth Century England (London: Verso, 1977), p. 70.

29 Landsman, 'One Hundred Years', p. 449.
30 Mary Clayton, 'Changes in Old Bailey Trials for the Murder of New-Born Babies, 1674–1803', *Continuity and Change* 24:2 (2009), pp. 337–359, here p. 348.
31 See Watson, *Medicine and Justice*.
32 *OBP*, Sarah Perry, February 1817, t18170219-31.
33 Allyson May, *The Bar and the Old Bailey, 1750–1850* (Chapel Hill: University of North Carolina Press, 2014), p. 78.
34 *Ibid.*
35 William Hunter, *On the Uncertainty of the Signs of Child Murder in the Case of Bastard Children* (Glasgow, 1783), digitised text available at www.gla.ac.uk/myglasgow/library/files/special/teach/murder/murder.html (accessed 2 January 2022), p. 14.
36 See Chris Milroy, 'Neonatal Deaths, Infanticide and the Hydrostatic (Flotation) Test: Historical Perspectives', *Academic Forensic Pathology* 2:4 (2012), pp. 338–345.
37 Mark Jackson, *New-born Child Murder: Women, Illegitimacy and the Courts in Eighteenth-Century England* (Manchester: Manchester University Press, 1996).
38 Stanley B. Atkinson, 'Life Birth and Live-Birth', *Law Quarterly Review* 20:2 (1904), pp. 134–159.
39 Watson, *Medicine and Justice*, Ch. 4.
40 Before 1803, most prosecutions for newborn child murder were brought under a 1624 statute by which if a mother concealed the birth of her bastard child, it was presumed to have been born alive; but by the 1760s it was customary to require 'some sort of presumptive proof' of live birth: William Blackstone, *Commentaries on the Laws of England* (1769) vol. 4, p. 198.
41 *OBP*, Maria Poulton, May 1832, t18320517-65; *R v Ann Poulton* (1835) 5 C. & P. 329.
42 The parish meeting or Vestry was the nineteenth-century equivalent of a local council.
43 'Parish of St Clement Danes', *Morning Advertiser*, 5 May 1832, p. 2, British Newspaper Archive (hereafter BNA). It may be the parish's initial support for the prosecution that explains the multiplicity of medical witnesses.
44 *R v Ann Poulton* (1835) 5 C. & P. 329, italics added.
45 *OBP*, Hannah Diana Connolly, September 1806, t18060917-48.
46 *R v Eliza Brain* (1834) 6 C. & P. 349; *R v Ann Crutchley* (1837) 7 C. & P. 814.

47 Ibid. For a more emphatic ruling in 1845 that killing a child in the course of birth was not murder see Behlmer, 'Deadly Motherhood', p. 411.
48 R v Elizabeth Sellis (1837) 7 C. & P. 850.
49 Ibid.
50 'Norfolk Circuit – Cambridge, March 24', London Courier and Evening Gazette, 27 March 1837, BNA. Both the law report and the newspaper report need to be read to understand the case clearly.
51 (1842) Car. & M. 650.
52 The cases of R v Richard Enoch and Mary Pulley (1833) 5 C. & P. 539 and R v Ann Crutchley (1837) 7 C. & P. 814 had suggested that an independent circulation was necessary, but might take place before the umbilical cord was cut.
53 James Oldham 'Informal Lawmaking in England by the Twelve Judges in the Late Eighteenth and Early Nineteenth Centuries', Law and History Review 29:1 (2011), pp. 181–220.
54 Duncan Kennedy, 'Freedom and Constraint in Adjudication: A Critical Phenomenology', Journal of Legal Education 36:4 (1986), pp. 518–562, here p. 518.
55 R v Ann Crutchley (1837) 7 C. & P. 814.
56 See Roger Chadwick, Bureaucratic Mercy: The Home Office and the Treatment of Capital Cases in Victorian England (New York: Garland, 1992).
57 Watson, Medicine and Justice, p. 188.
58 Ibid.
59 Patrick Atiyah and Robert S. Summers, Form and Substance in Anglo-American Law (Oxford: Clarendon, 1987), p. 38. See also Martin Wiener, Reconstructing the Criminal (Cambridge: Cambridge University Press, 1990).
60 Roger Smith, Trial by Medicine: Insanity and Responsibility in Victorian Trials (Edinburgh: Edinburgh University Press, 1981); Joel Peter Eigen, Mad-Doctors in the Dock (Baltimore: Johns Hopkins University Press, 2016).
61 Tony Ward, 'Law, Common Sense and the Authority of Science: Expert Witnesses and Criminal Insanity in England, ca. 1840–1940', Social & Legal Studies 6:3 (1997), pp. 343–362; Arlie Loughnan and Tony Ward, 'Emergent Authority and Expert Knowledge: Psychiatry and Criminal Responsibility in the UK', International Journal for Law and Psychiatry 37:1 (2014), pp. 25–36.
62 See Tony Ward, 'Legislating for Human Nature: Legal Responses to Infanticide, 1860–1938', in Mark Jackson (ed.), Infanticide: Historical Perspectives on Child Murder and Concealment, 1550–2000 (Aldershot: Ashgate, 2002), pp. 249–269.

63 https://en.wikisource.org/wiki/Dictionary_of_National_Biography,_1885–1900/Mitford,_John_Thomas_Freeman- (accessed 4 January 2022).
64 *House of Lords Debates* 221 (28 July 1874) col. 847.
65 Hilary Marland, 'Getting Away with Murder', in Mark Jackson (ed.), *Infanticide, Historical Perspectives on Child Murder and Concealment, 1550–2000* (Aldershot: Ashgate, 2002), pp. 168–192, here p. 171.
66 Ann Higginbotham, 'Sin of Age: Infanticide and Illegitimacy in Victorian London', *Victorian Studies* 32:3 (1989), pp. 319–337; Christien Krueger, 'Literary Defences and Medical Prosecutions: Representing Infanticide in Nineteenth-Century Britain', *Victorian Studies* 40:2 (1997), pp. 271–294; Josephine McDonagh, *Child Murder and British Culture, 1720–1900* (New York: Cambridge University Press, 2003).
67 George Eliot, *Adam Bede* (London: Penguin, 1985 [1859]), p. 455.
68 Rachel Dixon and Tony Ward, 'Manslaughter, Concealment of Birth and Infanticide, 1900–37', in Karen Brennan and Emma Milne (eds), *100 years of the Infanticide Act: Legacy and Impact* (Oxford: Hart Publishing, forthcoming 2023).
69 Brigitte H. Bechtold, 'Infanticide in Nineteenth Century France: A Quantitative Interpretation', *Review of Radical Political Economics* 33:2 (2001), pp. 165–187, here p. 168; see also Tracey Rizzo, 'Between Dishonor and Death: Infanticides in the *Causes Celebres* of Eighteenth Century France', *Women's History Review* 13:1 (2004), pp. 5–21.
70 Bechtold, 'Infanticide in Nineteenth Century France,' p. 168.
71 *Ibid.*
72 James Donovan, 'Infanticide and the Juries in France 1825–1913', *Journal of Family History* 16:2 (1991), pp. 157–176.
73 Smith, *Trial by Medicine*; Ward, 'Law, Common Sense and Science'; Loughnan and Ward, 'Emergent Authority'; Dixon, *Infanticide*.
74 *OBP*, Louisa Lunn, March 1904, t19040321-332.
75 *Ibid.*
76 *Ibid.*
77 *Ibid.*
78 Daniel Grey, 'Women's Policy Networks and the Infanticide Act 1922', *Twentieth-Century British History* 21:4 (2010), pp. 441–463, here p. 445.
79 This is acknowledged even by his admiring biographer: Gordon Lang, *Mr Justice Avory* (London: Herbert Jenkins, 1935).
80 *Nottingham Evening Post*, 28 July 1921.

81 We discuss this difficult issue in more detail in Dixon and Ward 'Manslaughter, Concealment of Birth and Infanticide, 1900–37'.
82 *Ibid.*
83 *Lincolnshire Echo*, 'Brigg Girl and Dead Baby', 6 November 1931, BNA (www.britishnewspaperarchive.co.uk).
84 *Ibid.*
85 *Ibid.*
86 *Nottingham Evening Post*, 'Charged with Murder', 25 November 1937, BNA (www.britishnewspaperarchive.co.uk).
87 *Nottingham Evening Post*, 'Charged with Murder', 2 December 1937, BNA.
88 *Lincolnshire Echo*, 'Lincoln Murder Charge', 2 December 1937, BNA.
89 *Hull Daily Mail*, 'Infant's Body in Box', 24 June 1931, BNA.
90 *Ibid.*
91 *Yorkshire Post and Leeds Intelligencer*, 'York Assizes, Londesborough Woman Acquitted', 26 November 1931, BNA.
92 *Hull Daily Mail*, 'Day-Old Baby Alleged Placed on Fire', 27 September 1944, BNA.
93 *Hull Daily Mail*, 'Sentence Postponed', 18 November 1944, BNA.
94 For the background to the 1938 Act see Ward, 'Legislating for Human Nature'.
95 'Sentence Postponed' (n. 93 above).
96 Ian Burney, *Bodies of Evidence, Medicine and the Politics of the English Inquest, 1830–1926* (London: Johns Hopkins University Press, 2000), p. 108.
97 *Ibid.*, p. 154.
98 Landsman, 'One Hundred Years of Rectitude'; for a recent example see Beth A. Bechky, *Blood, Powder and Residue: How Crime Labs Translate Evidence into Proof* (Princeton: Princeton University Press, 2020).
99 Watson, *Medicine and Justice*, Ch. 2.
100 Gary Edmond *et al.*, 'Model Forensic Science', *Australian Journal of Forensic Sciences* 48:5 (2016), pp. 496–537; Tony Ward, 'The Forensic Ethics of Scientific Communication', *Journal of Criminal Law*, 87:1 (2023), pp. 3–17.

8

Forensic physicians and the Francoist prosecution of infanticide, *c*. 1939–1969: The case of the haemorrhage of the umbilical cord as cause of death

Sara Serrano Martínez

Introduction

In the nineteenth and twentieth centuries many countries in Europe and Latin America enacted special laws for the crime of newborn child murder (hereafter, infanticide), establishing relatively lower penalties compared to other homicides.[1] It has been argued that medical testimonies often favoured practices of lenient sentencing in cases of infanticide, both before and after special laws were passed for this crime. In England and Ireland, from the seventeenth to the twentieth centuries, doctors showed their uncertainties, thus allowing juries' acquittals and lower sentences.[2] This also happened in nineteenth-century France.[3] Yet analyses of infanticide proceedings from other legal systems have started to change this historiographical narrative which associates the presence of medical evidence with lenient outcomes. Looking at European and Latin American contexts, Sara McDougall and Felicity Turner have argued that the 'criminalization of childbirth', including the prosecution of infanticide, hardened with modernity, and that 'the professionalization of medicine in the twentieth century' was a key factor in this shift.[4] Regarding Mexico, Nora E. Jaffary has argued that the late nineteenth century witnessed 'greater legal confidence in the reliability of medical assessments of mothers' criminal guilt or innocence'.[5] The present chapter adds to this increasingly complex comparative picture of the history of infanticide and justice, showing that in the first decades (1939–1969) of the Francoist dictatorship (1939–1975), when pronatalist policies were particularly important, medical testimonies also contributed to indicting and convicting suspects of infanticide. I show this by analysing one of the medical questions that arose in infanticide cases: the question of whether the newborn could have died due to the haemorrhage of their cut, but untied, umbilical cord.

The question of the umbilical cord's haemorrhage was not unique in Spain or the Francoist context; for instance, Kristin Ruggiero has suggested that the lack of tying of the umbilical cord was frequently the basis for the charge of infanticide in turn-of-the-century Buenos Aires.[6] In Spain, before the Franco regime there were also infanticide cases in which this was considered to be a newborn's cause of death.[7] Yet, the issue of the umbilical cord is a good case to analyse the role of medical evidence in the Francoist prosecution of infanticide, firstly because it came up recurrently in the first decades of the dictatorship, contributing to several indictments and convictions, and secondly because this practice contrasted with medico-legal literature that showed doubts about whether the haemorrhage could commonly be a cause of death in newborns. This discrepancy between theory and practice regarding the umbilical cord's haemorrhage becomes clear from the analysis I have carried out of a sample consisting of one hundred archival files belonging to court cases of infanticide from six provincial courts (Madrid, Ávila, Toledo, Guadalajara, Tarragona and Girona) from the 1940s and 1950s. Statistics suggest that some archival records are incomplete, and many cases were not traceable. From those files that were traceable in registers, I have consulted all the files available (Madrid, Ávila, Tarragona and Girona) or random samples (Toledo and Guadalajara). Moreover, I have studied twenty-four decisions from the Supreme Court coming from all around Spain from the 1940s to the 1960s.[8]

Moreover, in the few lines that historians have dedicated to infanticide in the Francoist dictatorship, it has been argued that women in other provinces (Murcia and Lugo) left their newborns' cords untied to make them bleed and die when they faced the impossibility of accessing abortions.[9] This inference becomes questionable if one takes into account that contemporary physicians doubted that the haemorrhage was necessarily fatal. What was at work in these cases of infanticide was not only a matter of reproductive control and its repression but also a significant event in the history of medicine: namely, a silence among doctors and legal practitioners alike regarding medico-legal debates about the umbilical cord's haemorrhage. Focusing on the case of the haemorrhage of the umbilical cord, thus, does not only show that medical evidence was not always associated with lenient outcomes in cases of infanticide, as stated in the current international literature, but also helps to counter some historiographical assumptions about infanticide as a practice of reproductive control in the Franco regime.

Clarifying why physicians who conducted the autopsy did not mention the debates in medico-legal literature, and why jurists – particularly defence lawyers – did not bring up the debate, raises historiographical questions about how medico-legal expertise worked and was conceptualised in the Francoist dictatorship. Historians have already shown how medical experts facilitated practices of torture and extra-judicial executions in Francoist military and political courts,[10] and provided theories contributing to justify detentions of those deemed 'socially dangerous', like Roma people, gay people and alcoholics.[11] Recently, Stephanie Wright has argued that, in cases of rape, medical experts brought in ambiguous theories that increased the already existing arbitrariness of Francoist criminal law courts.[12] This chapter elaborates on the embedding of medical expertise in the Francoist criminal law courts, identifying some important factors of the Spanish forensic culture in the dictatorship that explain why the fatal haemorrhage of the umbilical cord was in practice considered a cause of death in Francoist courts: its system of appeals, how medical expertise was conceptualised, how autopsies' reports were structured, and the epistemic ideals for forensic experts.

After examining how the medico-legal literature that circulated in Spain until the 1960s debated the fatality of umbilical cord haemorrhages, I will show that there was a contrast between the generalised doubts and cautions of the literature and the practices of both experts and legal practitioners in court: in practice the haemorrhage of the umbilical cord was accepted as cause of death, and this led to several indictments and convictions of suspects of infanticide. Next, I will briefly sketch how the fascist pronatalist context of the dictatorship determined indictments and convictions of infanticide. Finally, I will show how various cultural and institutional characteristics of the Spanish and Francoist forensic culture contributed to the absence of debate about the cord's haemorrhage, providing the pretext for several indictments and convictions.

The haemorrhage of the umbilical cord, a plausible cause of death?

In their popular *Treatise of Legal Medicine* (1961), the professors of legal medicine Leopoldo López Gómez and Juan Antonio Gisbert Calabuig argued that, at the time, haemorrhages of the umbilical cord in newborn children were 'judged to be completely exceptional, and even unbelievable'.[13] In their opinion, such an event could only occur on two rare occasions, namely, that the child was haemophilic, or that the cord had been ripped at the level of its abdominal insertion, that is, right by the navel. Otherwise, the physiological mechanism resulting from birth would have prevented any haemorrhage by itself: once the cord was cut, the new, independent respiration of the child was established, and with it the umbilical arteries would retract and their arterial pressure would lessen, which would all run counter to the production of a haemorrhage through the cord's section, even if it was left untied.

As it is clear from these authors' tone, there were other works that did not specify that a fatal umbilical cord's haemorrhage could only occur under certain conditions. In 1917, professor of legal medicine Antonio Lecha-Marzo stated that the haemorrhage of the umbilical cord could result from its lack of ligature[14] and, in 1942, the manual of the Lyon professor Étienne Martin, which did not discuss the frequency of the fatal haemorrhage of the cord either, was translated into Spanish.[15] These two texts were well known in Spain, and I have found concrete evidence that Martin's work was read by some forensic physicians practising during the Franco regime.[16]

However, before 1961 there was a second body of literature that was emphatic that the fatal umbilical cord haemorrhage was highly unlikely – and this line of scholarship was more available than the other strand. This body of literature had begun with two nineteenth-century works that were very influential in Spain, those of Pedro

Mata and of Ambroise Tardieu.[17] A similar stance was defended in a 1935 manual which was specifically directed at the education of prospective forensic practitioners, who would be practising in Spanish courts in the 1940s and 1950s,[18] and in later works.[19] López and Gisbert's treatise, with which this section opened, was reedited in 1967 and 1970, and according to various reviews, by 1969 it was 'considered to be the most complete and scientifically elevated among the texts about the topic [of legal medicine]'.[20]

In sum, although there were a few works that did not account for the low incidence of the fatal haemorrhage of the umbilical cord in newborns, Spanish physicians also had within their reach various medico-legal handbooks that did specify the likelihood of this cause of death. This latter strand of the literature argued that fatal haemorrhages of the umbilical cord were possible, but that they did not occur frequently or in normal conditions. Yet, as I will show in the next section, the fatality of the cord's haemorrhage was considered a more common event in Spanish forensic practice.

The umbilical cord's haemorrhage as a decisive element in court practices

In 1962, a maid working in Madrid was convicted of wilfully killing her newborn child, who had died, the autopsy report and the judges claimed, due to the umbilical cord's haemorrhage and anoxia (lack of oxygen). This judgment is in striking contrast with the contemporary medico-legal discussion regarding the umbilical cord and perinatal death. By 1961 many medical doctors and forensic practitioners in Spain could know that an umbilical cord's haemorrhage was rarely fatal. Yet, in this 1962 decision, this was ruled to be the cause of death of the child, while there was no sign of the conditions that, according to the literature, made this event more likely (neither haemophilia nor ripping close to the navel; the cord, indeed, had been ripped at 10cm from the navel). The doctors who conducted the autopsy could not identify any 'signs of mechanic violence' on the body of the child, but they did observe signs of anoxia and saw that the child's umbilical cord had been ripped but not tied. Their conclusion derived from this observation and from the premise that the lack of tying could lead to a fatal 'loss of blood'. They did not refer at all to the medico-legal discussions regarding the umbilical haemorrhage as cause of perinatal death.[21] This was far from being the only case in which forensic experts and judges of the Francoist regime deemed the haemorrhage of the umbilical cord to be the cause of death of a newborn child without referring to the medico-legal discussions about it. In twenty other infanticide cases investigated in nine different Spanish provinces from the 1940s to the early 1960s, the haemorrhage of the cord was also found as cause of death.[22] In most of these cases, prosecutors and judges did not come up with this conclusion by themselves, but built on the conclusion of the post-mortem.[23] Besides omitting any reference to medico-legal debates, none of the autopsy reports pointing at the haemorrhage of the cord as cause of death mentioned haemophilia and only one noted the cut to be ripped close to the navel.[24] Most autopsy reports based this conclusion on observing that some organs were bloodless or showed signs of anaemia, which were indeed signs to which some medico-legal manuals referred as possible indicators of the cord's haemorrhage.[25] Yet, three other autopsies did not justify the conclusion explicitly, noting that the cord was cut at 40cm, at 45cm, and at 'two transversal fingers' from the navel.[26] Thus, the justification of why the haemorrhage of the cord was deemed to be the cause of death was scant in several cases, and the medico-legal literature was not discussed.

What is more, in other cases where the autopsy specified that the cord was untied but did not say that this was the cause of death, some judges and prosecutors inferred the suspect's intent to kill the baby from this lack of tying. Some judges even concluded that the suspect had intentionally aimed for the untied cord to lead to a fatal bleeding. For instance, in a case from 1947, the medical doctors clearly stated that the causes of death were a neck fracture and a traumatic brain haemorrhage, both resulting from a harsh blow with an object or against the wall. Still, the deciding judges believed that hitting the baby was the second option of the suspects – the child's mother and grandmother – once they saw that, despite their intentional act of leaving the cord untied, the child was still alive.[27] Similarly, in 1964 the provincial court of Orense convicted a woman arguing that she had suffocated the child, and that, right after doing that, she had cut and not tied the umbilical cord, which, according to the court, 'if the baby would not have been asphyxiated would have realised her aim to kill her child'.[28] In several other cases, moreover, the failure to tie the umbilical cord was regarded as evidence suggesting that the accused did not want the child to survive.[29]

While two of the cases where doctors believed that the cord's haemorrhage was the cause of death were dismissed, and two suspects were acquitted, these outcomes did not result from doubts about whether the cord's haemorrhage was a sufficient cause of death.[30] Judging from the available data, it is clear that many indictments and convictions from the 1940s to the 1960s were based on the theoretical premise that the haemorrhage of a newborn's umbilical cord was likely to be fatal – either directly, by pointing at this as the cause of death, or more subtly, by referring implicitly to the untied cord ambivalently as either circumstantial evidence of intent or as one amongst other intended actions for taking the child's life.

In sight of the existing medico-legal debates about the fatality of the cord's haemorrhage, it is striking they were not brought up in most of the cases by any of the parties involved, given that this had the potential to counter a decisive factual element in indictments and convictions. The medical claim that the haemorrhage of the cord was the cause of death was only subject to specific scrutiny in two of the nineteen investigations where it came up, and it was not directly questioned in cassation appeals before the Supreme Court. Only one defence lawyer appointed new medical doctors – a gynaecologist and a generalist – to question the fatal haemorrhage hypothesis. In the other case, it was the prosecutor who, in the pre-trial investigation, pressed the physicians who had carried out the autopsy to specify the mechanisms of this cause of death, later on appointing other experts to confirm the opinion. In the first case, all physicians debated at trial whether the haemorrhage of the cord could have been the cause of death of the child, which the defence experts only accepted as a theoretical possibility.[31] In the other case, the new experts, two obstetricians, explained how the change from a maternal circulation to the pulmonary respiration occurred, and what consequences this had in terms of pressure in the umbilical vessels, and they argued that multiple studies had already demonstrated that the cord could be left untied without a subsequent bleeding. They admitted that fatal umbilical haemorrhages could occasionally happen, but stated that, ordinarily, they did not. At trial, before the questions of the parties, they claimed that, in the particular case in question, the untied cord could not be the cause of death.[32] In all other cases, by contrast, this medical claim was left unquestioned.

The influence of Francoist pronatalism

The discrepancy between medico-legal discussions and forensic practices regarding the issue of the fatal umbilical cord's haemorrhage was certainly shaped by the pronatalist context of the Franco regime. Experts' and judges' assumptions, together with circumstantial evidence, bolstered the conclusion that the death of the child had resulted from an intentional act, leaving the cord untied. For example, in the only two aforementioned cases where there was debate about the cord's haemorrhage, physicians' explanations that the fatal haemorrhages were infrequent did not translate decisively into the outcome of the two aforementioned cases, and the suspects were still convicted.

In some cases, experts and jurists accepted the haemorrhage as cause of death prima facie, since this confirmed their prejudices that unmarried mothers often killed their newborns. The Franco regime adopted pronatalist policies that, following the example of Fascist Italy, framed the need to raise the Spanish population as a remedy against the nation's decline.[33] Although the obligation of declaring pregnancies was never established legally, and although concealment of birth was not in itself criminalised as was the case in other countries, the police, local authorities and neighbours in practice controlled women's bodies, denounced them and gave testimony regarding suspects' putative concealments of pregnancy and birth. This kind of testimonial or circumstantial evidence regarding concealment of pregnancy and birth led some prosecutors and judges to infer a suspect's intent to kill the newborn. Typically these inferences were implicit, but when the decision of a provincial court was appealed some judges sent an explanation to the Supreme Court regarding their judgment. In one of these explanations, from 1943, the court of Albacete explained why they had deemed the cord's haemorrhage to be proven and attributable to the intent of the accused – despite the fact that the autopsy report had explicitly stated that the cause of death could not be determined. Essentially, the court explicated, they had built on the autopsy report; however, in fact their main reasoning hinged on circumstantial evidence about concealment of childbirth:

> that [expert] evidence is strengthened with the fact that the accused went to a stable to give birth and put the child in a sack and buried it, thus if the accused would not have wanted to kill the child to conceal her dishonour, she would have tied the umbilical cord and she would have held the childbirth in a more appropriate location.[34]

Whether the accused was already a mother was an important fact from which incriminating inferences were made, also concerning the tying of the cord. One of the main objectives of the pronatalist policies of the Franco regime was to provide Spanish women with knowledge regarding the care of infants. The aim of improving medical assistance in childbirth – since, at least until the late 1940s, in Spain the majority of deliveries were not medically assisted – was also embedded in pronatalism and its attribution of ignorance to lower-class women. Mothers (working-class mothers in particular) were believed to be responsible for child mortality, especially in children's first year of life, both due to the diet they gave to children and to their ignorance regarding childbirth, neonatal care and infants' healthcare.[35] Far from being seen as ignorant and thus not guilty, in infanticide cases mothers were judged to be knowledgeable and thus guilty of wilfully omitting perinatal care, including a proper tying of the child's umbilical cord – although this was not believed to be 'instinctual knowledge', as was the case in early-twentieth-century Buenos Aires.[36] Yet, if a suspect was already a mother, she was regarded as more knowledgeable in matters of perinatal care.[37] Particularly, the suspects' mothers – the children's grandmothers – were targeted in this regard. This was in line with the cultural expectation that they ought to take responsibility for their daughters' moral behaviour, and for the way their daughters practised motherhood: in the words of physician Roig Raventós, grandmothers had a 'classical mission as supervisors in the upbringing of [their] grandchildren'.[38] For example, in the only two cases of my sample where there was debate about the fatality of the cord's haemorrhage, but suspects were still convicted, the deliveries had been assisted by the grandmothers of the babies. That grandmothers had experience with childbirth appears to have been the main evidence from which prosecutors and judges, in these cases, inferred that the lack of tying of the cord was intentional.

However, while this pronatalist context offers a convincing explanation for why prosecutors and judges, as well as possibly some physicians, were inclined to accept the cord's haemorrhage as cause of death, this explanation falls short of explaining why lawyers did not use medico-legal debates to raise doubts in benefit of their defendants. Moreover, it does not explain whether, and under what understanding of expertise, it was common that autopsy reports avoided referring to medico-legal debates. Analysing the Spanish forensic culture, and its specific shape in the Francoist context, allows me to shed some light on these facts.

The importance of forensic culture

Besides prejudices against unmarried women and their mothers shaped by pronatalism, there are other factors that help to clarify why the medico-legal debate and distrust about this hypothesis was not brought up more frequently, particularly by defence lawyers. For instance, defence lawyers possibly did not know the medico-legal discussions, opted for other defence strategies, or did not dedicate much effort to infanticide defendants, given that the vast majority of them were poor and were defended by lawyers in state-aid duty (*turno de oficio*). Defences focusing on the legal conditions for proving intent, for example, were feasible without questioning autopsy reports.[39] Yet, what also could have facilitated the lack of questioning of the cord's haemorrhage hypothesis – and could have contributed to lawyers' ignorance in some cases – was the character of the Spanish forensic culture in the Francoist regime. As this section will show, some characteristics of this culture can be found in how medical expertise was conceptualised, the way autopsy reports were structured, the epistemic ideals held for forensic experts, and the continuity of the pre-Francoist Spanish system of appeals.

The Spanish system of appeals prevented discussion about the cord's haemorrhage at the post-trial stage. Although during the Civil

War there were jurists who advocated for a radical change in criminal procedure (following the Nazi example) this was not taken to practice in the dictatorship.[40] Instead, the configuration of the Spanish criminal procedure built in the late nineteenth century, with the 1872 and 1882 procedural laws, was kept in force in the dictatorship.[41] In this configuration, judges had a great deal of discretion in their evaluation of evidence. Revision of facts by a second court was impossible in Spain until the Second Republic, when the law was reformed to accept 'authentic documents' as evidence that could allow the Supreme Court to review matters of fact.[42] Many defence lawyers appealed to the Supreme Court because they believed that the provincial court judges had not properly assessed expert conclusions, arguing that expert reports could qualify as 'authentic documents', or appealing to scientific expertise as the exclusive purview of doctors to question the provincial court's assessment of evidence. This was unsuccessful because the term 'authentic documents' was interpreted as mainly referring to notarial scriptures.

In a case of infanticide from 1943, for example, a lawyer argued that his defendant was convicted by mere presumptions, and that judges had gone 'beyond the medical report of the case file'. While the physicians had concluded they could not determine the cause of death, the provincial court's judgment was ambiguous and claimed that the accused had 'provoked the newborn's death *in this way*' (my emphasis), stating that she had ripped the umbilical cord and buried the child; thus, the judges' words left open whether the burial or the ripping of the untied cord had killed the baby. Physicians, the lawyer argued, were 'the only professionals capable technically to make scientific statements'.[43] However, this and other similar appeals were systematically rejected, for the Francoist Supreme Court adhered to the pre-Francoist doctrine according to which the realm of facts was of the exclusive purview of the first instance judge and expert reports, even if pronounced under Catholic oath, were not binding. Thus, the Francoist Supreme Court appropriated the cultural and legal hierarchy of the system of free evaluation of evidence that the lawyer was trying to counter.[44] These precedents prevented defence lawyers from searching for medico-legal reasons to put forward in appeals – a task in which they could have come across doubts regarding the frequency of the umbilical cord's haemorrhage.

That judges arrived at the conclusion that the newborn's cause of death was an umbilical cord's haemorrhage, and possibly that some lawyers ignored how to question that narration of facts, was overall caused by experts' omissions of any medico-legal theories and debates from their autopsy reports. It is possible that some medical examiners were unaware of the medico-legal discussions themselves. This can be explained by the fact that forensic physicians, as well as generalists, were regarded by the courts as sufficiently competent in all matters of medicine, including obstetrics. While generalists' competence could stem from the fact that they used to assist childbirths, forensic physicians' expertise derived from their image as specialists in all medical sub-disciplines relevant for legal matters. Since the early twentieth century, in Spain the specialists in legal matters were the forensic physicians, that is, medicine graduates who had obtained a permanent position through a specialised state exam (they were civil servants forming a state Corps of Forensic Physicians) to practice attached to an investigating court.[45] Through the preparation for the state exam, they supposedly obtained a specific background in all medical specialities relevant for the legal realm. In this legal system medical doctors who were not specialised in obstetric matters were therefore regarded as experts in cases of infanticide. Except for the case from Girona, where the prosecutor appointed two gynaecologists to be certain about the fatality of the cord's haemorrhage, all other prosecutors and investigating judges did not appoint gynaecologists or ask midwives about any of these issues. In the two cases in which medical specialists – obstetricians – were appointed, medico-legal debates regarding the haemorrhage of the cord were brought in, and in both cases they questioned the autopsy report's conclusion that this was the cause of death. By contrast, non-specialists assumed that it was clear that the cord's haemorrhage could kill the baby.[46]

The epistemic ideals held by physicians shaped autopsy reports, and favoured the presentation of some medical statements, like the cord's haemorrhage, as more conclusive than in specialised literature. The form of Spanish autopsy reports did not aim at reflecting the theories behind experts' findings. Autopsy reports were rather conceived of as public documents containing a statement under oath, and by which the experts provided the court with only the strictly relevant information, their authority and expertise being assumed to be already verified through their credentials and the fact that they were permanently attached to the court. The structure of these reports as mandated by the 1882 procedural law included an organised description of the external and internal examination of the body. After that, they had to provide the court with the relevant conclusions and findings, including an individualised cause of death and their thoughts about the circumstances of the death.[47] Thus, theoretical discussions, assessments of likelihood of a certain pathological event, and didactic explanations did not have a predetermined place in the structure of autopsy reports. Experts were also supposed to indicate their examination techniques and results, but in practice the description of those techniques was typically superficial or left out of reports, which mostly indicated what experts had observed, but not how they had arrived at their observations.[48]

While some experts, like the forensic physician Gregorio Nieto, believed that it was convenient to include all the steps of their inferences as much as possible, others believed that 'reasoning is not necessary, since one [the expert] declares under oath', and thus, their word could be taken as truthful.[49] In practice, even those practitioners who detailed their inferences normally limited themselves to connecting pathological observations with their subsequent conclusions, but they did not mention which theoretical framework or methods they were adhering to. In this manner, in cases dealing with the umbilical cord's supposed haemorrhage, what would be included as a reasoning was that the cord presented a certain length, colour and cut, and that certain organs or vessels were bloodless, without any references to authors, debates or theories. This customary exclusion of theoretical considerations left room for concealing relevant information on purpose, which physicians could decide to do for various reasons. This was also the case in other countries where – like in Spain – written autopsy reports were mandated: Nicholas Duvall has argued that autopsy reports in Scotland functioned as Latourian black boxes, affirming experts' authority via the concealment of experts' uncertainty.[50] Indeed, the structure of autopsy reports in Scotland and Spain were apparently very similar, which suggests that this might be a common element of various European contemporary forensic cultures after nineteenth-century liberal reforms of criminal procedure.

Besides concealing uncertainties as performance of expertise, I argue, the structure of autopsy reports in Franco's Spain also allowed for emphasising conclusive and incriminating post-mortem reports. As Duvall has also shown to be the case in Scotland, mandatory written autopsy reports 'facilitated a system whereby additional medical expertise could be brought to bear in the investigation' without need for an exhumation and new autopsy and thus 'enabled' second experts' challenge of the initial conclusions of the autopsy.[51] In the aforementioned case in which a prosecutor from Girona appointed two specialist gynaecologists to clarify whether the cord's haemorrhage could be fatal, the specialists revised the autopsy report written by two general practitioners instead of performing a new post-mortem examination. However, even if written autopsy reports provided room for a differing second opinion, Duvall's argument about the potential for challenges must be nuanced, at least in the Spanish context. Revision of written reports, overall, could make disagreement explicit, but still, the autopsy report's lack of theoretical and methodological reflection did not allow for a two-way medical discussion per se if experts were not personally confronted. Confrontation had to take place after a direct order of the investigating judge for experts to testify together, or at trial – where, often, medical examiners were not present, because the parties only requested the autopsy report as documentary evidence. In the Girona case, the gynaecologists could engage with the medico-legal literature and question the written report of the two GPs by merely reading it, but it was only during the trial, when they could talk to one of these generalists, that it could become clear that the first medical examiners did not have a differing theoretical position to respond to the specialists.[52] In sum, the Spanish configuration of autopsy reports excluded theoretical decisions and disagreements, and this favoured the lack of debate about the fatality of the umbilical cord's haemorrhage.

The normative ideas about communication held by medical experts also impacted on the structure of autopsy reports. Similarly to what happened in Scotland, Spanish medico-legal guidelines regarded a good report and statement as a concise and plain one, which had to ideally avoid technical terms and discussions.[53] This implied, importantly, that experts were supposed to refrain from spontaneously discussing any data that the court had not requested and to avoid any information that could lead to confusion. Yet, some forensic physicians believed they had to actively try to identify perpetrators, their motives and the criminal actions.[54] Consistently with this ideal, in practice some medical examiners framed cases of suspected infanticide in which the only identifiable cause of death was the bleeding of the umbilical cord as criminal cases, by stating that they believed that the cord was left untied on purpose. A paradigmatic example is a 1941 post-mortem report from a forensic physician and a general practitioner from Madrid. These experts did not mention the fact that the cord was cut at the level of the navel for justifying the likeliness that the haemorrhage was the cause of death: instead, they mentioned it because they believed it 'obviously demonstrates that the lack of care was voluntary'. Besides this reconstruction of the deeds, they also went on to infer that the child's injuries around the mouth were 'without any doubt' a result of someone's attempt to silence the baby's cries. This, moreover, was for them evidence that besides the mother of the child someone else must have intervened in the delivery and crime.[55]

To these epistemic ideals could be added physicians' aim to show adherence to the regime and collaboration with Francoist courts. Colleagues and authorities of the dictatorship impelled forensic physicians to collaborate with the regime and act in coherence with its ideology and religion. This point was expressed by the Falangist Antonio de la Fuente with the lemma, 'We do not want mere technicians of legal medicine'.[56] This normative discourse meant to intimidate and set the tone for a renewed Francoist forensic culture, as direct ideological purges themselves did.[57] Given this context, forensic physicians and other medical doctors appointed as experts by the courts, could have regarded the task of helping the courts, and the legal mandate to find a cause of death, as a stricter demand than in other political contexts. Historians and STS scholars have discussed how impartiality – understood as experts' neutrality and independence regarding the interests of the parties – has been a key value of forensic expertise in criminal matters, particularly in legal systems in which some experts were appointed by the defence and others by the prosecution.[58] Medical examiners in the Franco regime were presented with an additional ideal: they were encouraged to mainly collaborate with the regime, which could be interpreted as an order to help in the prosecution of criminals.

In sum, while the Francoist forensic culture appropriated many elements of the nineteenth-century configuration of the Spanish forensic culture, shared by other European countries, its specific shape bolstered these continuities by explicitly framing them in the new dictatorial context. The outcome, the Francoist forensic culture, facilitated indictments and convictions that fitted in assumptions and prejudices in line with pronatalist policies and ideas. This led to a situation in which, despite the contemporary scientific state of the art, which denounced the hypothesis of the fatal haemorrhage as rare, this hypothesis was commonly found to apply in cases of infanticide, leading to indictments and convictions. Experts and jurists were already prone to accepting that unmarried mothers had killed their babies by not tying the cord, but arriving at such a conclusion was facilitated by the character of the Spanish forensic culture and its continuation and specific shape in the Francoist regime.

Conclusion

The specific medical issue of whether the umbilical cord haemorrhage was fatal came up in several infanticide trials in Spain in the period 1937–1969. When this happened, medical and legal practitioners accepted this possibility more often than researchers and leading authors in medico-legal literature. I have pointed to several factors that explain this discrepancy between theory and practice, which concern the shape of the Francoist forensic culture. One important factor was that courts regarded forensic physicians and generalists as sufficiently competent in obstetric matters. Both epistemic ideals and indirect political pressures to collaborate with the Francoist state could have encouraged medical experts to provide conclusive reports and exclude any discussion of theoretical debates and jargon. Thus, experts' specific assessments regarding the likelihood of a fatal umbilical cord haemorrhage were uncommon, and they could negatively impact the expert's image.

Moreover, the Francoist forensic culture, building on the previous Spanish configuration of criminal procedure, left little space for the questioning and discussion of factual evidence in appeals, making it impossible for defence attorneys to contest the factual decisions of courts. All this shaped a context in which previous decisions building on the haemorrhage of the cord as cause of death were likely to be repeated, and concrete attempts to question this repetition did not have a reasonable chance to succeed. This analysis shows how the application of the concept of forensic culture can help to add precision and complexity to the available historiography about medical evidence in cases of infanticide: in some contexts, medical evidence contributed to indictments and convictions, and did not only function as a vehicle to mete out lenient sentences.

But this example also demonstrates that it is necessary to consider medical experts as crucial agents of the Francoist justice in the criminal law jurisdiction. Previous works have already shown the importance of assessments of dangerousness, corruption, document forgery, and manipulation of scientific theories and conclusions in regard to medical expertise functioning in the dictatorship. The fact that medical expertise was also important in other types of cases shows that more research is needed about the mechanisms by which the Francoist justice, including the ordinary criminal jurisdiction, worked as a key means for repression. Indeed, the configuration of medical expertise and the specific shape of the Spanish forensic culture in the dictatorship contributed crucially to criminal investigations and trials in which the enforcement of pronatalist policies and ideas was at stake, as the case of infanticide and the umbilical cord has illustrated.

Notes

This project has received funding from the European Research Council (ERC) under the European Union's Horizon 2020 research and innovation programme (grant agreement no 770402).

1 Amongst others: Kerstin Michalik, 'The Development of the Discourse on Infanticide in the Late Eighteenth Century and the New Legal Standardization of the Offense in the Nineteenth Century', in Ulrike Gleixner and Marion W. Gray (eds), *Gender in Transition: Discourse and Practice in German-Speaking Europe, 1750–1830* (Michigan: The University of Michigan Press, 2006), pp. 51–71; Willemijn Ruberg, 'Travelling Knowledge and Forensic Medicine: Infanticide, Body and Mind in the Netherlands, 1811–1911', *Medical History* 57:3 (2013), pp. 359–376; Silvia Chiletti, 'Infanticide and the Prostitute: Honour,

Sentiment and Deviancy between Human Sciences and the Law', in Valeria P. Babini, Chiara Beccalossi and Lucy Riall (eds), *Italian Sexualities Uncovered, 1789–1914* (Basingstoke: Palgrave MacMillan, 2015), pp. 143–161.

2 See also: Karen M. Brennan, ' "A Fine Mixture of Pity and Justice": The Criminal Justice Response to Infanticide in Ireland, 1922–1949', *Law and History Review* 31:4 (2013), pp. 793–841; Rachel Dixon, *Infanticide: Expert Evidence and Testimony in Child Murder Cases, 1688–1955* (Abingdon: Routledge, 2021).

3 Simone Geoffroy-Poisson, 'L'infanticide devant la cour d'assises de la Haute-Marne au XIXe siècle', *Les Cahiers du Centre de Recherches Historiques* 35 (2005), online, p. 11.

4 Sara McDougall and Felicity Turner, 'Introduction: Rethinking the Criminalization of Childbirth: Infanticide in Premodern Europe and the Modern Americas', *Law and History Review* 39:2 (2021), pp. 225–228, here p. 228.

5 Nora E. Jaffary, 'Maternity and Morality in Puebla's Nineteenth-Century Infanticide Trials', *Law and History Review* 39:2 (2021), pp. 299–319, here p. 309.

6 Yet, she did not provide evidence showing that this was a generalised practice, and she did not analyse the role of experts. Kristin Ruggiero, 'Honor, Maternity, and the Disciplining of Women: Infanticide in Late Nineteenth-Century Buenos Aires', *Hispanic American Historical Review* 72:3 (1992), pp. 353–373, here pp. 360, 363–364.

7 Supreme Court of Spain, Judgment of 26 November 1928, ECLI:ES:TS:1928:844 (European Case Law Identifier, for metadata and full judgment search in: https://e-justice.europa.eu/430/EN/european_case_law_identifier_ecli_search_engine?clang=en).

8 My total sample (taking into account all kinds of sources) is biased towards the 1940s and 1950s, given that only six of 139 began in the 1960s. Besides fifteen cassation appeal dossiers from the 1940s (Archivo Histórico Nacional) and twenty-four judgments by the Supreme Court from 1939 to 1969 published in the database of the CENDOJ (www.poderjudicial.es), which cover all the Spanish territory, my sample consists of one hundred complete court files (pre-trial and court dossiers) from six provinces: all the cases available at the archives from Tarragona (investigations that began from 1936 to 1960), Ávila (1937–1945), Girona (1939–1952) and Madrid (1939–1959), and random selections from Guadalajara and Toledo from the 1940s and 1950s. This sample of complete court files includes investigations of newborn child murder that began as investigations of parricide, considering all files of parricide available from Girona,

and a random selection from the other provinces. This sample of complete court files includes dismissals and cases where suspects stood trial. To assess the representativeness of my sample of complete court files in concrete, it is useful to compare it with prosecutors' statistics, which are available for the period 1944–1959, not before. For the period 1944–1959 I consulted all the (twenty-five) cases that were registered in the inventories from Madrid's archive (*Archivo General de la Administración*). These only cover a small part (less than 1 per cent) of the cases that were allegedly investigated in that province (2,068), assuming that prosecutors' statistics of the time were certain. In provinces other than Madrid, albeit there are also some discrepancies between archival records and statistics, the total number of cases investigated was lower, so the cases available from the period 1944–1959 cover a larger percentage of the total than in the case of Madrid: eight of thirty-one (Girona), four of five (Ávila) and nine of thirteen (Tarragona). The sample for Toledo and Guadalajara was exploratory and randomly selected, covering (for the period 1944–1959) two of thirty-one (Toledo) and five of twenty-four cases (Guadalajara). Further details about my sample are available upon request. For the statistics, see the memos published each year from 1945 to 1960 by the chief prosecutors, available online: www.fiscal.es/documentaci%C3%B3n?sort=publishDate%2B&q=memoria.

9 Juan Francisco Gómez Westermeyer, 'Historia de la delincuencia en la sociedad española: Murcia, 1939–1949: Similitudes y diferencias en otros espacios europeos' (PhD thesis, Universidad de Murcia, 2006), p. 346; Tamara López Fernández, 'Aunque me cueste la vida. El aborto en el Partido Judicial de Lugo (1945–1960)', in Ismael Saz Campos *et al.* (eds), *X Trobada Internacional Investigadorxs del Franquisme* (València: Comissions Obreres del País Valencià and Universitat de València, 2021), pp. 781–796, here p. 795.

10 Adrián Sánchez Castillo, 'La "justicia" de Franco en Calera y Chozas (Toledo) falsificación documental y en-cubrimiento de asesinatos extrajudiciales en la posguerra española', *Revista Universitaria de Historia Militar* 17:8 (2019), pp. 229–254; César Lorenzo Rubio, 'La máquina represiva: la tortura en el franquismo', in Pedro Oliver Olmo (ed.), *La tortura en la España contemporánea* (Madrid: *Catarata*, 2020), pp. 131–198.

11 Carolina García Sanz, ' "Disciplinando al gitano" en el siglo XX: regulación y parapenalidad en España desde una perspectiva europea', *Historia y Política* 40 (2018), pp. 115–146; Ricardo Campos Marín, 'La construcción psiquiátrica del sujeto peligroso y la Ley de Vagos y Maleantes en la España franquista (1939–1970)',

Culturas Psi 7 (2016), pp. 9–44; Abel Díaz, 'Afeminados de vida ociosa: Sexualidad, género y clase social durante el franquismo', *Historia Contemporánea* 65 (2021), pp. 131–162.

12 Stephanie Wright, '"Caballeros mutilados" y mujeres "deshonradas": cuerpo, género y privilegio en la posguerra española', *Historia y Política* 47 (2022), pp. 163–192, here pp. 182–183.
13 Leopoldo López Gómez and Juan Antonio Gisbert Calabuig, *Tratado de medicina legal*, vol. 1 (Valencia: Saber, 1961), p. 214. Original: 'se consideran completamente excepcionales, e incluso inverosímiles'.
14 Antonio Lecha-Marzo, *Tratado de autopsias y embalsamamientos: el diagnóstico médico legal en el cadáver* (Madrid: Los Progresos de la Clínica, 1917), p. 363.
15 Étienne Martin, *Manual de Medicina Legal*, trans. Wilfredo Coroleu (Barcelona: Salvat, 1942), p. 657.
16 Spain, Tarragona, Arxiu Històric de Tarragona (AHT), Audiència Provincial de Tarragona, 'Sumari 280/1950', Installation unit 3253, Correlative unit 486; Guillermo Uribe Cualla, *Medicina Legal y Psiquiatría Forense* (Madrid-Bogotá: Ediciones Guadarrama S.L., 1957, 7th edn), p. 484.
17 Pedro Mata, *Tratado de medicina y cirugía legal*, vol. 1, 2nd edn (Madrid: Imprenta de Don Joaquin Merás y Suarez, 1846), pp. 438–439; Ambroise Tardieu, *Étude médico-légale sur l'infanticide* (Paris: Ballière et Fils, 1868), pp. 189–193.
18 Antonio Piga, José Águila Collantes and Blas Aznar, *Manual Teórico Práctico de Medicina Forense. La presente obra contesta al programa de médicos forenses. Tomo I* (Madrid: Instituto Reus, 1935).
19 Albert Ponsold, *Manual de Medicina Legal*, trans. Manuel Sellés (Barcelona: Salvat, 1954), p. 317.
20 Luis C. Rodríguez Ramos, 'LÓPEZ GÓMEZ, Leopoldo y GISBERT CALABUIG, Juan Antonio. "Tratado de Medicina legal". Editorial Saber, Valencia, 1967, T. I., 843 págs.; T. II., 583 págs., T. III., 595 págs.', *Anuario de Derecho Penal y Ciencias Penales. Fascículo 2. Revista de Libros* (1969) pp. 401–402, here p. 401. Original: 'considerado [...] como el más completo y el que alcanza un mayor rango científico entre los textos dedicados al tema'. Vicente Moya Pueyo *et al.*, *Medicina Legal y Forense*, vol. 1 (Madrid, 1972), p. 4.
21 Spain, Alcalá de Henares, Ministerio de Cultura y Deporte, Archivo General de la Administración (hereafter AGA), Catalog (07) 51_00, Catalog number 26/12298, Audiencia Provincial de Madrid, 'Sumario 8/1959', fol. 22 rear. Original: 'signos de violencia mecanica [sic]', 'pérdida de sangre'.

22 AGA, Catalog (07) 01_13, Catalog number 41/00708, Audiencia Provincial de Madrid, 'Sumario 342/1941, Rollo 6860/1941'; AGA, Catalog (07) 01_23, Catalog number 41/01334, Audiencia Provincial de Madrid, 'Sumario 40/1941'; AGA Catalog (07) 01_ 28, Catalog number 41/06319, Audiencia Provincial de Madrid, 'Sumario 150/1943'; AGA Catalog (07) 01_36, Catalog number 41/ 07192, Audiencia Provincial de Madrid, 'Sumario 231/1944, Rollo 31/1945'; AGA Catalog (07) 01_36 41/07228. Audiencia Provincial de Madrid, 'Sumario 106/1944'. AGA Catalog (07) 01_55, Catalog number 41/15213, Audiencia Provincial de Madrid, 'Sumario 341/ 1947'; Spain, Ávila, Archivo Histórico Provincial de Ávila (hereafter AHPAv), Catalog number 037405, Audiencia Provincial de Ávila, 'Sumario 10/1937, Rollo 61/1937'; AHPAv, Catalog number 037433, Audiencia Provincial de Ávila, 'Sumario 10/1939, Rollo 33/ 1939'; Spain, Toledo, Archivo Histórico Provincial de Toledo (hereafter APHTO), Catalog number 70241/2, Audiencia Provincial de Toledo, 'Sumario 37/1943, Rollo 692/1943'; Spain, Guadalajara, Archivo Histórico Provincial de Guadalajara (AHPGU), Catalog number J-001214, Audiencia Provincial de Guadalajara, 'Sumario 32/1945, Rollo 180/1945', AHPGU, Catalog number J-001234, Audiencia Provincial de Guadalajara, 'Sumario 230/1948', and AHPGU Catalog number J-000250, Audiencia Provincial de Guadalajara, 'Sumario 40/1949, Rollo 128/1949'; Spain, Girona, Arxiu Històric de Girona (hereafter AHG), Catalog number 129/6, Audiència Provincial de Girona, 'Causa 86/1943, Rotlle 505/1943', AHG, Catalog number 247/1, Audiència Provincial de Girona. 'Causa 87/1950, Rotlle 386/1950'; Spain, Madrid, Ministerio de Cultura y Deporte, Archivo Histórico Nacional (hereafter AHN), ES.28079/6//FC-TRIBUNAL_SUPREMO_PENAL (Supreme Court of Spain, Criminal Law), Box 10, Case file 1126; Box 5, Case file 965; Box 61, Case file 148; Box 149, Case file 1436. Supreme Court of Spain, Judgments of 3 March 1949 (ECLI:ES:TS:1949:803), 21 April 1951 (ECLI:ES:TS:1951:1242), and 12 June 1957 (ECLI:ES:TS:1957:422).

23 In one case judges concluded this while the physicians had claimed they could not determine a cause of death (AHN, ES.28079/6//FC _ TRIBUNAL_SUPREMO_PENAL Box 5, Case file 965). In other cases the autopsy report was missing (because the investigation dossier was unduly destroyed: AGA, Catalog (07) 01_36, Catalog number 41/ 07192) or was not kept in the archive I consulted.

24 AGA, Catalog (07) 01_23, Catalog number 41/01334, Audiencia Provincial de Madrid, 'Sumario 40/1941'.

25 AHPTO, Catalog number 70241/2, Audiencia Provincial de Toledo, 'Sumario 37/1943, Rollo 692/1943'; AHG, Catalog number 129/6, Audiència Provincial de Girona, 'Causa 86/1943, Rotlle 505/1943', AHG, Catalog number 247/1, Audiència Provincial de Girona. 'Causa 87/1950, Rotlle 386/1950'; AGA, (07) 01_23, 41/01334, Audiencia Provincial de Madrid, 'Sumario 40/1941'; AGA (07) 01_36, 41/07228, Audiencia Provincial de Madrid, 'Sumario 106/1944'; AHPAv Catalog number 037405, Audiencia Provincial de Ávila, 'Sumario 10/1937, Rollo 61/1937'; AHG Catalog number 129/6, Audiència Provincial de Girona, 'Causa 86/1943, Rotlle 505/1943'; López Gómez and Gisbert Calabuig, *Tratado*, 1, p. 214 Martin, *Manual*, p. 657.

26 AGA, Catalog (07) 01_28, Catalog number 41/06319, Audiencia Provincial de Madrid, 'Sumario 150/1943'; AGA Catalog 01_13, Catalog number 41/00708, Audiencia Provincial de Madrid, 'Sumario 342/1941, Rollo 6860/1941'; AHPGU, Catalog number J-1234, Audiencia Provincial de Guadalajara, 'Sumario 230/1948'. Original: 'a dos traveses de dedo'. This autopsy report, though, indicated that once opened there was no 'clot' in the cord (Original: 'cohágulo' [sic]).

27 AHT, Audiència Provincial de Tarragona, 'Sumari 80/1946', Installation unit 3524, Correlative unit 182.

28 Supreme Court of Spain, Judgment of 27 February 1967, ECLI:ES:TS:1967:2370. Original: 'en el supuesto de no haberle asfixiado conseguiría dar muerte a su nacido hijo'.

29 AGA Catalog (07) 01_36, Catalog number 41/07209, Audiencia Provincial de Madrid, 'Sumario 99/1944, Rollo 685/1944', AHN, ES.28079.AHN/6//FC-TRIBUNAL_SUPREMO_Penal, Box 5, Case file 965; Supreme Court of Spain, Judgments of 10 March 1949 (ECLI:ES:TS:1949:803), 8 May 1959 (ECLI:ES:TS:1959:1107), 24 March 1960 (ECLI:ES:TS:1960:1637), 27 February 1967 (ECLI:ES:TS:1967:2370), 3 June 1967 (ECLI:ES:TS:1967:2827), 15 January 1968 (ECLI:ES:TS:1968:1129), and 3 June 1969 (ECLI:ES:TS:1969:1027).

30 Only two cases were dismissed, one because the suspect was found to be unaccountable and the other because no suspect could be identified. AHPAv, Catalog number 037433, Audiencia Provincial de Ávila, 'Sumario 10/1939, Rollo 33/1939'; AGA, Catalog (07) 01_55, Catalog number 41/15213, Audiencia Provincial de Madrid, 'Sumario 341/1947'. We cannot rule out the possibility that there were cases in which someone – including the police or peace courts – decided not to report a case for thinking that the untied cord was not suspicious of

criminality, but these decisions would either leave no trace or would only be traceable through municipal archives throughout Spain, out of the scope of my sample. For the acquittal see: AHPAv, Catalog number 037405, Audiencia Provincial de Ávila, 'Sumario 10/1937. Rollo 61/1937'.
31 AHPAv, Catalog number 037405, Audiencia Provincial de Ávila, 'Sumario 10/1937, Rollo 61/1937'.
32 AHG, Catalog number 129/6, Audiència Provincial de Girona, 'Causa 86/1943, Rotlle 505/1943'.
33 Laura Sánchez Blanco, 'Las políticas demográficas italiana y española: l'Opera Nazionale per la protezione della Maternità e dell'Infanzia y la Obra Nacional-Sindicalista de Protección a la Madre y al Niño', in Patrizia Botta et al. (eds), *Rumbos del hispanismo en el umbral del Cincuentenario de la AIH*, vol. 7 (Roma: Bagatto Libri, 2012), pp. 227–236.
34 AHN, ES.28079/6//FC _TRIBUNAL_SUPREMO_PENAL Box 5, Case file 965. Original: 'esta prueba se robustece con el hecho de ir a dar a luz la procesada a la cuadra y meterlo en un saco y enterrarlo, de suerte que si la inculpada no hubiera querido matar al niño para tapar su deshonra, hubiera ligado el cordón umbilical y el acto del parto lo hubiese celebrado en sitio más adecuado'.
35 Irene Palacio Lis, *Mujeres ignorantes: madres culpables. Adoctrinamiento y divulgación materno-infantil en la primera mitad del siglo XX* (Valencia: Universitat de València, 2003). Salvador Cayuela Sánchez, 'La biopolítica en la España franquista' (PhD thesis, Universidad de Murcia, 2010).
36 Ruggiero, 'Honor, Maternity', p. 363.
37 Supreme Court of Spain, Judgment of 18 October 1962, ECLI:ES:TS:1962:530.
38 Palacio Lis, *Mujeres ignorantes*, p. 199. Original, as cited by Palacios: 'clásica misión fiscal en la crianza de los nietos'.
39 AGA, Catalog (07) 01_28, Catalog number 41/06319, Audiencia Provincial de Madrid, 'Sumario 150/1943'.
40 Mónica Lanero Táboas, 'Proyectos falangistas y política judicial (1937–1952): dos modelos de organización judicial del Nuevo Estado', *Investigaciones históricas: Época moderna y contemporánea* 15 (1995), pp. 353–372.
41 Regarding the nineteenth-century reform of procedural laws in Spain see: Enrique Álvarez Cora, 'La evolución del enjuiciamiento en el siglo XIX', *Anuario de Historia del Derecho Español* (2012), pp. 81–112.
42 'Ley disponiendo que los artículos que se mencionan de la ley de Enjuiciamiento criminal queden redactados en la forma que se indica', *Gazeta de Madrid* 188 (7 July 1933), pp. 139–140.

43 AHN, ES.28079/6//FC _TRIBUNAL_SUPREMO_PENAL Box 5, Case file 965. Original: 'más allá que el dictamen médico del sumario'.
44 Amongst others: Supreme Court of Spain, Judicial Decree of 9 April 1951, ECLI:ES:TS:1951:47A.
45 Juan Manuel Jiménez Muñoz, *Historia legislativa del cuerpo de médicos forenses* (Valladolid: Universidad de Valladolid, 1974).
46 AHG, Catalog number 129/6, Audiència Provincial de Girona, 'Causa 86/1943, Rotlle 505/1943'. Whether the cord was customarily tied is unclear, since some manuals appear to have doubted this was the case, aiming at teaching women to tie the cord: A. Frias Roig, *Lo que deben saber las madres* (Madrid: Publicaciones "Al servicio de España y del Niño Español", 1946), p. 11. Moreover, that custom or medical advice did not assume the haemorrhage's fatality: as the gynaecologists appointed by the prosecutor in the case from Girona said, blood loss through the cord was not fatal, but it was not good for the child, especially if added to other health conditions or lack of care in general.
47 'Ley de Enjuiciamiento Criminal', *Gazeta de Madrid*, 274 (1 October 1882), p. 3.
48 'Ley de Enjuiciamiento Criminal', *Gazeta de Madrid*, 274 (3 October 1882), p. 19.
49 Gregorio Nieto Nieto, *La autopsia médico-legal* (Soria: Imp. Casa de Observación, 1947), pp. 10 and 14; López Gómez, Gisbert Calabuig, *Tratado* 1, p. 62. Original: 'No se precisan razonamientos, ya que se declara bajo juramento'.
50 Nicholas Duvall, 'Reporting Violent Death: Networks of Expertise and the Scottish Post-mortem', in: Alison Adam (ed.), *Crime and the Construction of Forensic Objectivity from 1850* (London: Palgrave, 2020), pp. 211–229, here p. 213.
51 Duvall, 'Reporting Violent Death', p. 214; Nicholas Duvall, 'Forensic Medicine in Scotland, 1914–39' (PhD thesis, University of Manchester, 2013), p. 34.
52 AHG, Catalog number 129/6, Audiència Provincial de Girona, 'Causa 86/1943, Rotlle 505/1943'.
53 López Gómez, Gisbert Calabuig, *Tratado*, 1, p. 62.
54 López Gómez, Gisbert Calabuig, *Tratado*, 1, p. 78; Nieto, *La autopsia*, pp. 85–89; Eduardo Guija Morales, *Introducción a la metódica funcional para el diagnóstico medicoforense* (Barcelona: Ediciones BYP, 1950).
55 AGA, Catalog (07) 01_23, Catalog number 41/01334, Audiencia Provincial de Madrid, 'Sumario 40/1941', fol. 11 front. Original: 'demuestra evidentemente que esta falta de cuidado fue hecha voluntariamente', 'sin género de duda'.

56 Alfonso de la Fuente Chaos, *Los valores morales del nacional-sindicalismo y la medicina legal* (Madrid: Ediciones de la Vicesecretaría de Educación Popular, 1942). Original: 'No queremos simples técnicos de la medicina legal'.

57 As was also the case with other public servants, medical doctors and forensic physicians were purged if they were regarded as ideologically contrary to the new Regime, or if they had held important political or administrative positions in the Second Republic. Mónica Lanero Táboas, *Una milicia de la justicia. Política judicial del franquismo (1936–1945)* (Madrid: Centro de Estudios Constitucionales, 1996).

58 For instance: Christopher Hamlin, 'Scientific Method and Expert Witnessing: Victorian Perspectives on a Modern Problem', *Social Studies of Science* 16:3 (1986), pp. 485–513; Sheila Jasanoff, *Science at the Bar: Law, Science, and Technology in America* (Cambridge, MA: Harvard University Press, 1997); Barbara J. Shapiro, 'Testimony in Seventeenth-Century English Philosophy: Legal Origins and Early Development', *Studies in History and Philosophy of Science* 33:2 (2002), pp. 243–263; Alison Adam, *A History of Forensic Science: British Beginnings in the Twentieth Century* (Abingdon: Routledge, 2016); Riccardo Montana, 'Prosecution in Action in the Italian Justice System: The Amanda Knox Case', in Lieve Gies and Maria Bortoluzzi (eds), *Transmedia Crime Stories* (Basingstoke: Palgrave, 2016), pp. 167–188.

9

Doing law, psychiatric expertise and 'crimes of passion' in the Netherlands and Russia in the twentieth century

Volha Parfenchyk and Willemijn Ruberg

Introduction

In recent years, feminist activists have called for renewed attention for and solutions to 'femicide' or the killing of women because they are women, by men, often their (ex-)partners. They proposed the term 'femicide' also as a replacement for the older notion of 'crimes of passion', regarding the latter term as a euphemism, that glamourised violence against women while also condoning or mitigating male aggression. As a legal term 'femicide' has been included as a separate crime in Latin American countries in the early twenty-first century.[1] This coining of new terms in relation to gendered crime does justice to the harrowing facts of violence to women. It dovetails with the aims of feminist legal studies, which demonstrate that the power of law – and the naming of crimes is one aspect of that – is not neutral and often works to the disadvantage of women and ethnic or LGBT+ minorities.

At the same time, legal scholars have pointed to the difficulties in defining femicide and to the way this term may also obscure the different motives for crimes against women.[2] From a historical perspective we can add that the term 'femicide' seems to describe an ahistorical, asymmetrical relationship between violent men and female victims. Arguably this term neglects both the historical and cultural variability of femicide and dealing with it. In this chapter we provide an historical and cross-cultural analysis of how different actors, such as the legislature, the judiciary and psychiatrists, together shaped the definition and prosecution of the precursors of femicide, i.e. the 'crime of passion', as they were called in most Western European countries, and 'a homicide motivated by jealousy' in Russia. Taking a cultural-historical perspective, we use as a working definition a crime that revolved around an intimate relationship between adult men and women, and in which particularly love and jealousy played a role, including both male and female perpetrators and victims. Although this crime could be committed by both men and women, in the vast majority of cases the perpetrator was male, and the victim female. We provide two case studies – the Netherlands and Russia – to show how these crimes of passion have been defined by the law and prosecuted in practice in the twentieth century. We follow Rebekka Habermas's anthropological approach of 'doing law':

> Developments in the legal system result in fact from the constantly changing interaction of norms, actors, and institutions. Thus, the idea that justice is 'set' or 'established' is replaced by the concept of a dynamic process involving a multitude of entities, which, endowed with varying degrees of power, repeatedly renegotiate justice.

'Doing law' entails looking at justice as a 'process of negotiation involving many participants rather than a process of assignment'.[3] In this way, through this cultural comparison and historical analysis, we aim to show that what a 'crime of passion' is, is not self-evident: it is continually debated and negotiated by multiple actors, both through time and space.

Building on our cross-cultural comparison, we conclude that both in Russia and the Netherlands the image of 'crimes of passion' revolved around 'othering': these crimes were seen as typical of other countries or classes, thus confirming a certain self-image. In the Netherlands, cultural and legal discourse claimed that the crime of passion, in which honour was central, was typically French and that the French legal system and press were lenient in their judgment of this crime, in contrast to the sensible, rational and emancipated Dutch. In Russia, political and legal discourse opposed socialism against capitalism, perceiving jealousy at the core of the crime of passion as a pernicious element of the capitalist mentality connected to private property and possessiveness.

However, we demonstrate that this cultural-political image did not always dovetail with legal and forensic practice; the latter was much more complicated than a seemingly consistent cultural discourse surrounding crimes of passion. In the Netherlands, despite the claim that this country was not familiar with the crime of passion, in practice lawyers, prosecutors and psychiatrists regarded the pathology underlying this criminal behaviour as a serious diagnosis, potentially serving to mitigate the sentence of the (often male) perpetrator. In Russia, legal practice did not only connect an act of killing out of jealousy to 'capitalist' greed, but also to the offender's illiteracy and lack of poor education or due to his mental abnormalities. Thus, whereas the cultural and political discourse on crimes of passion clearly identified certain ('other') perpetrators with specific motives, legal practice did not always correspond to this cultural-political imagery, and sometimes even contradicted it. Comparing Russian and Dutch forensic cultures can therefore inform us on the discrepancy between cultural-political images of a certain crime and forensic and legal practice.

Historiography of crimes of passion: national variability

Before we discuss the Dutch and then the Russian case, it is important to sketch how modern European legal systems and forensic psychiatry have responded to the 'crime of passion'. In the fledgling field of forensic psychiatry, doctors explored the relationship between insanity and emotions. From the early nineteenth century, mostly French and German physicians and psychiatrists had coined diagnostical concepts such as 'affective monomania', 'moral insanity' and later – around 1900 – 'psychopathy', notions which were not characterised simply by loss of reason but by the impact on the feelings or morals of the suspect. A perpetrator could display either a total lack of emotion or extreme feelings and yet not be diagnosed as completely insane.[4] This question of the boundaries between normal and pathological emotions, and their connection to insanity, reverberated in the legal and psychiatric discussions on crimes of passion.

The term 'crime of passion' has always been a popular, rather than a legal concept, in the sense that it never was a separate article in the law. However, some legal codes included it as a defence of honour and hence as a mitigating factor. This can be seen first and foremost in the French Code Pénal from 1810, which was also imposed on other countries such as the Netherlands. Its article 324 stated that when a husband murdered his wife and her lover after catching them in adultery in the matrimonial home, his sentence would be reduced. This article was repealed in France in 1975. As Ute Frevert shows, these laws excusing (mostly) men acting out of wounded honour were not limited to southern-European countries.[5] Even if legal codes did not explicitly refer to adultery or honour, the notion of 'temporary insanity' could be used in judicial practice to refer to the emotional condition of the perpetrator serving as an excuse for the crime and possibly to a more lenient sentence. Emotions as part of the 'heat of passion' argument could thus act as a cover for honour.[6] Thus, throughout the twentieth century and in different legal systems, legal codes have allowed for a specific, possibly more lenient treatment for perpetrators of crimes of passion either implicitly or explicitly.

Historians have furthermore pointed to the presence of a jury and the influence of forensic psychiatrists as factors leading to an allowance of mitigating circumstances for perpetrators of crimes of passion. The jury is regarded as championing a popular acceptance of 'just' violence when gender norms were violated, leading to more lenient sentences for (male) perpetrators of crimes of passion, particularly relating to adulterous wives. A closer look at the empirical findings of historians, however, shows that the role of the jury in several countries has been variable.[7] Juries could also be out of step with a shifting popular opinion and cultural circumstances impacted variously in different countries.[8]

In most countries, the participation of forensic psychiatrists in court cases increased in the twentieth century. Psychiatrists themselves devoted numerous studies to the crime of passion, to sketch perpetrator profiles and explain the motives behind this deed. The infamous Italian criminal anthropologist Lombroso in the 1870s regarded perpetrators of crimes of passion as lofty and honourable in contrast to common criminals.[9] In contrast, one of Lombroso's followers, the doctor Léon Rabinowicz, saw the perpetrator of crimes of passion in the 1930s as abnormal and ill.[10] Historian Joëlle Guillais therefore argues that after 1930, criminologists and psychiatrists viewed these crimes as dangerous, testifying to a bloodthirsty temperament.[11] However, this pathologisation had started earlier. As Maurice Cottier mentions, already in the first decade of the twentieth century German and French doctors addressed pathological jealousy.[12] Generally, forensic doctors and psychiatrists were increasingly involved in many European countries, but they were not all-powerful or overruling the judiciary.[13] The influence of forensic psychiatry in the legal system showed many national variations.

To summarise, nearly all modern European legal systems in the twentieth century allowed for some kind of lenient treatment of perpetrators of crimes of passion, either via the law or via forensic psychiatry. In the following analysis we explore which actors were involved in 'doing law' regarding these crimes and what roles specific cultural-political imagery played in the Netherlands and Russia.

The image of the crime of passion in the Netherlands

In the Netherlands – which had an inquisitorial system without a jury – the crime of passion never existed in the law but was prosecuted as murder or homicide. Nevertheless, in judicial practice prosecutors, lawyers and forensic psychiatrists did refer to 'crimes of passion'. Before we explain what role this notion played in judicial practice, we will address the Dutch cultural image of the crime of passion and the ways psychiatry defined this type of crime.

Dutch texts written by criminologists and psychiatrists as well as Dutch newspapers testify to a representation of crimes of passion as 'French' and 'other', mostly in regard to its judgment, though sometimes also in regard to the motive and the type of perpetrator. Especially during the first half of the twentieth century, the crime was associated with typical French or southern-European passion and 'traditional French clemency towards a crime passionnel'[14] because of the French jury system. The jury as well as the French sensationalised press were seen to contribute to popular understanding of this crime.[15] In 1938, a prosecutor in a court case stated that: 'The general precaution demands, that in our country a "crime passionnel" is not given a conditional sentence.'[16] In 1947 psychiatrist Gerrit Kempe elaborated that 'although it is correct that generally southern peoples are more violent than northern', the main difference was caused by the legal system: the French jury treated especially female perpetrators of crimes of passion leniently. A lay jury, according to Kempe, was different from 'experienced, cool, and critical professional judges'. Moreover, these types of cases gave eloquent lawyers the chance to 'shine', which, in combination with a sensationalised press, made the crimes in France more conspicuous, in contrast to the 'decent' Dutch newspapers.[17] In short, the French legal system and press were seen to lead to leniency and contrasted with the sober Dutch newspapers and the more professional and distanced Dutch judges.

In other respects, as well, the crime of passion offered an opportunity to compare the Dutch self-image to that of other countries. Firstly, Dutch criminologists and psychiatrists regarded this crime as typical for the lower classes. Sometimes, this was contrasted to the glamorous, more elitist, image of the French crime of passion. In France, psychiatrist Symon Tammenoms Bakker speculated in 1951, perpetrators frequently came from 'intellectual and society' circles. In contrast, the Dutch perpetrators he studied derived from the labouring classes, whom he saw as uninhibited and 'primitive'. Tammenoms Bakker thought that culturally and scientifically educated people held women in higher regard.[18] The connection between class and gender was also made by criminologist Samuel Philips, who found in his 1938 book that most male perpetrators belonged to the working classes.[19] The criminologist argued that it was clear that in the lower classes (he spoke of 'bad milieus') women were less appreciated than in the higher echelons of society. The reaction to disappointed love was regarded as more dangerous in the lower classes because they generally used aggression faster and had not yet grasped the woman's right to self-determination in regard to love. Therefore, Philips found it important to stimulate women's emancipation.[20] The crime of passion could also bolster a nationalist discourse, exemplified in a 1928 murder case in which an Italian man shot his twenty-year-old girlfriend after she had rejected him. During the trial the public prosecutor demanded freedom of choice for Dutch girls regarding fiancés, claiming they should not be terrorised by their male lovers.[21]

Secondly, the national self-image came to the fore in Dutch court cases in which the suspects were immigrants from countries in which honour was paramount. In 1966 an Italian miner killed his Dutch blond, 'Northern'-looking wife after he had caught her with another man, in the presence of his own father. His lawyer pled for clemency since the man was from Sardinia 'where the wife is still considered to be a possession of the man'; and he had been hurt in his honour and manhood before the eyes of his father. The lawyer requested the court take into account that the man was overwhelmed by passion.[22] Foreign honour was also discussed in a case from 1965, in which a man from the Indonesian Kei-island, but living in the Netherlands, had killed his wife's lover. Dutch newspapers applied an orientalist discourse in their reports of the court case. The lover and his son had attacked the husband with a knife and kicked him, to which the latter had retaliated. Therefore the lawyer of the defence argued for self-defence and asked: 'Can a Western person understand this? There are Dutch legal scholars who argue that a sense of honour can prevent a suspect to run away so that resistance [self-defence] can be acceptable.' The prosecutor argued for manslaughter but stated that in fact it was a crime of passion. He pled that 'we should take into account different habits and ideas'. The suspect was sentenced to four years in prison.[23]

In these two court cases honour was presented as a quality that belonged to southern-European or eastern men, not to the Dutch. More generally, the crime of passion as described in Dutch newspapers and psychiatric texts could serve to distinguish the sensible, rational, emancipated Dutch from the passionate Other – often French, or Italian – for whom (male) honour mattered more. This representation dovetailed with the Dutch self-image of a sober, moderate, middle-class and civilised nation.[24]

Dutch psychiatrists and the profile of the criminal of passion

As in other European countries, in the Netherlands, psychiatrists throughout the twentieth century were keen to find the boundaries between normal and pathological jealousy.[25] By mid-century, psychiatrists noted a change in the attitude of criminologists and judges towards crimes of passion: romance was no longer emphasised and the perpetrator had come to be seen as a selfish, mentally unstable human being, who gained personally from his crime.[26] Psychiatrist Tammenoms Bakker noted in 1951 that the perpetrator's aggression was mostly directed at the object of his affection, rather than the lover of his ex. Other hallmarks included partial amnesia and suicidal thoughts and attempts.[27] Nearly all perpetrators had a problematic emotional life, having a strong sense of self-worth and being 'vain, narcissist, selfish and egocentric'. The majority showed a heightened sensitivity about being hurt themselves but less receptive for pain afflicted to others. Tammenoms Bakker concluded: 'The perpetrator of the crime passionnel is irritable, aggressive, suspicious, and jealous.'[28] He divided this crime into two types: the 'normal' characterological crime and the 'abnormal' psychopathological passionate crime, evenly divided over the sixty-four cases of crimes of passion (in three of which the perpetrators were women) he studied in the Amsterdam prison in 1928–1951. His research was based on psychiatric and new 'psychological-experimental' research, yet exactly how Tammenoms Bakker made this distinction remains unclear. In fact, he often underlined that the dividing line between the two groups was vague and that only gradation and intensity of certain mental aberrations determined whether perpetrators belonged to one group or the other.[29] The difficulty of distinguishing 'normal' from 'pathological' perpetrators of crimes of passion thus comes to the fore in psychiatric studies.

In addition to the pathologisation of the criminal of passion, the psychiatric profiles of the perpetrators show both consistency and change. Psychiatrists all saw similar elements in the profile of this criminal: a jealous, selfish person with emotional or mental problems, who acted from disappointed love. Throughout the twentieth century, Dutch forensic psychiatrists and criminologists found that most perpetrators stemmed from the lower classes and the vast majority were male. The number of female perpetrators, however, was seen to increase: whereas criminologist Philips found that 5.46 per cent of perpetrators (over the period 1915–1934) of crimes of passion were female,[30] in de Boer's study of partner killings over the period 1950–1980 17 per cent were women.[31]

Psychiatrists tried to distinguish 'reasonable' from abnormal behaviour. In regard to the gender of the victim, interestingly, Tammenoms Bakker added a table dividing the behaviour of the victim (the vast majority of whom were women) into good, bad and 'questionable' behaviour, since the victim's abominable behaviour could lead to sympathy for the perpetrator, whose acts should otherwise be disapproved of.³² That older cultural ideas on gender continued to exist also surfaces in Dutch newspapers. Some women who were the victims of men who committed 'crimes of passion' were blamed for their –often adulterous– behaviour. In 1972, a twenty-six-year-old male student had shot his rival in love, the husband of the woman he was having an affair with. The prosecutor reprimanded this woman for her behaviour: she 'had to assess for herself to what extent she was on trial here, too'. He pled for diminished accountability for the suspect and for manslaughter, not murder, since during the crime there was no calm deliberation. The suspect was sentenced to six years' imprisonment for murder. In the verdict a mitigating circumstance was 'his passion for the woman and the long-lasting stress resulting from her attitude towards him'. The court accepted the psychiatric reports but saw no connection between the suspect's mental illness and his crime.³³ In other cases in which men were the suspects, adulterous women were blamed as well. In the early twenty-first century women have come to be regarded more as victims. This increasing attention to female victims can thus be added to the most consistent trend since the mid-twentieth century: the pathologisation of the criminal of passion, for which psychiatrists tried to demarcate abnormal from normal perpetrators. Experts thus participated in 'doing law': the process of negotiation that produces justice.

Sentences and treatment in Dutch practice

Considering the fact that the crime of passion never existed in the Dutch legal code and that Dutch cultural and psychiatric discourse distanced itself from this 'foreign' crime, it is remarkable that in practice the term 'crime of passion' was not only used in newspapers covering court cases, but also by prosecutors, defence lawyers and psychiatrists in the courtroom. Throughout the twentieth century prosecutors and lawyers for the defence argued for clemency based on the fact that the crime was committed out of passion, that is from strong, sudden emotions or in a bout of insanity, which could imply (partial) unaccountability or mitigating circumstances. Interestingly, psychiatrists called in as expert witnesses were sometimes literally asked whether they considered the act a crime of passion, even though that was neither a specific crime listed in the criminal code, nor an official psychiatric label. For instance, in his 1962 psychiatric report on the case of a twenty-five-year-old Italian factory employee who had stabbed a female colleague, professor Pieter Baan wrote there was no *crime passionnel*. However, he did conclude that even though the man was not suffering from a mental illness, in the weeks before the crime he had an increasing 'strong pathological aberration of the mind' and at the moment of the crime he was 'in a quiet pathological condition'. Therefore, Baan concluded that he was unaccountable and on the basis of his report and that of a psychologist, the man was held unaccountable by the court, sent to an asylum and given TBR (Ter Beschikking van de Regering) or psychiatric treatment as punishment.[34]

The TBR (later TBS) system was established as part of the Dutch psychopath laws in 1928. These laws gave judges the power to send fully and partially irresponsible criminals to an asylum for psychopaths after their potential prison sentence. This TBR status could be indefinitely extended by the judge every two years and was intended to provide treatment for the perpetrator and protection from dangerous delinquents for society.[35] The role of forensic psychiatry was expanded in later decades. Especially the first decade after the Second World War testified to increased institutionalisation of Dutch forensic psychiatry and witnessed a strong trust in the latter by the judiciary.[36]

In cases of crimes of passion, the Dutch judiciary often followed the expert advice of forensic psychiatrists, testifying to a cooperation between the law and psychiatry and leading to a high percentage of convictions which included both prison sentences and psychiatric treatment. In his 1938 study criminologist Philips, based on a total of 183 cases, concluded that crimes of passion accounted for 18 per cent of convictions for murder and manslaughter and 27.8 per cent of all murder convictions for the period 1915–1934.[37] In regard to punishment, these criminals received high sentences. Even though Philips' research is not based on the psychiatric reports made for the court cases, he was convinced that the number of psychiatric reports made for this type of crime was higher than for other crimes: 44 per cent were examined psychiatrically (only one woman); for 34 per cent of the examined men a ground for diminished accountability was found.[38]

This high level of psychiatric involvement in and impact on punishment was confirmed in the 1951 study on the period 1928–1951 by psychiatrist Tammenoms Bakker. He divided the perpetrators of crimes of passion into normal and abnormal ones. Of the thirty-two 'normal' perpetrators, seven (22 per cent) were sentenced while taking mitigating circumstances into account. Of the thirty-two 'abnormal' perpetrators, twenty-two were found less accountable, three unaccountable, seven received psychiatric treatment as sentence and were sent to a psychiatric institution (all showed signs of paranoid psychoses).[39] Thus, for nearly all of the 'abnormal' ones their mental condition determined the kind of treatment and punishment they received, but it is striking that even 22 per cent of the 'sane' perpetrators were given lower sentences.

The significant influence of psychiatric experts in the Netherlands is confirmed by the 1990 study by forensic psychiatrist de Boer, covering 124 partner killings in the period 1950–1980, for which the suspects were psychiatrically examined in the Pieter Baan Centrum (PBC), the foremost centre for forensic examination in the Netherlands. In 122 out of the 124 cases there were 'sickly mental aberrations'; not the classical psychiatric illnesses, but serious personality disorders.[40] In the vast majority of cases the PBC psychiatrists concluded that the suspects who had killed their partner were less accountable or unaccountable (only two were fully accountable).[41] In 85 per cent of cases the PBC report formed the basis for the judges' decision on (un)accountability, so they very often followed the psychiatrists' advice.[42] The stronger the gradation of unaccountability, the lower the prison sentence given. The length of the prison sentence was overall the same for men and women, but women more often received only a prison sentence, while men were more often convicted to both a prison sentence and treatment.[43]

These criminological and psychiatric studies all conclude that the influence of forensic psychiatric expertise on sentencing practices was considerable and that a high percentage of perpetrators was found (partially) unaccountable or benefitted from mitigating circumstances. In short, perpetrators of 'crimes of passion' in practice were sometimes judged more leniently on the basis of personality disorders, and often received treatment as punishment regardless of the absence of this crime as such in the legal code and the vehement Dutch cultural distancing from the 'French' crime of passion and their milder form of judgment by the French jury system and press.

To conclude, the Dutch treatment of crimes of passion is paradoxical. On the one hand, this crime did not exist in the criminal code and culturally the Dutch regarded it as typically French, both in character and regarding the more lenient treatment by the French legal system and jury and the sensationalised French press. In practice, however, the term 'crime of passion' continued to be used regularly throughout the twentieth century in Dutch court cases, by prosecutors, lawyers and psychiatrists. The latter also acknowledged that it was a crime mostly committed by the Dutch lower classes. From the beginning of the twentieth century, the crime of passion was often considered as pathological behaviour and perpetrators were frequently regarded as (diminished) accountable by forensic psychiatrists, receiving more lenient sentences or psychiatric treatment. The influence of Dutch forensic psychiatry on the judiciary was consistent and considerable. We therefore see a Dutch legal system in which forensic psychiatry is an important element, but judicial practice also unveils a Dutch forensic culture that revolved around an older notion of a crime that actually did not exist in the law; moreover this forensic culture was built on a self-image of a rational and emancipated nation.

Crimes of passion in Russian criminal law

'Crimes of passion' had a powerful cultural-political image in Soviet Russia as well. However, and similarly to the Netherlands, this image did not always dovetail with how different actors of criminal investigation practices, including the judiciary and psychiatrists, interpreted the nature and the gravity of this crime.

As such, the term 'crimes of passion' was used neither in Russian law, nor in the doctrine. Instead, the term 'homicide committed out of jealousy' became a standard legal term. The first Russian Criminal Code that was adopted in 1922 (amended in 1926) after the October Revolution thus explicitly referred to jealousy as a motive for homicide.[44] Similarly to many other legal systems, in

Russian law a motive did not form an element of the '*mens rea*', so it did not have to be established to prove *that* the crime was committed. However, it had to be established to determine *how* the perpetrator had to be punished for the crime committed. As we will show later, when a jealousy motive was established, it had a great influence on the offender's sentence.

In addition, the Criminal Code from 1922, as well as the next Criminal Code from 1960, had a provision on 'sudden mental disturbance' that was similar to the 'provocation' defence stipulated in criminal laws of many common law systems.[45] According to this provision, a homicide committed in a state of 'sudden mental disturbance' caused by 'violence or grave insult' on the part of the victim carried a less severe sentence. Although this article did not specifically refer to jealousy or 'heat of passion', it was occasionally applied to homicide committed after a sudden discovery of spousal infidelity. However, this provision had been applied extremely sparingly. For example, according to Kharitonova, in the 1960–1980s only 3.8 per cent of homicide cases committed with the motive of jealousy were prosecuted as homicide committed in a state of 'sudden mental disturbance'.[46] The analysis of court cases adjudicated by the Moscow regional court in the 1920s also shows that the application of this provision to 'crimes of passion' was extremely rare.[47] One reason explaining this could be that such a 'mental disturbance' had to be sudden to justify the application of this provision, while in practice the sudden onset of this 'mental disturbance' was missing, for example, in situations of prolonged mental agitation caused by jealousy. Furthermore, whether adultery was a 'grave insult' was heavily debated, which might also cause a more hesitant application of this provision by the judiciary.[48] The most important consequence of this approach was that 'crimes of passion' carried long and severe sentences throughout the entire period we study. Even though, as we will show, the judiciary started to apply the provision on mitigating circumstances after the entry into force of the Criminal Code in 1960 and treat them much more differentially, the eventual sanctions were nevertheless more severe than those foreseen for homicide committed in the state of 'sudden mental disturbance'.[49]

The image of jealousy in the official Soviet Russian legal and political discourse

As stated above, in Dutch culture crimes of passion were regarded as crimes that were alien to Dutch society. This distancing was done alongside a cultural line; it was assumed that there was an association between a crime and a particular cultural context in which this crime was committed. This cultural context had a great influence on this crime's acceptability within society, as well as on the sentencing practices. This attempt to distance oneself from 'crimes of passion' was pertinent also to the Russian legal and political discourse. However, rather than opposing Russian culture against other cultures, the opposition between socio-economic systems, namely bourgeois capitalism and socialism, was at the basis of this distancing.

The association between jealousy and capitalism was particularly noteworthy in the 1920s when the newly appointed Bolshevik government was busy drafting new socialist laws, including the new Criminal Code. The latter stipulated that a homicide committed out of jealousy was an aggravated homicide, as jealousy was an 'ignoble motive', similar to revenge and greed. Hence, the motive of jealousy due to its 'ignoble' nature was an aggravating factor, automatically implying a more severe sentence. Many legal scholars and ideologists praised this approach. Well-known Russian scholar Andrei Piontkovskii argued that this article was an illustration of the 'new legal consciousness of proletariat' that was embedded in the new Russian laws and that distinguished them from the 'bourgeois laws'.[50] Legal scholar Iakov Staroselskii, referring to the articles of the new Criminal Code, stated that a 'proletarian point of view was in a particular way implemented in each of its articles', not only in those that related to the counterrevolutionary crimes, but also to 'the smallest crimes against the person, where for the first time in world history jealousy, for example, figured as a factor aggravating guilt, rather than mitigating it'.[51] Hence, for these scholars the imposition of a severe sentence on those accused of 'crimes of passion' was precisely what characterised the new proletarian (legal) consciousness and the new laws that reflected this new consciousness. It also distinguished these new proletarian laws from the bourgeois ones.

This approach to jealousy as a motive of crime was to a large extent present throughout the following decades. Similar to the discourse revolving around 'crimes of passion' in the 1920s, Russian legal scholars continued emphasising the importance of severe sentencing for 'crimes of passion'. They argued that jealousy was an element of capitalist mentality, a 'private property instinct', making it by definition 'an ignoble motive'.[52] According to legal scholar Mikhail Aniiants, jealousy was 'a disgusting relic of the past' justifying severe sentencing.[53] However, in the 1960s slightly diverging points of view started to appear. For example, legal scholars Pobegailo and Zagorodnikov argued that jealousy as such was not an 'ignoble' motive; however, it could give rise to such 'ignoble' motives as revenge and anger.[54] Therefore, these scholars argued, offenders committing murders out of jealousy were not always dangerous and their severe sentencing was not always justified.

As we will show in the next section, the emergence of these different points of view in the official legal discourse might have been a reflection of how 'crimes of passion' were approached in judicial practice. More specifically, judges saw it as a much more complex emotion, caused by multiple factors, manifesting differently, and leading to variable (legal) consequences. Furthermore, jealousy as a motive for homicide alone did not seem to be sufficient to consider 'crimes of passion' as particularly dangerous. Eventually this recognised complexity of jealousy as an emotion and the violent behaviour triggered by it also affected the official legal and political discourse. The jealousy motive was eventually excluded from the scope of aggravating factors in the Russian Criminal Code, and the 'crime of passion' became 'ordinary' homicide. Jealousy as a feeling was still disapproved of, and homicide committed out of jealousy continued to carry long sentences. However, a seemingly consistent narrative that saw jealousy predominantly in its connection to capitalism that by definition justified a severer sentence gave way to a more casuistic approach to the prosecution of this type of crimes.

Crimes of passion in Soviet Russian judicial practice

The first sign that the influence of capitalism was not the only reason why individuals commit 'crimes of passion', and that the latter therefore should not carry high sentences, came from judicial practice. A selection of court records adjudicated by the Moscow regional court from the 1920s and early 1930s shows that courts treated the offenders accused of 'crimes of passion' differentially. In some cases, they indeed saw the motive of jealousy as an aggravating factor due to its presumed link to capitalism, eventually imposing long prison terms on the offender. For example, in a case heard by the Moscow Regional Court in 1931 the court convicted the offender for killing the lover of his wife out of jealousy to the maximum term of deprivation of liberty.[55] In explaining its verdict, the court stated:

> The accused, despite living for so long among the Bolsheviks, coming from a petty bourgeois environment, has not overcome his petty bourgeois ideology, in particular his views about women. He sees them not as the fighters for socialism but as objects needed to satisfy his so-called 'aesthetic', 'erotic' and other needs which reflect his possessive individualistic ideology. All this was clearly demonstrated in how he treated his wife; his jealousy and his behaviour, including the crime itself, very clearly reflect his entire mean petty bourgeois nature.[56]

Hence, this case illustrates the link that the judiciary drew between capitalism, possessiveness, jealousy and delinquent behaviour.

Yet, the judges did not always mete out strict punishments to individuals accused of 'crimes of passion'. For example, courts were more inclined to impose a lenient sentence on individuals who were born and raised in the rural environment and who were carriers of a 'backward peasants' consciousness'. In such cases, jealousy was often regarded as a character trait that the offenders had due to their backwardness and lack of proper education.[57] As these characteristics were mitigating circumstances according to the Russian Criminal Code, in many instances courts imposed lenient sentences, often less than half of what they would otherwise have imposed.

The discontent that the judges had about the Criminal Code's one-size-fits-all approach to crimes of passion might have affected the legislator's approach to it. Whereas jealousy as an emotion was still disapproved of, it was questioned whether it was sufficient to qualify the 'crime of passion' as a particularly serious crime. Jealousy as a feeling and as a motive for an action, it was argued, could be healthy or pathological, caused by real or imaginary infidelity, and all these factors should be given attention by the judiciary to decide on the appropriate sentence.[58] As legal scholar Sergei Borodin wrote, the experience (which probably meant judicial practice) showed that treating jealousy as an aggravating factor and imposing severe sentences on the offenders convicted of killing their partner out of jealousy simply was not justified.[59] A similar point of view was voiced by Eduard Pobegailo.[60] This criticism might have been taken into account in the deliberation of the new Russian Criminal Code from 1960. It removed jealousy from the list of aggravating circumstances. As a general rule, a killing out of jealousy became 'ordinary' homicide and the form and degree of punishment were to be decided by the judiciary in each individual case.

The differential treatment of the offenders accused of killing their partner or a beloved out of jealousy that was made possible with the adoption of the new Criminal Code was further reinforced in judicial practice. For example, according to some sources, in the period from the 1960s until the 1980s in around 30 per cent of cases they were punished severely and in 16 per cent they were punished leniently.[61] Among the factors aggravating punishment were mostly recidivism, alcohol intoxication and the immoral behaviour of the offender. The mitigating circumstances included confession, first-time crime, 'immoral behavior of the victim' (infidelity) and, as shown in the following section, mental disorders of the offender. In other words, in judicial practice the acknowledgement of jealousy as a motive of the crime was not regarded by the judges as a factor that automatically turned this crime into a particularly dangerous one. Jealousy might have been still disapproved of, yet it was not seen as exclusively linked with bourgeois capitalism and thus by definition warranting a more severe punishment.

Crimes of passion and the role of psychiatric expertise in Soviet Russia

Alongside the judiciary, psychiatrists acting as forensic experts in criminal investigations might also have played a role in bringing about these changes. As early as the 1920s, Russian psychiatrists – similarly to the judges – saw jealousy not only in its association with capitalism.⁶² For psychiatrists, jealousy was also a possible symptom of the offender's mental disorder. They did acknowledge that connecting jealousy with mental illness might be legally problematic: this could lead to the conclusion about the offender's partial unaccountability and as a result justify the imposition of a less severe sentence. At the same time, they were still inclined to connect jealousy, violent behaviour and mental disorders. Furthermore, the assumption that delinquency could be a symptom of one's mental pathologies was also seen as ideologically 'correct'. Explaining violent behaviour with scientific (that is, medical) arguments was consistent with the teaching of Lenin's dialectical materialism that recognised the importance of scientific evidence for law-making and legal practice.⁶³

In the following thirty years the role of psychiatrists in criminal investigation became more limited. Whereas the praising of science as the right basis for legal decisions remained, the reference to biological explanations was no longer considered correct, leading to psychiatrists being accused of 'lombrosianism' (the term became a standard one to accuse psychiatrists of the deviation from the 'correct' science; 'correct' from then on could only be the socio-economic explanations of criminality).⁶⁴ As a result, until the late 1950s the role of psychiatrists in criminal investigation was limited to providing expert assessment on the classical issue of legal insanity, rather than on determining a causal link between the crime and the offender's biological predisposition to it.⁶⁵

However, in the late 1950s, the latter again became possible. The requalification of homicide committed out of jealousy into an 'ordinary' homicide and the possibility for a more individualised treatment of offenders accused of it reinforced this practice, enabling a more medicalised approach to dealing with such offenders. For example, in the period from the 1960s until the 1980s in 40 per cent of homicide cases committed out of jealousy in which borderline mental abnormalities such as psychopathy or mental retardation were diagnosed, these disorders were taken into account in the determination of punishment as mitigating circumstances.⁶⁶ The only exception was chronic alcoholism that was mostly considered as an aggravating factor and, if diagnosed, was the ground for the offender's forced hospitalisation. The evidence demonstrating the exact role that psychiatrists played in changing the approach to sentencing the offenders convicted of killing their intimate partner out of jealousy in Russia is scarce. Yet it does suggest that psychiatrists further contributed to weakening the connection between jealousy, and the crimes motivated by it, exclusively with capitalism, by associating the former also with the offender's psychological abnormalities.

To conclude, similarly to the Dutch case, the crime of passion was a contradictory phenomenon in Russia. In the official political and legal discourse, particularly in the first half of the twentieth century, jealousy was seen as an emotion alien to the socialist society that the Soviet Union was building, as it was associated with capitalism, private property and egoism. In addition, due to this association with capitalism, jealousy-driven violent behaviour was seen as particularly dangerous to the socialist legal order, thus justifying severer legal sanction. Parallel to this official discourse, however, killing out of jealousy became a rather 'normal' and a somewhat 'typical' crime. Whereas indeed it could be committed due to the offender's capitalist possessiveness and greed (and thus seen as alien to the socialist mores), it could also be an outcome of the offender's illiteracy and lack of poor education or due to his mental abnormalities. The eventual exclusion of the jealousy motive from the scope of aggravated factors from the 1960 Criminal Code could be seen as a way to (partially) resolve this paradox, even though jealousy to a large extent continued to be condemned in the official public discourse.

Conclusion

In this chapter, we have applied the approach of 'doing law' to compare the cultural and legal constructions of 'crimes of passion' in Russia and the Netherlands in the twentieth century to demonstrate that the nature of that crime was continually debated and negotiated by multiple actors, such as the legislature, the judiciary and psychiatrists. In both countries a political and cultural discourse on this crime underlined a self-image by contrast with an Other: the Soviet socialist discourse framed 'capitalist' jealousy as its opposite and the 'moderate' and 'rational' Dutch contrasted themselves with the passionate French and Italian who were more lenient towards perpetrators trying to uphold their honour. However, in the Netherlands this cultural discourse was not an official part of the legal system, as it was in the Soviet Union; it belonged to a broader forensic culture.

Comparing these political, cultural and psychiatric discourses to legal practice, however, we found that these discourses became more complicated. Although Dutch prosecutors, lawyers, psychiatrists and commentators claimed that the 'crime of passion' and its lenient punishment were foreign, in practice this notion was used to mitigate sentences and forensic psychiatrists were asked whether certain murders belonged to this category. In Russia, 'crimes of passion' in practice were not only associated with 'capitalist' greed, but also with the offender's illiteracy, mental abnormalities and poor education. Thus, although our comparison highlighted major differences in the contents of the political and cultural discourses on 'crimes of passion', and the involvement of forensic psychiatrists was more frequent and influential in the Dutch legal system than in Russia, in both countries several actors together constructed the contents of this particular crime in legal practice, demonstrating its cultural and historical variability. We therefore suggest that a comparative approach to different forensic cultures in practice is fruitful to lay bare how crimes are defined and prosecuted. This might also imply that establishing that the old-fashioned concept of 'crimes of passion' is glamourising violence against women and replacing it by 'femicide' is not enough to unveil its character: the term femicide in turn might obscure historical change and differences between national or regional cultural constructions of this crime, or between these discourses and the practices of prosecution.

Notes

This project has received funding from the European Research Council (ERC) under the European Union's Horizon 2020 research and innovation programme (grant agreement no. 770402).

1 Jill Radford and Diana Russell (eds), *Femicide: The Politics of Woman Killing* (Buckingham: Open University Press, 1992).
2 Marieke Liem, 'Femicide: een kritische reflectie op het gebruik van de term', *Boom Strafblad* 5 (2021), pp. 164–166.

3 Rebekka Habermas, *Thieves in Court: The Making of the German Legal System in the Nineteenth Century* (New York: Cambridge University Press, 2016 [German original 2008]), pp. 8–11.
4 David W. Jones, 'Moral Insanity and Psychological Disorder: The Hybrid Roots of Psychiatry', *History of Psychiatry* 28:3 (2017), pp. 263–279, here p. 265.
5 Ute Frevert, 'Honour and/or/as Passion: Historical Trajectories of Legal Defenses', *Rechtsgeschichte/Legal History* 22 (2014), pp. 245–255, here pp. 248–249.
6 Frevert, 'Honour and/or/as Passion', pp. 246–248.
7 Eliza Earle Ferguson, 'Judicial Authority and Popular Justice: Crimes of Passion in fin-de-siécle Paris', *Journal of Social History* (Winter 2006), pp. 293–315, here pp. 294, 309. Ruth Harris, *Murders and Madness: Medicine, Law, and Society in the Fin-de-Siècle* (Oxford: Clarendon Press, 1989), pp. 208, 226. Rebecca Crites, 'Husbands' Violence against Wives in England and Wales, 1914–1939: A Review of Contemporary Understandings of and Responses to Men's Marital Violence' (PhD thesis, University of Warwick, 2016), pp. 109–110; Ginger Frost, ' "He Could Not Hold His Passions": Domestic Violence and Cohabitation in England (1850–1905)', *Crime, History and Societies* 12:1 (2008), pp. 45–63. Efi Avdela, 'Emotions on Trial: Judging Crimes of Honour in post-Civil-War Greece', *Crime, History & Societies* 10:2 (2006), pp. 33–52, Nerea Aresti, 'El crimen de Trubia. Género, discursos, y ciudadanía republicana', *Ayer* 64:4 (2006), pp. 261–285, here pp. 274–276.
8 Avdela, 'Emotions on Trial', p. 11.
9 Maurice Cottier, *Fatale Gewalt. Ehre, Subjekt und Kriminalität am Übergang zur Moderne: Das Beispiel Bern 1868–1941* (UVK Verlagsgesellschaft: Konstanz and Munich, 2nd edn, 2019 [2017]), p. 227.
10 Léon Rabinowicz, *Le crime passionnel* (Plon: Paris, 1931).
11 Joëlle Guillais, *La chair de l'autre: Le crime passionnel au 19e siècle* (Paris, 1986), pp. 281–286, quoted by Harris, *Murders and Madness* (1989), p. 303, note 37.
12 Cottier, *Fatale Gewalt*, p. 132, note 199; Max Friedmann, 'Über die Psychologie der Eifersucht', *Grenzfragen des Nerven- und Seelenlebens* 82 (1911), pp. 76, 85.
13 Crites, 'Husbands' Violence against Wives in England and Wales, 1914–1939', pp. 175–179; Earle Ferguson, 'Domestic Violence by Another Name', p. 33; Harris, *Murders and Madness*, p. 125; Efi Avdela, 'Emotions on Trial'. Cottier, *Fatale Gewalt*, pp. 139–141.
14 *Algemeen Indisch dagblad: de Preangerbode*, 8 November 1952. On the same case, see also *De Volkskrant*, 6 November 1952.

15 Samuel Henri Philips, *Het passioneele misdrijf in Nederland* (L. J. Veen's Uitgevers Mij. N.V.: Amsterdam, 1938), pp. 1, 118.
16 *Soerabaijasch Handelsblad*, 8 November 1938.
17 Gerrit Th. Kempe, *Misdaad en wangedrag* (Amsterdam 1947), pp. 128–130, here pp. 148–149.
18 Symon P. Tammenoms Bakker, *Het passionele misdrijf*, Voordracht voor het Psychiatrisch Juridisch Gezelschap (Van Rossen: Amsterdam, 1951), pp. 10–13, 22–23.
19 Philips, *Het passioneele misdrijf in Nederland*, p. 82.
20 *Ibid.*, pp. 84, 114, 116.
21 Noord-Hollands Archief, Archive Gerechtshof Amsterdam (access no. 29) inv. no. 145 (case N. 1928); *De Tribune*, 24 September 1928.
22 *Limburgsch dagblad*, 9 November 1966.
23 *De Volkskrant*, 8 January 1965; *Gereformeerd Gezinsblad*, 23 January 1965.
24 J. C. H. Blom, *Burgerlijk en beheerst: Over Nederland in de twintigste eeuw* (Amsterdam: Balans, 1996).
25 Three extensive psychiatric studies exist: by Philips (1938) based on crimes of passion committed in 1915–1935; by Tammenoms Bakker (1951) based on the period 1938–1951, and by de Boer (1990) based on partner killings in 1950–1980.
26 Kempe, *Misdaad en wangedrag*, pp. 131, 134; Franciscus Marinus Havermans, *Opstellen over forensische psychiatrie* (2nd edn, Roermond: Romen en Zonen, 1956 [1951]), p. 85.
27 Tammenoms Bakker, *Het passionele misdrijf*, pp. 10–13.
28 *Ibid.*, pp. 20–21.
29 *Ibid.*, pp. 5–6, 18–21.
30 Philips, *Het passioneele misdrijf in Nederland*, pp. 42, 63–64.
31 A. P. de Boer, *Partnerdoding: een empirisch forensisch-psychiatrisch onderzoek* (Arnhem: Gouda Quint, 1990) p. 165. De Boer states that one out of three partner killings were passionate killings: De Boer, *Partnerdoding*, pp. 84–85.
32 Tammenoms Bakker, *Het passionele misdrijf*, p. 20.
33 *Het Vrije Volk*, 24 August 1972.
34 *Leeuwarder Courant*, 16 May 1962; *Algemeen Dagblad*, 30 May 1962.
35 Harry Oosterhuis, 'Treatment as Punishment: Forensic Psychiatry in The Netherlands (1870–2005)', *International Journal of Law and Psychiatry* 37 (2014), pp. 37–49, here p. 41.
36 Ido Weijers and Frans Koenraadt, 'Toenemende vraag naar expertise – een eeuw forensische psychiatrie en psychologie', in Frans Koenraadt, Constantijn Kelk and Joost Vijselaar (eds), *Tussen behandeling en straf. Rechtsbescherming en veiligheid in de twintigste eeuw* (Deventer: Kluwer 2007), pp. 1–74, here p. 60.

37 Philips, *Het passioneele misdrijf*, pp. 50–51.
38 *Ibid.*, p. 115.
39 The three who were held unaccountable were sent to a mental institution. Of the twenty-two less accountable, seven received TBR, of whom five were diagnosed as psychopaths.
40 De Boer, *Partnerdoding*, p. 159.
41 *Ibid.*, p. 76.
42 *Ibid.*, p. 159.
43 *Ibid.*, pp. 116, 110.
44 Article 136 Criminal Code 1922 (article 143 Criminal Code 1926).
45 Article 144 Criminal Code 1922 (article 138 of the amended Criminal Code 1926). The provision on 'sudden mental disturbance' remained in the Criminal Code 1960 (article 104).
46 T. Kharitonova, 'Motiv revnosti I ego znachenie dla otvetstvennosti pri umyshlennom ubiistve po sovetskomu ugolovnomu pravu' (Unpublished dissertation, Kazan, 1983), p. 88.
47 Tsentralnyi gosudarstvennyi arkhiv Moskovskoi oblasti, Central State Archive of the Moscow Oblast (TsGAMO), fond 5062.
48 For a review see Kharitonova, *Motiv revnosti*, pp. 100–101.
49 Kharitonova, p. 128.
50 A. Piontkovskii, 'Prestuplenie v sotsialisticheskom obschestve', *Sovetskoe pravo* 2:5 (1923), pp. 1–32, here p. 22.
51 Ia. Staroselskii, 'Principy postroienia ugolovnoi repressii v proletarskom gosudarstve', *Revolutsia prava* 2 (1927), pp. 83–105, here p. 93.
52 B. Volkov, *Motiv i kvalifikaciia prestuplenia* (Kazan: Kazan University Press, 1968) p. 97.
53 M. Aniiants, *Otvetstvennost za prestuplenia protiv zhizni po deistvuiuschemu zakonodatelstvu soiuznykh respublik* (Moscow: Juridicheskaia literatura, 1964), p. 122.
54 E. Pobegailo, *Umyshlennye ubiistva i borba s nimi: ugolovno-pravovoie i kriminologicheskoie issledovaniie* (Voronezh: Izdatelstvo Voronezhskogo Universiteta, 1965), p. 127; N. Zagorodnikov, *Prestuplenia protiv zhizni po sovetskomu ugolovnomu pravu* (Moscow: Gosiurizdat, 1961), p. 141.
55 The name of the perpetrator has been pseudonymised for privacy reasons.
56 TsGAMO, fond 7335, opis 1, delo 138, p. 267.
57 TsGAMO, fond 5062, opis 3, delo 749.
58 S. Borodin, *Prestuplenia protiv zhizni* (Saint-Petersburg: Juridicheski tsentr Press, 2003), pp. 104–105.
59 S. Borodin, *Otvetstvennost za ubiistvo: kvalificacia i otvetstvennost po rossiiskomu ugolovnomu pravu* (Moscow: Juirst, 1994), p. 10.

60 E. Pobegailo, *Izbrannye trudy* (Saint-Petersburg: Juridicheski tsentr Press, 2008), p. 358.
61 Kharitonova, *Motiv revnosti*, p. 127.
62 A. Buneev, 'O vmeniaemosti (K postanovke vorposa)', *Zhurnal nevropatologii i psikhiatrii* 5 (1931), pp. 104–108.
63 V. Lenin, *The State and Revolution*, trans. Robert Service (London: Penguin Books, 1992), p. 81.
64 T. Feinberg, *Psikhopatii i ikh sudebno-psikhiatricheskoe znachenie* (Moscow: Sovetskoe zakonodatel'stvo, 1934); Dan Healey, 'Russian and Soviet Forensic Psychiatry: Troubled and Troubling', *International Journal of Law and Psychiatry* 37:1 (2014), pp. 71–81.
65 D. Dianov, 'Formula nevmeniaemosti i praktika ee primenenia v sovetskii period razvitia sudebnoi psikhiatrii' (Unpublished dissertation, Moscow, 1997).
66 Kharitonova, *Motiv revnosti*, pp. 140–141. See also Daniil Lunts, 'Otsenka sudom psuhicheskih anomalii obviniaemogo, ne iskluchaiuschih vmeniamosti', *Pravovedenie* 2 (1968), pp. 86–94.

10

A culture of consensus: Organising expertise in Norwegian forensic psychiatry, late nineteenth to early twentieth century

Svein Atle Skålevåg

Introduction

In 2012, the man behind the biggest mass killing in Norwegian history, who had killed seventy-seven people in two politically motivated terror attacks in Oslo and on the island of Utøya the previous year, was put on trial in Oslo. The question of the criminal responsibility of the defendant dominated the trial that attracted enormous attention nationally and internationally. Two forensic psychiatrists, appointed by the court, found that the defendant was and had been psychotic. By Norwegian legal tradition this should imply that he was not to be held legally accountable for his acts. The conclusion triggered a public uproar, and a second pair of forensic experts, also psychiatrists, were appointed by the court. They came to a different conclusion – that the defendant was not psychotic but had a personality disorder.[1] Surely, this was not the first time in the history of forensic psychiatry in Norway that different forensic experts came to different conclusions. But never before had forensic psychiatry been subjected to this level of intense scrutiny by the public gaze. What the public seem to have been surprised to see exposed was that there was seemingly so little consensus among the members of the forensic psychiatric community, and of the legal culture in a broader sense, about what constituted psychosis and what constituted irresponsibility. It was demonstrated that psychiatrists did not agree with each other, and that many legal professionals held divergent views on the question of criminal responsibility. It was as if a culture of consensus had been cracked open.

The court case arguably marked the end of a long period of consensus around the question of criminal responsibility in Norway – among psychiatrists, but also between psychiatrists and legal professionals. This consensus was procedural as much as it was doctrinal. It had come about as the product of a particular way of organising the forensic expertise that was meant to elucidate the problem of criminal responsibility. It was due to a legal system that shied away from party-based expertise, a legal rule that equated 'mental illness' with 'irresponsibility', and a forensic commission that sought to homogenise the performance of psychiatric expertise, by formulating norms of how to frame an expert opinion.

This system was the product of a number of legal changes in the late nineteenth and early twentieth centuries, which included a reform of the criminal code and of the rules of criminal procedure, and a transformation of the way that forensic expertise was organised. Crucial among these reforms were the establishment of a permanent Commission for Forensic Medicine (*Den Retsmedicinske commission*) in 1900. All these legal reforms happened at a time when the different versions of a 'positivist school' of criminal law gained traction in Europe.[2] In particular Franz von Liszt and his idea of a multidisciplinary science of crime (*gesamte Strafrechtswissenschaft*) and his emphasis of a goal-oriented criminal law (the *Zweckgedanke*), was an important influence on the Norwegian reform.[3] The Norwegian adherents of Liszt wanted to transform criminal law from a system for the distribution of justice, for retribution against wrongdoings, to a machine for an efficient defence of society.

In this chapter I will first make some historiographical observations. Then in the first section, I will trace the background for the transformation of the early twentieth century in the trajectory of early psychiatry in Norway. In the second section I will discuss this transformation, and in the third section I will use two examples from forensic psychiatric practice from the first decade of the twentieth century to show what the practical work of a forensic expert consisted of, and that the nature of this work was also conducive to a consensus between legal professionals and medical professionals.

Medicalisation, topography and forensic culture

The literature on the history of European forensic psychiatry has portrayed the legal system as an arena that the emerging psychiatry set out to conquer, and that this whole field consequently was shaped by professional interests.[4] For example, Jan Goldstein's very persuasive account of French psychiatry in the nineteenth century, *Console and Classify* (1987), argues that a search for professional prestige brought French psychiatrists into the courts of law in the 1820s.[5] Specifically, the concept of homicidal monomania, according to Goldstein, was used as a veritable battering ram by early psychiatrists (or alienists) to gain a foothold in criminal law. Their main argument was that there were forms of mental illness that only the trained eye could spot. This attempt to medicalise – to use a more modern term – criminal law, created much hostility and conflict between the small group of alienists and the larger community of legal professionals. This hostility was played out in the public sphere, in newspapers and medical and legal periodicals.

A different history emerges through Michel Foucault's writings on forensic psychiatry.[6] He argued that what happened in the nineteenth century was not that a profession set out to conquer the territory of another, but that there was a profound transformation of criminal law through which its new stated goal was to protect society from the 'dangerous individual'. The transformation was not, according to Foucault, a product of wilful reform of a legal system, but should be seen as the unintended result of circumstances that are heterogeneous, i.e. both institutional, technological and discursive. This heterogeneous ensemble of factors provoking a change is also identified by the Foucauldian neologism 'dispositive'.[7] The positivist school of criminal law, in Foucault's view, was not the dynamo in this transformation, but a discourse that finally was able to codify changes already taking place.

More recent historical scholarship is similarly cautious to overemphasise the importance of professional interest. Harry Oosterhuis, speaking of the Netherlands, states that 'Forensic psychiatry was not a product of a univocal professional urge to expand.'[8] Eric Engstrom, expanding on an observation by Richard Wetzell, speaks of 'a second wave of research on criminology and forensic psychiatry in Germany'. These studies have taken a 'more subtle' approach to the law-psychiatry relationship, seeking to overcome what Engstrom refers to as the 'paradigms of medicalization'. Engstrom (who partly identifies with this second wave), seeks to achieve this by emphasising the importance of 'forensic practice' as opposed to criminological 'theories'. What emerges from highlighting the practical work of forensic experts and legal professionals is a particular 'topography' of forensic practice.[9] Engstrom does not disregard interprofessional disputes, but he directs our attention to the ways that these disputes are dispersed in a very specific institutional landscape. This conceptualisation – emphasising practice and spatial distribution – seems suited to identify also national and regional differences in forensic psychiatry.

This chapter does not aim at a complete forensic psychiatric topography, nor at a systematic international comparison, but the goal is to identify a forensic culture that is nationally specific. Following Foucault's emphasis on the heterogeneous circumstances, and Engstrom's emphasis on practice and spatial specificity, I will show that the Norwegian forensic culture was characterised by a high degree of consensus.

The role of the forensic expert was significantly different within the adversarial legal system on the one hand and the inquisitorial system on the other. In the former case experts were typically pitted against each other, whereas in the latter the expert was considered the court's objective advisor. Though there was a tendency of combining features from both systems in the nineteenth century, the principled opposition remained.[10] Hence, to a certain degree, the very design of the legal system on the continent was conducive to a consensus among forensic experts. It is also significant in this context that in the German states, for example, medical faculties had traditionally been close to the state and delivered expert opinions since the eighteenth century, in a way that was not the case in anglophone countries.[11] The Norwegian legal system of the nineteenth century shared features with both the continental and the Anglo-American systems with regards to the role of experts. It stands out, I will suggest, as a particularly strong consensus culture was created, which both relied on institutional innovations and on a consistent medical doctrine of criminal responsibility.

The emergence of forensic psychiatry in nineteenth-century Norway

The early occurrence of forensic medical expertise in Norway is not very well documented, but there is evidence that medical experts acted as witnesses in court to elucidate the question of criminal responsibility at least as early as in 1818.[12] The medical experts were in the early cases general physicians, and not experts on mental illness. There are also recorded examples, beginning in the 1830s, that a court of law (in appeal cases) would ask a *second* opinion from the medical faculty at the only university of the kingdom (Det kongelige Frederiks Universitet, established in 1811).[13] This university, and hence Norway as a whole, did not have any chair in psychiatry until 1915. The practice of acting as a consulting body for the government in certain cases was probably inherited from the University of Copenhagen, where it had been practised since the eighteenth century. The professors would give their opinion based on the documents in the case, not on personal examination of the defendant. For example, in a case against a woman accused of domestic violence in 1837, the faculty found that the defendant was suffering from periodical mania, and the supreme court consequently regarded her as irresponsible for her actions.[14] The custom of soliciting a second opinion set forensic medicine apart as a field of forensic expertise. As physician Paul Winge later pointed out, in no other forensic questions was a 'secondary expertise' routinely sought.[15]

The role of the medical faculty may be understood in terms of a hierarchy of knowledge, as opposed to a system of specialisation. The professors were considered well placed to offer an opinion because they were professors, not because they had a specific experience in this field. From the mid-nineteenth century, they were challenged by the alienists who regarded themselves as specialists.

Before the mid-nineteenth century there were only a few small institutions for the insane in the country.[16] In 1848 the parliament passed an act that regulated the treatment and care for the mentally ill. The Mental Illness Act regulated already existing institutions for the mentally ill, but more importantly it laid the foundation for the construction of public mental asylums under medical control. The first of these, the Gaustad asylum, opened outside Christiania

(Oslo) in 1855, and it was followed by other state institutions in the 1870s and 1880s. These new institutions created career opportunities for a small group of aspiring alienists. They also provided the new specialists with observatories of sorts, a research material for further studies through the day-to-day activities of the asylum. It would take another half century to establish a chair in psychiatry and gain recognition as an academic specialty. But the director at the Gaustad asylum would take an informal role as the leader of Norwegian psychiatry. That does not mean that all physicians recognised that psychiatry was a branch of medicine that required a special knowledge and experience. In the second half of the nineteenth century there were occasional signs of friction between the physicians in the asylum and the professors in medicine at the university, most notably in matters pertaining to forensic psychiatry.[17]

The new psychiatrists/alienists did not fit easily in the hierarchy of knowledge of its time. Asylum doctors formed opinions based on familiarity with hundreds of psychiatric cases which they had the possibility to observe over extended periods of time. They therefore argued that they possessed knowledge of quite a different order from that of ordinary physicians, who might see a handful of mentally ill patients in their career, and even then, only for brief consultations.[18] The professors of the medical faculty also lacked this crucial experience with psychiatric cases, in the alienists' view. Due to the absence of a chair in psychiatry, the new, small group of trained alienists came into existence at the margins of the medical hierarchy.

A discord between the alienists and the medical faculty in matters of forensic medicine thus emerged soon after the establishment of the first Norwegian institution for the mentally ill, the Gaustad asylum. Already in 1856, one year after its opening, the medical superintendent Ole R. Sandberg met with the professors at the faculty to lecture them about the nature of melancholia, a subject about which he found their knowledge lacking.[19] Three years later, and directly related to this meeting, a series of open meetings were held in the Medical Society of Christiania, the most important medical society in the country, where the professors from the faculty traditionally were a dominant force.

At these meetings, superintendent Sandberg attacked the professors for not recognising his superior expertise in matters of forensic psychiatry. Remarkably, he also laid out a strategy for preserving the authority of the medical expert. The medical expert in matters of criminal responsibility, Sandberg suggested, should never be tempted to speculate on 'responsibility'; his only task was to shed light on the question of mental illness before the legal authorities. The existence or absence of illness was in his opinion a scientific question, not open to lofty speculations, and it was as a scientist that the forensic expert claimed authority: expert conclusions should be based on positive knowledge. Only within these boundaries would the expert appear as a true medical expert; as such it would be far more difficult to ignore his opinion than if he speculated on free will or responsibility. Sandberg thus pointed out a strategy that would be foundational for the Norwegian forensic culture for a century to come, or more.

To summarise, in the latter half of the nineteenth century there was a tension within the medical community around matters of forensic psychiatry. The medical community as such can hardly be said to have had an interest in 'conquering' the arena of criminal law. But for the alienists, the legal arena became an arena to assert their competency vis-à-vis the rest of the medical community. The differences between the alienists on the one hand, and the general physicians and professors of medicine on the other, were not rooted in different medical theories. All of them held a shared understanding of mental illness: mental illness was understood as a condition of mental derangement that followed from physiological anomalies. But Sandberg went beyond this common organicist concept in laying out a practical strategy to enforce discursive discipline: the forensic expert should not let himself be distracted by awkwardly phrased questions from the judge, but only give his opinion on the medical question: Is the defendant suffering from mental illness? If he did not stick to strict discipline here, he risked undermining the very authority of medicine.

Restructuring the field of forensic expertise

It is noteworthy that Sandberg already in the 1850s interpreted the criminal code as allowing for a strict 'medical' interpretation, in line with what would later be referred to as a 'biological principle'. This medical interpretation pointed towards a possibility for creating a consensus based on a strict division of labour between medical experts and legal professionals. It also implied, for the physicians, that mental illness was a question of 'either/or': either the defendant was insane, or he/she was not. However, the problem remained, as a legal commission pointed out in 1896, that there was no real uniformity in the judgment of physicians who acted as forensic experts.[20] This lack of uniformity would have to be addressed in order to arrive at something that resembled a culture of consensus.

It came to be addressed in the broad reform of criminal law and social policy that was implemented in Norway at the turn of the century, a cornerstone of which was a new law of criminal procedure (1887) as well as a new penal code (1902). The reform was conceived of as part of the democratisation of public life, of which legal matters were considered an important element. But it went further, in producing a series of reforms that expanded the scope for governmental action. For example, a new act for the protection of children was part of this new progressive agenda.[21] The reform of criminal procedures that introduced the jury into Norwegian criminal law was a major step. This reform in turn triggered a reform of the criminal code itself. The new code was passed in 1902. In this code, the medical interpretation of criminal responsibility was strengthened. As part of this broader set of legal reforms, the government also established the permanent Commission for Forensic Medicine, giving the field of forensic expertise a more formal structure.

The liberals had long wanted to introduce the jury in criminal procedures as a means to reduce the power of the legal professionals. In 1884, when a new liberal government came to power, their chance came. The criminal procedure act of 1887 followed the adversarial model, similar to that of the common law nations: the defence and the prosecution argued their respective cases orally before a presumedly impartial judge. The principle of orality was furthermore introduced as a means of opening the court to public scrutiny.[22] In this system, the expert witnesses in forensic medicine were as a general rule not appointed by the parties but by the courts. The question of criminal responsibility could be handled by the authorities in two ways: either the prosecutorial authorities decided not to pursue a case, if they found that the insanity of the defendant had been proven before the case was put on trial, or it was left to the court to decide the matter. In the latter case, the court would appoint two experts to examine the defendant and consecutively present their findings during the legal proceedings. A result of this way of organising a trial and the forensic psychiatric expertise in it was that the courts of law, or the public for that matter, rarely came to hear opposing arguments around the responsibility of the defendant. It facilitated the construction of consensus in expertise, as the experts generally spoke with one voice.

But for the forensic experts in matters of psychiatry, this reform was not enough to secure consensus. What was further needed was a rule on criminal responsibility that let the medical expert speak the language of medicine, also in court. The code of 1902 was, as already mentioned, conceived under the influence of the international criminalist movement, or 'the positivist school', and their call for a more solid scientific foundation for criminal law. These scholars and reformers distanced themselves from the old idea of punishment as retribution, and instead regarded criminal law in a social perspective. Crime was for them a social fact, rather than an immoral act. And criminal law should seek to have a specific impact on the fabric of society, instead of being a pedagogical tool to teach people how to behave. In Norway these ideas were mainly channelled through legal scholars who were also politicians, most significantly Bernhard Getz and Francis Hagerup, both representing the conservative party. In 1892 they founded a Norwegian branch of the Internationale Kriminalistische Vereinigung (International Criminalist Association), the association founded by Franz von Liszt and collaborators.[23] This association also attracted a few physicians interested in criminal anthropology, but the medical influence was rather exercised through the Physicians' Association that was founded in 1886. In 1900 this association presented the parliament with a set of medical considerations regarding the criminal code. They were written by police physician Paul Winge, and the future professor of psychiatry Ragnar Vogt. They embraced the general principles of the criminalists, most importantly that society needed a variety of ways to respond to crime, in addition to punishment.

For the most consistent followers of the new thinking in criminal law, such as the Italian legal scholar Garofalo, 'responsibility' was an idea that belonged to the old legal paradigm.[24] It had a metaphysical tint to it that did not harmonise well with the new positivist thinking. Garofalo argued that the very distinction between the responsible and the irresponsible criminal had to go. Instead, the courts should focus solely on the question of what danger the criminal represented to society. Only a minority among the adherents of the new criminal law followed this stringent application of a positivist perception of criminal law though. In Norway the reformers considered the option only in passing. Instead, they focused closely on the choice of words in the revised rule on criminal responsibility.

The intense scrutiny of the rule of criminal responsibility came out of a concern also for how medical expertise was organised in court: for Vogt and Winge, writing on behalf of the Association for physicians, the courts needed to ask questions that the experts could answer.[25] That meant that the code needed to employ a terminology that made sense in a medical discourse. This led to a proposal to make the 'biological principle' more explicit in the code than it hitherto had been, that is, to state in so many words that the mentally ill should not be held criminally responsible.[26] This point of view was partly heard in 1902, but it was fully implemented in the next revision of the code, in 1929.

The criminal code of 1842 had also contained a clause on criminal responsibility, which did not use any specifically medical terms in determining who were to be regarded as irresponsible. The code had recognised that there existed mental states that excluded criminal responsibility. But the law makers had left it to the judges to decide whether a criminal individual was in such a state of mind at the time of the crime. Nevertheless, many commentators in the second half of the nineteenth century, especially physicians, interpreted it medically, as expressing the 'biological principle', that is, to simplify things: to hold that the mentally ill could under no circumstances be held legally responsible for their acts. When the rule in the 1890s was up for revision, the forensic experts meant that the new version should express this principle more unambiguously, that is, that the code should specifically mention the biological or medical conditions that were to be recognised by the courts of law as criteria for responsibility (most importantly the condition of mental illness).

The medical or biological principle was by no means a new, nor was it a Norwegian, invention. In Sweden it had been an accepted legal doctrine since 1826.[27] Depending on interpretation, it could also be said to inhabit the influential French code penal of 1810, the Portuguese penal code of 1852, the Belgian code of 1867 and the Spanish code of 1848 and 1870.[28] The name of the qualifying medical condition varied between different countries. The alternative to this doctrine was that the letter of the law omitted references to medical (biological) states, and instead referred to psychological states (states of mind). This was in the 1890s referred to as a 'psychological principle' and it was implemented for instance in the Austrian code of 1852. Yet other codes used a combination of these principles. This was the case in the German code of 1871, which posed the absence of free will as well as the presence of mental illness as conditions for irresponsibility.[29]

We have seen that Ole Sandberg, the medical superintendent of Gaustad asylum, already considered the medical principle to be law in Norway in the 1850s. By the 1890s this interpretation was being argued forcefully by Paul Winge, who has already been mentioned. He was the first Norwegian psychiatrist to devote his full attention to matters of forensic psychiatry, and the first Norwegian psychiatrist who did not work in an asylum. He qualified for the doctoral degree in 1896 with a dissertation on the forensic examination of the insane criminal, and he wrote extensively on legal and medical history to produce evidence that the medical principle was firmly anchored in the Norwegian legal tradition.[30] His work for the police included a variety of tasks, of which performing mental evaluations of offenders was an important part. In the 1890s Winge took it upon himself to push for a reorganisation of forensic medicine. By 1900, his expertise was recognised when the Physicians' Association engaged him to contribute with his expertise. By the 1920s the medical doctrine on criminal responsibility was unequivocally expressed in the criminal code.

The choice between a medical (or biological) and a 'psychological' doctrine of criminal responsibility had consequences also for the role of the expert, as was implied by Vogt and Winge, writing for the Association of physicians in 1900.[31] According to the medical principle, the role of the expert would be to exclusively point out to the courts whether any of the relevant biological states were present in the defendant. In practice this would mean declaring whether the defendant suffered from a mental illness or not. It was always implied that this was a matter of positive fact, and not of interpretation. It was in this sense that the biological principle could be regarded as a 'positivist' principle. The psychological principle, on the other hand, would make the division of labour between the professionals in the court much less clear cut. It would require the experts to weigh in on a question that was *not* regarded as a matter of fact, but as a matter of law, which was the question whether the defendant was 'responsible'. In such a situation the statement of the medical expert would be just another opinion on the question of responsibility. This was a situation that the architects of the Norwegian forensic culture would seek to avoid.

It was clear that it would take some disciplining of the corps of forensic experts in order to avoid judgment and interpretation, and stick to positive, medical facts. As we have seen, forensic medicine had for a long time been organised fairly loosely. A remedy for this was therefore also sought in the 1890s, resulting in the establishment of the Commission for Forensic Medicine.[32] This was first proposed by Paul Winge in the 1890s. His goal was to produce the 'uniformity of judgment' that was seen as lacking among forensic experts, a uniformity that would be the expression of a culture of consensus. Winge envisaged a commission that would be equipped with a number of facilities that could actually carry out forensic work demanded by the courts, be it pathological, toxicological or psychiatric examinations. One of these facilities would be a psychiatric 'observation station', an '*Observationsanstalt*'.[33] Such institutions were indeed erected in Germany in the 1890s.[34] In the Netherlands they were discussed, but seem not to have been realised.[35] This institution, had it been built, would have concentrated much of the forensic medical work in the country in a few hands, securing a uniformity of medical judgment and further production of knowledge.

Winge's ambitious design for a set of new forensic institutions, set up to professionalise forensic medicine and perform more reliable forensic observations, was, however, never realised in Norway. What instead was created was a two-level system: on the first level, the court would continue to appoint forensic experts who would examine the defendants. They would also produce written records that were to be filed with the new Commission for Forensic Medicine. This commission constituted the second level in this system. It consisted of five permanent members (later to be expanded), who would examine the examination files, looking for sub-standard opinions, and react to them. The Commission was composed of three experts in pathology and two psychiatrists, selected by the government for a period of ten years. For the first two decades of its existence, Paul Winge and Harald Holm were its psychiatric members. The latter was director of the psychiatric asylum in the capital. Winge worked for the police as police physician, but with his doctorate and his literary production he may have been the closest thing there was to an academic psychiatrist. When he suddenly died in 1920, he was replaced by the professor in psychiatry at the university in Christiania, Ragnar Vogt, whose chair was not associated with an asylum, but with a university clinic. Holm, who retired the same year, was replaced by Hans Evensen, an asylum director. Hence the Commission was composed to comprise both academic and asylum psychiatrists; except for Winge, none of its members represented a narrow expertise in forensic psychiatry.

This composition meant a recognition of psychiatry as a distinct medical specialty, at a time when psychiatry was still not represented with a chair at the university. The new Commission for Forensic Medicine implied a restructuring of the Norwegian forensic culture and the knowledge structures associated with it. Transcripts of all forensic expert opinions from legal experts of the entire country were to be communicated to the Commission, which was to ensure that they held satisfactory quality. These reports fell into two groups: autopsy reports and forensic psychiatric reports. The latter group for the most part regarded the question of criminal responsibility. The Commission's two psychiatric members were solely responsible for auditing the forensic psychiatric reports. Hence, the Commission functioned as a kind of medical supreme court: it examined the activity of the lower courts based on documents produced by them. In the capacity of commissioners, they did not examine the defendants themselves. But the same experts were not excluded from being commissioned as experts for the court, in which case they would examine the defendants.

A *culture of consensus* 253

The Commission that was established in 1900 laid the foundation for a consensus produced within the medical community in forensic matters, but only indirectly did it lay the foundation for professionalisation: the actual forensic 'observation' was still in many cases performed by physicians who were *not* psychiatrists. But their activities were supervised from a distance, by the Commission which facilitated a medical community speaking with one voice, and even a consensus between the medical and the legal communities.

The normalising work of the Commission

The Commission published an annual report, aimed at the forensic community. It contained statistics, and a selection of forensic expert opinions on specific cases. These opinions, which make up the bulk of the published pages, had been presented in courts of law, and they were now spotlighted for the whole community to see. In the years from 1900 to 1927 a total of thirty-seven opinions were published by the Commission, of which Paul Winge co-authored twenty-two (he died in 1920). Until 1922 all these paradigmatic opinions were written by one or two members of the Commission.[36] They would homogenise the practice of forensic medicine by proposing a specific style of reasoning.

To get a clearer view of what the practice of individual forensic psychiatric experts looked like, a closer look at the early reports of the Commission for Forensic Medicine is informative. The report from the year 1902 provides two psychiatric examples. The first case from 1902 dealt with a dipsomaniac – an alcoholic – whom the experts regarded as mentally ill and a danger for public safety.[37] The report is twenty pages long, with only the final three pages constituting a discussion of the case. The rest of the report consists of quotations from witnesses about the mental state of the defendant. This is then followed by a discussion of how the defendant reacted to alcohol, which concludes thus: 'Dipsomania is a mental illness or maybe rather a symptom of mental illness, which under circumstances such as in this case, makes the patient dangerous for the public safety when he suffers an attack.'[38] In this conclusion the two crucial forensic questions of the time were addressed: the question of illness and the question of dangerousness. Legally speaking these were two separate questions, but in this case, experts were able to tie them together: it was due to his illness that this man was dangerous.

The second case in the report from 1902 was also related to alcohol. The case report consists of a long list of the many infractions committed by the defendant in the past: sexual assaults on children, serial thefts and excessive drinking. He had been in and out of institutions and prisons and had been declared insane previously. Due to his life in various institutions, the forensic experts had access to information presumably of higher quality than the hearsay they were often forced to rely on. For example, the defendant's reaction to alcohol had been examined by a physician at some point along the road when the defendant was served copious amounts of brandy. According to the information, he responded 'typically', which is to say, normally, on alcohol. During another stay in a mental asylum, his intelligence had been tested by means of a questionnaire regarding history, geography and arithmetic. In the concluding discussion, the experts presented the opinion that this was a degenerate individual and a 'moral imbecile'. They concluded from this that he was to be regarded as mentally ill, and as a danger to public safety. Based on this conclusion, the case against this defendant was dismissed, and he was sent to a mental asylum.

These two cases illustrate two points. Firstly, that the kind of clientele that the forensic experts in matters of psychiatry were introduced to made it inevitable that they addressed questions beyond the restricted question of mental illness. In both cases, the most important part of the assessment regarded the defendant's dangerousness in the future. This was all the more important as it opened a different repertoire of societal reactions, as in the second case, the mental asylum. The experts mapped the entire career of these multiple offenders, and the offences they were charged with seemed almost coincidental in this broader picture. They demonstrate how crucial the apparatus of forensic psychiatry was in order to make a new epistemic object visible: though the occasion for the examination is a crime, the object that becomes visible through the forensic examination is the criminal.[39]

A culture of consensus 255

Secondly, the publication of these cases in the annual report of the Commission for Forensic Medicine, without any further comments, demonstrates that the Commission, in practice, was performing a certain kind of silent normativity. In a later edition, the Commission promised to publish all cases of general interest, but they never explained why exactly these cases would be of interest for the readers. That is presumably because they were never meant to illuminate any specific legal or medical questions, but they were proposed in order to homogenise the practice of forensic medicine by proposing a specific style of reasoning.

The Commission for Forensic Medicine worked for a 'uniformity of judgment' among forensic psychiatrists. This uniformity would be built on the 'biological principle', that is, that forensic experts would advise the courts on matters of medicine. But the two early cases show that the matters of forensic psychiatry in many cases were less medical than they might appear. The dangerous individual is a most striking example of this.

Despite this tension in the epistemology of forensic expertise, the general impression would be that the criminal courts were very much bound by the judgments of the forensic experts. Technically this was not the situation. Both in questions of responsibility and of dangerousness, the courts had the final word. But in legal practice, many felt that it was outside the courts' discretion to question the experts' judgment. In a high-profile trial of a case of attempted murder in 1963, the jury did not abide with the forensic psychiatrists' opinion that the defendant was mentally ill. In the aftermath of the case, Johs Andenæs, a professor and leading expert in criminal law, reminded the public that in Norwegian legal tradition, the courts had 'in practice' been bound by the opinion of the forensic experts.[40] And the chairman of the Commission for Forensic Medicine, Gabriel Langfeldt, suggested on the basis of this case that it was now time to formalise this precedent and make it an obligation for the courts to conform to the opinion of the experts, as long as the experts were in agreement with each other.[41] His advice was not followed up, however, maybe because the general opinion was that the culture of consensus in the legal system was strong enough to make a formalisation superfluous. That seems to have been the case until the early 2000s and the Utøya trial.

Conclusion

This chapter has discussed the legal and institutional changes in the late nineteenth and early twentieth century that lay the foundation of a culture of consensus in Norwegian forensic psychiatry. I have referred to the result of these changes as a 'forensic culture' and suggested that a characteristic of this culture is that it was more conducive to creating consensus, both among psychiatric experts and between psychiatric and legal professionals. Key factors of the architecture of this culture were the fact that the courts rarely heard opposing expert opinions, the fact that experts regularly worked in pairs, and the establishment of a Commission for Forensic Medicine that sought to control but also to homogenise the work of forensic experts. Moreover, the biological or medical doctrine of criminal responsibility was a crucial part of this structure. For the next hundred years, the Commission would function as a guarantor for a 'uniformity of judgment' based on this biological principle.

On this principle, or the idea of this principle, it was possible to build a culture of consensus. It was mobilised in the encounter between two different professional groups in the late nineteenth century: legal professionals and medical professionals. There are certainly aspects of this debate that can be understood as a struggle of competence between these two professions. The cases from forensic practice that I have presented in this chapter, on the other hand, illustrate how in this practice something different from responsibility was also at stake: the dangerous individual as an object of knowledge. The dangerous individual was hardly a product of professional interest. Rather the legal and professional specialists responded to him/her with a concerted effort to protect society.

In the early twenty-first century, there were signs that the long-standing consensus was cracking. Most spectacularly this was exposed in the trial against the Utøya murderer. In the aftermath of the trial, the parliament started a process to revise the rule of responsibility. The political winds were now blowing against the long-standing medical principle in criminal law.

Notes

1 Colin Jacobsen and Daniel Maier-Katkin, 'Breivik's Sanity: Terrorism, Mass Murder, and the Insanity Defense', *Human Rights Quarterly* 37:1 (2015) pp. 137–152.
2 The literature on this school is abundant, see e.g. Peter Becker and Richard F. Wetzell (eds), *Criminals and their Scientists: the History of Criminology in International Perspective* (Washington, DC, Cambridge: German Historical Institute, Cambridge University Press, 2006).
3 Ragnar Hauge, *Straffens begrunnelse* (Oslo: Universitetsforlaget, 1996). It was part of the self-understanding of the reformers that they channeled the influence from the positivist school. In recent times it has been argued that the resulting criminal code was less influenced by the positivists than what is generally conceded. Jørn Jacobsen, ' "I selve Dybderne af den mennesklige Bevidsthed om Ret og Moral": Straffelova av 1902 og den tyske skulestriden', in Sverre Flaatten and Geir Heivoll (eds), *Straff, lov, historie. Historiske perspektiver på straffeloven av 1902* (Oslo: Akademisk publisering, 2014).
4 For a more thorough discussion of the historiography, see Harry Oosterhuis and Arlie Loughnan, 'Madness and Crime: Historical Perspectives on Forensic Psychiatry', *International Journal of Law and Psychiatry* 37:1 (2014), pp. 1–16.
5 Jan Goldstein, *Console and Classify: The French Psychiatric Profession in the Nineteenth Century*, 2nd edn (Chicago and London: University of Chicago Press, 2001 [1987]).
6 Michel Foucault, 'About the Concept of the "Dangerous Individual" in 19th Century Legal Psychiatry', *International Journal of Law and Psychiatry* 1 (1978), pp. 1–18; Michel Foucault, *Les anormaux: cours au Collège de France, 1974–1975* (Paris: Gallimard; Seuil, 1999). A similar perspective is to be found in Patrizia Guarnieri, 'Alienists on Trial: Conflict and Convergence between Psychiatry and Law (1876–1913)', *History of Science* 29:4 (1991), pp. 393–410.
7 For a definition of dispositive, see 'Le jeu de Michel Foucault', in Michel Foucault, *Dits et écrit, II (1976–1988)* (Paris: Gallimard, 2001), p. 299.
8 Harry Oosterhuis, 'Treatment as Punishment: Forensic Psychiatry in The Netherlands (1870–2005)', *International Journal of Law and Psychiatry* 37:1 (2014), pp. 37–49, here p. 40.

9 Eric J. Engstrom, 'Topographies of Forensic Practice in Imperial Germany', *International Journal of Law and Psychiatry* 37:1 (2014), pp. 63–64. Engstrom expands on an argument of Wetzell, who was speaking more broadly of a 'second wave' of scholarship of science under Nazism. Richard F. Wetzell, *Inventing the Criminal. A History of German Criminology, 1880–1945* (Chapel Hill: University of North Carolina Press, 2000), p. 303.
10 For a detailed description of an Italian case that shows such a combination, see Patrizia Guarnieri, *A Case of Child Murder: Law and Science in Nineteenth-Century Tuscany* (Cambridge: Polity Press, 1993).
11 Katherine D. Watson, *Forensic Medicine in Western Society: A History* (London and New York: Routledge, 2011), p. 54.
12 Svein Atle Skålevåg, *Utilregnelighet: en historie om rett og medisin* (Oslo: Pax, 2016), pp. 35–37.
13 Formally, the professors individually had the obligation to give advice to the state, but informally it passed over to the collegium over the years. Paul Winge, *Den retsmedicinske undersøgelse af den sindssyge lovovertræder* (Kristiania: Alb. Cammermeyers forlag, 1896).
14 Skålevåg, *Utilregnelighet*, pp. 71–72.
15 Paul Winge, *Den norske sindssygeret. Historisk fremstillet.* vol. 3 (Kristiania: Dybwad, 1917), p. 277.
16 Wenche Blomberg, *Galskapens hus. Internering og utskilling i Norge 1550 – 1850* (Oslo: Universitetsforlaget, 2002).
17 Skålevåg, *Utilregnelighet*, pp. 70–75.
18 Paul Winge proposed this argument time and again, see e.g. Winge, *Den retsmedicinske undersøgelse*, p. 105.
19 Professor Faye quotes from the minutes of this meeting in the debate that followed in the Medical Society. The minutes from the meeting in the Society were published as an appendix to the medical journal *Norsk Magazin for Lægevidenskaben* (1859), p. 661.
20 The report of the legal commission of 1896 is quoted in Straffelovkomiteen, Innstilling fra den av Justisdepartementet 11. mai 1922 opnevnte komité til revisjon av Straffeloven, 52 (Oslo 1925).
21 Tove Stang Dahl, *Barnevern og samfunnsvern. Om stat, vitenskap og profesjoner under barnevernets oppkomst i Norge*, UniPax (Oslo: Pax forlag, 1978).
22 Rune Slagstad, *De nasjonale strateger* (Oslo: Pax, 1998), p. 123; Dahl, *Barnevern og samfunnsvern*, p. 87.
23 Hauge, *Straffens begrunnelse*, p. 217. For the *kriminalistische vereinigung*, see Richard F. Wetzell, 'About the Concept of the "Dangerous Individual" in Turn-of-the-Century Penal

Reform: Debates on Recidivism, État Dangereux, Indeterminate Sentencing, and Civil Liberty in the International Union of Penal Law, 1889–1914', GLOSSAE. *European Journal of Legal History* 17 (2020), pp. 119–149.
24 Raffaele Garofalo, *Criminology*, trans. Robert Wyness Millar (Boston: Little, Brown and Company, 1914).
25 Skålevåg, *Utilregnelighet*, p. 113.
26 Skålevåg, *Utilregnelighet*, pp. 109–115.
27 Roger Qvarsell, *Utan vett och vilja: Om synen på brottslighet och sinnessjukdom* (Stockholm: Carlsson, 1993), p. 87.
28 The various codes are discussed in Straffelovkomiteen, *Innstilling fra den av Justisdepartementet 11. mai 1922 opnevnte komité til revisjon av Straffeloven*. For a more recent international overview, see Oosterhuis and Loughnan, 'Madness and Crime'.
29 Engstrom, 'Topographies of Forensic Practice in Imperial Germany', p. 64.
30 Paul Winge, *Samfundet og den sindssyge lovovertræder* (Kristiania: Alb. Cammermeyers forlag, 1898). Paul Winge, *Den norske sindssygeret: Historisk fremstillet*. Vol 1 (Kristiania: Dybwad, 1913).
31 Skålevåg, *Utilregnelighet*, p. 113.
32 See Birsen Erkmen, 'Den rettsmedisinske kommisjon', in Pål Grøndahl and Ulf Stridbeck (eds), *Rettspsykiatriske beretninger: Om sakkyndighet og menneskeskjebner* (Oslo: Gyldendal Akademisk, 2015).
33 Winge, *Den retsmedicinske undersøgelse*, p. 118.
34 Engstrom, 'Topographies of Forensic Practice in Imperial Germany', p. 65.
35 Oosterhuis, 'Treatment as Punishment', p. 40.
36 The annual reports of the commission were published regularly from 1900 to 1914. Then there was a hiatus until the publication was taken up again in 1920–1927, and then another long break before it resumed in 1968. It is still published, though less regularly. They have continued to provide examples of forensic cases to this day.
37 *Den retsmedicinske kommissions beretning*, vol 1.
38 'Dipsomanien er en sindsygdomsform eller maaske rettere et sindssygdomssymptom, der under omstændigheder som i nærværende tilfælde gjør de syge under paraoxysmerne (anfaldene) farlig for den offentlige sikkerhed', *Den retsmedicinske kommissions beretning*, vol. 1, p. 59.
39 Foucault, 'About the Concept of the "Dangerous Individual" in 19th Century Legal Psychiatry'.

40 Johs Andenæs, 'Giftsaken på Hamar: Juridiske randbemerkninger', *Lov og rett* 4:4 (1965), pp. 289–302.
41 Gabriel Langfeldt, 'Rettspsykiatrisk kommentar til professor Andenæs' artikkel om Hamar-saken', *Lov og rett* 4:5 (1965), pp. 429–432.

11

The 'key' to the crime: Criminal cases and the projection of expectations about forensic DNA technologies in the Portuguese press

Filipe Santos

Introduction

DNA technologies have been at the forefront of a renewed enthusiasm surrounding forensic science and its promises and expectations for crime fighting.[1] In the early 2000s, Portugal was starting to discuss the possibility of building a universal DNA database.[2] However, considering the threats to individual rights and civil liberties that this implied, the adopted legislation in 2008 would become one of the most restrictive in the European Union.[3]

In parallel to the discussions regarding the use of DNA technologies for forensic purposes in Portugal, forensic science started to be featured in the coverage of criminal cases in the Portuguese media. In this sense, newspapers became a source for understanding how representations about forensic science could be constructed and be made accessible to lay audiences, particularly in terms of its promises and potential for solving crimes. The choice to study mediatised criminal cases has to do with their potential to endure in the collective memory[4] and, thus, to shape the public representations of forensic science, crime and justice, but also citizens' understanding and acceptance of DNA technologies in criminal investigation.[5]

This chapter is divided into two main parts. I start by exploring the cultural and historical context for the emergence of different claims surrounding the so-called 'CSI effect', providing context on some aspects of the Portuguese forensic culture. This first part also introduces the five criminal cases used in this study that were selected from 1995 to 2010 based on the reported use of forensic DNA technologies, and the factors for their prolonged newsworthiness and coverage in daily newspapers.

The second part draws on extracts from the newspaper coverage of the criminal cases, exploring the senses and meanings about forensic science that are portrayed. The emerging popularity of the *CSI – Crime Scene Investigation* – series around the same time provided journalists with a sort of fictional metaphor to translate and convey to their audiences the 'novelty' and 'complexity' of forensic science that was used in the covered criminal cases.

I argue that the recurrent connotations with *CSI* generate a form of *journalist effect*, by which the fictional imagery of *CSI* influences the media's production of representations about police work, forensic science and criminal investigation. The analysis of the news articles suggests the prevalence of two dominant types of media discourse about forensic science in general, and DNA technologies in particular: on the one hand, a more popular discourse that celebrates the potential of DNA technologies as a 'truth machine'[6] that explores the use of fictional metaphors to convey the idea that science can produce the desired justice; on the other hand, a more sceptical and critical discourse that ponders the actual value and relevance of forensic science against the actual forensic practices and contingencies of individual and institutional actors within the judicial system.

Both discourses can be situated within the social, geopolitical and historical positioning of Portugal in what Boaventura de Sousa Santos called 'imagination of the centre'.[7] This can be useful to understand how the production of collective representations about forensic science in the context of newspaper crime coverage can be framed by underlying notions of an idealised efficient and sophisticated centre, as portrayed on *CSI*.

CSI, its 'effects', and the Portuguese context

Mediatised criminal cases usually expose the general public to the functioning of the justice system and criminal investigation, and it is possible that public representations and beliefs are constructed, at least in part, through the media's discourses. In parallel, crime fiction in its many shapes and formats also exposes the general public to a diversity of culturally influenced portrayals of the functioning of justice.[8]

The twenty-first century brought a new focus to the crime fiction genre, much more centred on forensic science and the apparent pervasiveness of surveillance technologies, like biometric databases, CCTV, tracking devices or facial recognition. The premiere of *CSI* in 2000 was the inception of a worldwide popularity phenomenon, which resulted in several spin-offs, with the original series running until 2015. The new 'heroes' in these stories suggest a shift in policing and crime fighting models. The cultural emphasis of the use of science and technology in fiction to fight and prevent crime is also visible in the enthusiasm with which governments and criminal justice systems have since adopted DNA profiling and databasing and other surveillance systems and infrastructures.[9]

Following the trends of the scientification of police work,[10] which describes how the use of science and technology by the police enables a power source that can provide an appearance of rationalisation and legitimacy in the fulfilment of their roles, the *CSI* series can be understood in popular culture as a metaphor for scientific and technological progress, but also for the political, social and cultural developments of the early twenty-first century. The emergence and availability of new forensic technologies like DNA profiling[11] at the turn of the century has impacted social representations about police work, criminal justice and forensic science. As Jasanoff recalls,[12] in the USA there were several landmark criminal cases where forensic genetics and scientific credibility played a key role, prompting the 'genetic age' of forensic identification.[13] In broad terms, *CSI* draws on these developments to render a fictional portrayal of forensic science as a sort of 'truth machine' that will use evidence, logic and reasoning to identify the real offender and exonerate the innocent.[14]

Fuelled by claims of the supposed impact of TV forensic science fiction on real-world beliefs, reports about a 'CSI effect' started to appear in the American media in 2002.[15] In the context of an adversarial justice system, like in the USA, where the role of the judge is that of an arbitrator between the parties, and where verdicts are reached by a jury of lay citizens, it is natural to have concerns about external factors that may influence the fairness of the trial. There have been multiple academic inquiries into the phenomenon of the

CSI effect and, even if it is not new that juries in real cases may be affected by the media,[16] this particular effect voices concerns of both lawyers and prosecutors surrounding forensic evidence. In short, legal actors worry that jurors may acquit when they should convict, or convict when they should acquit, due to either not enough 'scientific' evidence, or to an overestimation of expert testimonies or evidence. Simon Cole and Rachel Dioso-Villa have explored the developments of the CSI effect,[17] describing a typology consisting of six 'effects' that are found in the media. Besides the supposed influence in juries, lawyers and prosecutors, the authors found claims that, because of the series, people are better prepared to understand forensic science (*producer's effect*), students are interested in enrolling in forensic science courses (*professor's version*), and that CSI can teach criminals to avoid detection (*police chief's version*), as a form of forensic awareness.[18]

In addition to providing a typology[19] of the different claims surrounding the effect and finding that in the USA there are no higher or lower acquittal rates that could be attributed to a CSI effect, Cole and Dioso-Villa argued that, if anything, there is a CSI effect *effect*, that is, the increase of the media's discourses about the CSI effect on criminal trials.

While several empirical studies[20] did not find support for the idea that the fictional series influences the standard of reasonable doubt, or the expectations and attitudes of ordinary citizens serving in juries, they also focused on adversarial legal contexts, like the USA, where there is a higher probability that lay jurors may be asked to assess forensic evidence and testimonies.

In Portugal, the criminal justice system is based on the inquisitorial principle. In other words, the role of the court is to establish the material truth of the facts, in which the role of the judge is to conduct the inquiry and to ensure the impartiality and objectivity of the proceedings. In this sense, the Public Prosecution, the Judiciary Police and the forensic laboratories[21] are all legally conceived as neutral and impartial entities working towards the common goal of establishing the truth. Law 49/2008[22] defines the organisation of criminal investigation, assigning competences and coordination among police forces. The criminal investigation is carried out by the Public Prosecution, assisted by the Judiciary Police and/or other police forces, and supervised by a judge of instruction. However, as

Costa notes,[23] first responders to crime scenes, usually proximity police forces like the *Polícia de Segurança Pública* (in urban areas) or the *Guarda Nacional Republicana* (in rural areas), tend to shape the criminal narratives based on their 'selective professional vision' which may affect further developments, as other actors are called to intervene. If the case reaches trial, the judge can freely assess the credibility of witnesses and their testimonies. However, forensic examinations, technical or artistic expertise are presumed to be excluded from the free appreciation of the judge. For instance, if judges disagree with the content of a forensic report, they must provide arguments for the decision. Jury trials are rare and can only be requested by the prosecution or the defendant, in cases where the potential sentence equals eight or more years in prison.

In the Portuguese forensic culture, there is no record of public controversies over scientific credibility, which is expected in an inquisitorial system where two certified public institutions provide forensic services to the courts – the Laboratory of Scientific Police and the National Institute of Legal Medicine and Forensic Sciences. The absence of adversarial contests and the monopoly over forensic examinations reinforces the institutional objective of judicial neutrality. As argued by Costa, this culture of implicit trust and institutional neutrality can lead judges to see forensic science, and especially complex forensics like DNA analyses, as a sort of 'ready-made evidence' that can be accepted and trusted as it arrives in court as far as it stands on robust scientific authority.[24] Furthermore, previous studies described the Portuguese forensic culture as a 'bubble culture' or 'epistemic distancing', whereby experts seek to isolate themselves and the evidence from external contaminants, cognitive or otherwise.[25] In court, the experts' testimonies tend to circumvent expressions of opinion or interpretation of evidence, often stating what is written in reports. Therefore, given the relative distance of the lay public from courtroom proceedings, and the presumed neutrality of state forensic laboratories, the prosecution and the judiciary, the occurrence of the common types of CSI effects (e.g. expecting more scientific evidence or exaggerating its probative value) is unlikely to be found within the Portuguese justice system. Nevertheless, the media coverage of criminal cases may allow insights into the cultural influence of forensic science fiction, or the shaping of the CSI effect beyond the courtroom.

Criminal cases and newsworthiness factors

The analysis of crime reporting constitutes an opportunity to study the production of collective symbols, e.g. who are the heroes and the villains, through the dissemination of discourses and cultural meanings that contribute to the definition of social issues and threats to society.[26] Newspaper stories tend to be constructed according to frames that resonate with the audience's collective values, with the press acting as the broadcaster of dominant understandings about crime and offenders, capable of mobilising social energies in the reinforcement or change of prevailing norms and consensuses.[27]

This chapter draws from a larger study on the uses of DNA technologies for forensic purposes in Portugal.[28] The selection criteria for criminal cases were ample mediatisation, that is, regular news coverage for more than one year, and the use of DNA technologies in the course of the investigation. The selected timeframe for the research was set between 1995, around the time that DNA technologies became routinely used in Portugal, and 2010, since the cases had to be closed in order to access judicial files for the start of the research in 2011. The collection of news articles in online and printed issues was as thorough as possible, from the publication of the first item until the judicial closure of the case.

The choice of four daily newspapers that maintained activity for the selected period of research is justified by the need to achieve both diversity and saturation. The four newspapers include two 'reference' or 'quality' newspapers (*Público* and *Diário de Notícias*) and two 'tabloid' or 'popular' newspapers (*Jornal de Notícias* and *Correio da Manhã*). The quality press seeks the acceptance of the public and journalist peers by privileging the production of longer news items on complex political and economic subjects of national and international scope, accompanied by in-depth expert commentary. The correct use of language and the accuracy of reporting is also a staple in this type of press.[29] On the other side of the axis, as Sparks[30] would put it, the tabloid press aims for a readership interested in daily events. The style tends to be vivid and often sensationalist, using a colloquial approach to language and impacting headlines. In this type of press, there is an abundance of graphics and photographs, accompanied by short texts and opinion columns that often have demagogical tendencies.[31] On this distinction, Bourdieu[32] also mentions a division in the journalistic field between a 'commercial' and an 'intellectual' pole, elaborating on the differences between newspapers focused on the production of novelty and sensation and the newspapers that privilege broad commentary and in-depth analyses, while affirming the value of objectivity.[33]

The selected cases stood out from daily news routine. Jewkes systematised a list of twelve factors that may configure the newsworthiness of a given crime. Some are self-explanatory and most criminal events that include one or more factors are more likely to be newsworthy. These can be immediately found in the selected cases, like *sex*, *violence*, *celebrity or high-status persons* and *children*. The *Meia Culpa* case (1997) was a violent attack on a nightclub that caused thirteen deaths. Its coverage had thematic ramifications into prostitution and human trafficking, as well as illegal security in nightclubs. The *Tó Jó* case (1999) refers to a crime where António Jorge stabbed his parents, killing them and making attempts to destroy the bodies. Besides the violence, this case was particularly newsworthy because of possible connections to black metal bands and satanic rituals. The case of the *Serial Killer of Santa Comba Dão* (2005) involved the disappearance and murder of three young girls over the course of one year. The perpetrator was found to be a retired police officer and a highly regarded member of the community. He was said to be very religious and an admirer of Salazar.[34] Both the *Joana* (2004) and the *Madeleine McCann* (2007) cases relate to small children that mysteriously disappeared in the Algarve, leaving no trace or evidence. The latter of these cases received the most media coverage, even on a global scale. This is because of the convergence and combination of several newsworthiness factors which can be used to predict which criminal cases will have more media coverage. Jewkes's list also includes *proximity* (geographical or cultural), *predictability*, *threshold*, *simplification*, *individualism*, *risk*, *conservative ideology* and *political diversion*. These newsworthiness factors, isolated or combined, can be found in the five criminal cases that were selected for the analysis described in more detail in the next section.

CSI and fictional metaphors

Even before the popularisation of forensic science fiction, there were already signs of what Shelton and colleagues called a *tech effect*.[35] The case that would become known as *Tó Jó* happened on 12 August 1999, coinciding with a total solar eclipse. A 23-year-old man named António Jorge (abbreviated to Tó Jó) who was on vacation with his wife, travelled to his parents' house in Ílhavo and stabbed both to death. There were attempts to set fire to the house and to destroy the bodies. The coincidence with the solar eclipse and the fact that the suspect played in a black metal band and was interested in satanism led the authorities to suspect that the crime involved more than one offender, possibly motivated by some sort of satanic ritual, as Tó Jó had friends with similar interests.

Reporting on the 1999 *Tó Jó* case, a *Público* article about the arrest of Nuno, a friend of Tó Jó who had recently spent a weekend at Tó Jó's parents' house, expressed a tone of awe in view of the identification of the unknown element present in the blood stains found at the crime scene:

> To everyone's surprise, Nuno was arrested last Friday, almost a year after the events. The DNA tests were fatal for the young man from Porto. The technical conclusions achieved by the IMLC experts corroborated some clues and provided consistency to the police's thesis. And it is certain that one of the profiles individualised by the experts from the IMLC was perfectly compatible with the young man's.[36]

In a rarely used resort, additional DNA analyses were requested by the defence. The new examinations would acquit Nuno during trial, but this was not so prominent in the news.[37] Even in the earliest analysed case (*Meia Culpa*, 1997), the same newspaper includes a smaller explanatory text explaining the novelty of 'genetic fingerprinting':

> Unless we have a twin sibling, there is no one else in the world that has fingerprints like ours. Similarly, each one of us has, in the big molecule of DNA that contains our hereditary patrimony, a pattern of genetic fragments that is ours and only ours – and which distinguishes us from the rest of our kin. It is this particular and personal genetic pattern that is usually called a genetic 'fingerprint'.[38]

The *Meia Culpa* case refers to a crime that resulted in the highest ever number of mortal victims in Portugal. In April 1997, three hooded men invaded a nightclub called *Meia Culpa* in Amarante and, using a firearm to intimidate the customers and staff, poured gasoline on the furniture and set it on fire. They escaped in a stolen car that was found abandoned the following day. Because the emergency exit was blocked, the smoke and fire led to the death of twelve people at the scene, causing serious injuries in nine people, and one additional death resulting from injuries.

The underlying message from the news extract above was that these 'genetic fingerprints' could be used to identify the suspects from the balaclavas worn during the attack on the nightclub *Meia Culpa*. The following extract gives credit to the 'scientific police', highlighting the relevance and contribution of forensic science for the resolution of criminal cases:

> The investigation of the *'Meia Culpa'* case was a sort of test of the Judiciary Police itself, to which it responded effectively. Despite the pressures from the public opinion and the Government, the scientific police worked over ten consecutive days and nights, in order to arrive at some important conclusions on the 12th day.[39]

The analysis of the *Meia Culpa* case's judicial files reveals that there was much police work involved and that the analyses of the hairs found on the balaclavas were matched to only one of the suspects. The laboratory communicated with the police stating that they would compare any DNA profiles as soon as they were sent the reference profiles of any suspects, which eventually happened. The DNA reports were delivered a week before the investigation was concluded. By that time, all suspects had been quickly identified and arrested thanks to information from the mother of one of the boys who stole the car that would be used by the attackers. This information was extracted from the judicial files and had not appeared in the news. Although forensic science had made little or no contribution to finding the suspects, the established media narrative had already presented science as a determining factor for success.

The media coverage of later cases would be notoriously marked by the emerging popularity of *CSI*, which appeared as a cultural reference for a TV show and as a fictional metaphor for the expectations surrounding the role of forensic science for the investigation of criminal cases, as a protagonist that portrays a quick, impartial and neutral justice. References to *CSI* tend to convey a scenario of sophistication and crime-solving capabilities that can sometimes overshadow traditional police investigative work. The newspapers' narratives tend to fit into a 'mediated witness'[40] model that presents a criminal case in a way that elicits emotional responses from the readers. Since narratives have to be adapted to the audiences, there is always room for excessive simplification or even distortion of the facts.[41] From this perspective, it is expected that cultural references to fiction are included either as explanatory metaphors or as a way to support and lend credibility to the police's side of the story. In line with Cole and Dioso-Villa's typology, the tendency to rely on fictional and popular cultural metaphors to convey a story could be framed as a sort of *journalist effect*. The following extract from a tabloid newspaper does this in a way that glosses over the police's efforts by attributing the success to the police-scientist hybrid that is common in fictional series:[42]

> The investigation was, in fact, similar to a mix of two television series – 'CSI – Crime Scene Investigation', where the analysis of the most insignificant piece of evidence is fundamental, and 'Bones', where the analysis of corpses is a crucial element. It turns out that, during trial …, it's not enough to have a confession, and not even the reconstitution of the homicides … [43]

The case that would later become known as the *Serial Killer of Santa Comba Dão* had its first occurrence on 31 May 2005, when the dead body of a young girl was found by a fisherman on the beach in Figueira da Foz. While efforts to identify the girl were still being made, two other girls were reported missing in Santa Comba Dão, about 90km from Figueira da Foz: one in November 2005, and another in May 2006. All girls had their phones turned off and there was no indication that they had plans to travel or run away. The Judiciary Police was able to identify the first girl who was a neighbour of the other two missing girls.

The case of the *Serial Killer of Santa Comba Dão* was solved thanks to the investigative and organisational capabilities of the case's investigators that discovered the associations between the disappearance of the three victims and found the traces and evidence to confront the suspect (found to be a retired member of GNR – the Republican National Guard – a local police force in rural areas), leading to a confession and to the location of the bodies. The suspect was convicted and ordered to serve a prison sentence of 25 years, which is the maximum prison sentence in Portugal, and to pay compensation to the victims' families.

The *Joana* and *Madeleine* cases, because they involved children, were particularly newsworthy. The international scope of the *Madeleine McCann* case, in conjunction with other prominent factors, explains the different volumes of news production between these two particular cases.

The *Joana* case began on 12 September 2004, when an eight-year-old girl from a small village near Portimão, in the Algarve, was sent to the shop for some milk and canned tuna. Her mother reported to the local authorities that Joana did not come home, and searches were initiated. The Judiciary Police became involved when, reading the news about the case and watching an interview with Joana's mother on TV, the coordinating inspector began suspecting that the child had not run away, and that this could be a more serious crime that fell under the jurisdiction of the Judiciary Police. Following several questionings, Joana's mother and uncle

Table 11.1 Total news items published in the selected newspapers, related to the Joana Cipriano and Madeleine McCann cases

Newspaper	Collection dates	*Joana* case (total items)	Collection dates	*Madeleine McCann* case (total items)
Público	18/09/2004–16/11/2005	32	05/05/2007–22/07/2008	213
Correio da Manhã	15/09/2004–13/11/2005	113	04/05/2007–23/07/2008	384
Jornal de Notícias	17/09/2004–12/11/2005	77	04/05/2007–31/07/2008	380
Diário de Notícias	24/09/2004–12/11/2005	78	05/05/2007–28/07/2008	228

became official suspects for the murder of Joana. At the trial, little or no material evidence was produced. The child's body has not been found.

The disappearance of three-year-old Madeleine McCann is probably one of the most mediatised criminal cases of all time. In May 2007, a British couple was on vacation in the Algarve with their three children. They had travelled with friends and were staying in a holiday resort. On the evening of 3 May, the group of adults were having dinner at the resort's restaurant and would periodically check on the children who were sleeping in the apartments nearby. At around 22:00, Madeleine's mother discovered her daughter's disappearance. The authorities (GNR) were called in and searches for the child were initiated. One year later, and after Madeleine's parents were made official suspects, the investigation against them was closed for lack of evidence. Like in the case of Joana's disappearance, to this day no trace or evidence has been found that might explain the disappearance of Madeleine McCann.

Perhaps because of the growth of *CSI*'s popularity, but also because the investigations became immediately mediatised and there were no early results, the newspapers' coverage of the disappearances of Joana Cipriano and Madeleine McCann were strongly focused on the investigative uses of forensic science and DNA technologies in particular. In both cases, the existence of material evidence was questioned throughout the coverage and journalists had access to abundant information about the investigation. This meant that a large portion of the news articles about these cases, particularly in *Correio da Manhã*, concern searches, forensic examinations and laboratory reports, speculating about the significance for the cases' resolution.

The sensationalist style of the tabloid press underlying the coverage of the *Joana* and *Madeleine McCann* cases, influenced by the *CSI* imagery, results in a rhetoric style that places the reader as a sort of investigator of the facts, clues and evidence that are compiled throughout the inquiry, while at the same time it elicits emotional identification with the victims. This is enacted through the recurrent use of anonymous sources 'close to the investigation' and the speculations about the possible consequences for the course of the investigation, like in the following extract about the *Madeleine McCann* case:

> It is not only the fact that traces have been found that match Madeleine's DNA that leads the investigators to believe that this is a case of death. It is also the places where the traces were found ... The English dogs detected cadaver odours in the bedroom, in the boot of the car, and on the clothes that Kate [Madeleine's mother] wore that night. Then, there were traces of blood, not visible to the naked eye, that indicated the presence of the little girl behind a sofa in the bedroom and in the boot of the car rented 22 days after the disappearance [...] It was also there that the animals found biological traces of DNA that matches the English girl's and which rejects the possibility that they belong to [Madeleine's] twin siblings.[44]

As illustrated by this extract, DNA technologies came to play a leading role in this sort of media crime narrative, echoing the recent fictional portrayals of criminal investigation where forensic science offers the ultimate 'key to the crime'. Nevertheless, it becomes apparent that the use of modern forensic technologies is infused into traditional tools, procedures and ways of thinking and seeing, upon which criminal investigation continues to operate. In this scenario, evidence that is produced in a laboratory by scientists is perceived to bear a status of certainty, which can also contribute to reinforce the police's 'moral authority'.[45] This was also emphasised during the *Madeleine McCann* case, where the Judiciary Police was subjected to criticism, mainly in the foreign press.

Hence, this type of discourse can be associated with the infotainment features that characterise modern media. In the Portuguese semi-peripheral context, this creates a sort of mistranslation through an imaginary by which it is 'science' and not the police that solves the problem of crime. This is a feature which ultimately illustrates a cultural effectiveness of the 'imagination of the centre' and a consequence of the scientification of police work, insofar as the police's legitimacy is reinforced for using similar techniques and scientific methods as the police forces in 'central' countries which are seen as more advanced and sophisticated, as part of the narrative of the imagination of the centre that also appears in the discourse of the quality press in the following section.

Distancing and scepticism

Besides the allusions to *CSI* to describe the sophistication and effectiveness of forensic science that marked the narratives of the tabloid *Correio da Manhã*, the other analysed newspapers mention the *CSI* series in order to evoke the contrasts and the distance from reality to forensic science fiction. For example, mentions in the *Diário de Notícias*[46] are from an opinion column of a retired criminal investigator and from a statement by the president of the criminal investigation workers' union. Both compare reality to the fictional portrayals, stating the differences between the time that analyses take to produce results, and remarking that it is not normal that the same person who collects traces at crime scenes will analyse them in the laboratory. The *Jornal de Notícias* also published an opinion column by the president of the National Institute of Legal Medicine, who likewise asserts the distance between fiction and reality: 'However, regrettably, this type of exam has its limitations. They do not always provide the spectacular, clear, and unequivocal results that are seen in currently very successful television series, like CSI.'[47]

A reference to the *CSI* series appears in the quality newspaper *Público* as a metaphor for an ideal model of criminal investigation, albeit in an editorial written after the case was closed, directing criticism at the way the Judiciary Police conducted the investigation, but also to the sensationalist and speculative coverage by the media: 'It is not even necessary to expect that the PJ performs with the effectiveness of "CSI like" investigators to realise the number of mistakes made in the first hours and days.'[48]

The appeal to the fictional metaphor with recurrent mentions of the *CSI* series works in two different directions. On the one hand, the tabloid press resorts to the series' high-tech imagery and the power of science for criminal investigation purposes as a way to bolster public confidence in the Judiciary Police, and also to translate the complexity of criminal investigation into more familiar images. On the other hand, the quality press uses the metaphor of *CSI* as a contrast between the ideal and the actual technologies and resources in a semi-peripheral context like the Portuguese case, thus projecting the hyper-real scenario of *CSI* as an aspirational motif.[49] This discourse of the quality press about *CSI* could then be a symptom of what Boaventura de Sousa Santos described as the *imagination of the centre*,[50] or a Portuguese way of being semi-peripheral, insofar as the distance to the 'centre' is acknowledged, while simultaneously sensing a collective awareness that the gap may be bridged.[51]

Conclusion

The present analysis focused on understanding of how popular fictional metaphors, like the *CSI* series, can be enacted by journalists to convey information and project expectations about forensic science, DNA technologies and criminal justice in Portugal. The main concern underlying the CSI effect (or the *strong prosecutor effect*) was that people were being acquitted when they should be convicted because lay citizens in juries expected more scientific evidence. In an inquisitorial judicial system where jury trials are infrequent, and public controversies surrounding forensic evidence are almost non-existent, the media can often contribute to shape public adversarial narratives. When covering a shocking crime, this tendency can reproduce what Tyler[52] has called the *reverse CSI effect*, and Cole and Dioso-Villa called the *defendant's effect*. In other words, a psychological need to punish alleged offenders may lead lay jurors or, in this case, journalists, to place undue weight or significance on expert evidence. This sort of effect can be enhanced by pre-trial media coverage, or even by what is referred to as a trial by media.[53] Trials by media can be harmful to suspects' presumption of innocence and social reputation. In this context, exaggerated inferences from the existence of forensic evidence in a given case can be particularly damaging.

Although praise for the novelty of forensic genetics could be seen in the quality press in earlier cases (*Meia Culpa*, 1997 and *Tó Jó*, 1999), the use of fictional metaphors to support a narrative where forensic science would produce the definitive evidence to solve criminal cases was particularly featured in the tabloid *Correio da Manhã*. Taking Cole and Dioso-Villa's CSI effect typology as a reference, I would suggest that the inclusion of recurrent references to *CSI* in the tabloid press configures a *journalist effect*. This would be an effect on the modulation of journalistic discourse and style, by which the cultural and socio-legal references shared with the audiences are grounded on a fictional imaginary or dramatic genre as an explanatory metaphor. However, this may be a twofold effect. While the popular press uses references to *CSI* mainly to praise and legitimise police work, quality newspapers tend to mobilise the fictional metaphor of *CSI* as a critique and a contrast with projections of idealised ways of using forensic science for criminal investigation purposes.

Notes

1 Helena Machado and Susana Silva, 'Portuguese Forensic DNA Database: Political Enthusiasm, Public Trust and Probable Issues in Future Practice', in Richard Hindmarsh and Barbara Prainsack (eds), *Genetic Suspects: Global Governance of DNA Profiling and Databasing* (Cambridge: Cambridge University Press, 2010), pp. 218–239.
2 Maria João Boavida, 'Portugal Plans a Forensic Genetic Database of its Entire Population', *NewropMag* 10 April 2005, https://web.archive.org/web/20140712164838/http://www.newropeans-magazine.org/content/view/2063/121/lang,english/.
3 Filipe Santos, Helena Machado and Susana Silva, 'Forensic DNA Databases in European Countries: Is Size Linked to Performance?', *Life Sciences, Society and Policy* 9:12 (2013), pp. 1–13. doi: 10.1186/2195-7819-9-12.
4 Martin Innes, 'Crime as a Signal, Crime as a Memory', *Journal for Crime, Conflict and the Media* 1:2 (2004), pp. 15–22.
5 Brewer and Ley have suggested that the media are a privileged source of information about DNA technologies for lay publics. Paul R. Brewer and Barbara L. Ley, 'Media Use and Public Perceptions of DNA Evidence', *Science Communication* 32:1 (2010), pp. 93–117. doi: 10.1177/1075547009340343.
6 Michael Lynch et al., *Truth Machine: The Contentious History of DNA Fingerprinting* (Chicago: University of Chicago Press, 2008).
7 Boaventura de Sousa Santos, 'State, Wage Relations and Social Welfare in the Semiperiphery: The Case of Portugal', *Oficina do Centro de Estudos Sociais (CES)* 23 (1991), pp. 1–49. The expression 'imagination-of-the-center' was coined by Santos to describe the Portuguese political and economic transitions that combined the wake of the 1974 revolution, post-colonialism and its relations with former African colonies, with the membership of the EEC in 1986, placing Portugal as an intermediary between the core and the periphery.

8 Gray Cavender and Sarah K. Deutsch, 'CSI and Moral Authority: The Police and Science', *Crime, Media, Culture* 3:1 (2007), pp. 67–81. doi: 10.1177/1741659007074449. Another good example of the pervasiveness of surveillance technologies in crime fighting would be the 2011 CBS series *Person of Interest*.
9 Richard Hindmarsh and Barbara Prainsack (eds), *Genetic Suspects: Global Governance of Forensic DNA Profiling and Databasing* (Cambridge: Cambridge University Press, 2010).
10 Richard V. Ericson and Clifford Shearing, 'The Scientification of Police Work', in Gernot Böhme and Nico Stehr (eds), *The Knowledge Society: The Growing Impact of Scientific Knowledge on Social Relations* (Dordrecht: D. Riedel, 1986), pp. 129–159.
11 Murphy calls DNA typing the *archetypical second generation science*, Erin Murphy, 'The New Forensics: Criminal Justice, False Certainty, and the Second Generation of Scientific Evidence', *California Law Review* 95:3 (2007), pp. 721–797. See also Michael J. Saks and Jonathan J. Koehler, 'The Coming Paradigm Shift in Forensic Identification Science', *Science* 309:5736 (2005), pp. 892–895.
12 Sheila Jasanoff, 'DNA's Identity Crisis', in David Lazer (ed.), *DNA and the Criminal Justice System: The Technology of Justice* (Cambridge, MA: MIT Press, 2004), pp. 337–355.
13 Helena Machado and Barbara Prainsack, *Tracing Technologies: Prisoners' Views in the Era of CSI* (Farnham, UK: Ashgate, 2012).
14 'Arguments highlighting the benefits of forensic DNA technologies assume a hegemonic position in public discourses, where crime is typically assumed to be the problem and tools to fight crime are proposed to be the answer. Surveillance is seen as a necessary evil that needs to be accepted for a greater good' (p. 1129). Barbara Prainsack and Victor Toom, 'The Prüm Regime: Situated Dis/empowerment in Transnational DNA Profile Exchange', *British Journal of Criminology* 50:6 (2010), pp. 1117–1135.
15 See, for example, Richard Willing, ' "CSI effect" has Juries Wanting More Evidence', *USA Today*, 8 May 2004.
16 Valerie P. Hans and Juliet L. Dee, 'Media Coverage of Law: Its Impact on Juries and the Public', *American Behavioral Scientist* 35:2 (1991), pp. 136–149. doi: 10.1177/0002764291035002005.
17 Simon Cole and Rachel Dioso-Villa, 'Law and the Lab: Do TV Shows Really Affect how Juries Vote? Let's Look at the Evidence', *The Wall Street Journal* (New York, 2005), www.wsj.com/articles/SB111594466027532447; Simon Cole and Rachel Dioso-Villa, 'CSI and its Effects: Media, Juries, and the Burden of Proof', *New England Law Review* 41:3 (2007),

pp. 435–470; Simon Cole and Rachel Dioso-Villa, 'Investigating the "CSI Effect" Effect: Media and Litigation Crisis in Criminal Law', *Stanford Law Review* 61:6 (2009), pp. 1335–1374; Simon Cole and Rachel Dioso-Villa, 'Should Judges Worry about the "CSI Effect"?', *Court Review* 47 (2011), pp. 16–27.

18 Eric Beauregard and Martin Bouchard, 'Cleaning up Your Act: Forensic Awareness as a Detection Avoidance Strategy', *Journal of Criminal Justice* 38:6 (2010), pp. 1160–1166. doi: 10.1016/j.jcrimjus.2010.09.004.

19 See Cole and Dioso-Villa, 'CSI and its Effects: Media, Juries, and the Burden of Proof'.

20 Young S. Kim, Gregg Barak and Donald E. Shelton, 'Examining the "CSI-Effect" in the Cases of Circumstantial Evidence and Eyewitness Testimony: Multivariate and Path Analyses', *Journal of Criminal Justice* 37:5 (2009), pp. 452–460. doi: 10.1016/j.jcrimjus.2009.07.005; Shelton, Kim and Barak, 'A Study of Juror Expectations and Demands Concerning Scientific Evidence: Does the "CSI Effect" Exist?'; Ian Hawkins and Kyle Scherr, 'Engaging the CSI Effect: The Influences of Experience-Taking, Type of Evidence, and Viewing Frequency on Juror Decision-Making', *Journal of Criminal Justice* 49: March–April (2017), pp. 45–52. doi: 10.1016/j.jcrimjus.2017.02.003; Nicholas J. Schweitzer and Michael J. Saks, 'The CSI Effect: Popular Fiction about Forensic Science Affects the Public's Expectations about Real Forensic Science', *Jurimetrics Journal* 47 (Spring 2007), pp. 357–364.

21 Law 45/2004, that regulates medical-legal and forensic procedures, confers the monopoly of forensic activities to two public entities: the Laboratory of Scientific Police and the National Institute of Legal Medicine and Forensic Sciences. Lei 45/2004, *Regime Jurídico Das Perícias Médico-Legais e Forenses* (Portugal: Diário da República, 1.a série A — N.o 195., 2004).

22 Law n.º 49/2008 which approves the law for the organisation of criminal investigation. Available at: https://dre.pt/dre/legislacao-consolidada/lei/2008-67191210-67192945.

23 Susana Costa, 'Visibilities, Invisibilities and Twilight Zones at the Crime Scene in Portugal', *New Genetics and Society* 36:4 (2017), pp. 375–399. doi: 10.1080/14636778.2017.1394835.

24 Susana Costa, 'DNA as "Ready-Made Evidence": An Analysis of Portuguese Judges' Views', *International Journal of Evidence and Proof* 26:2 (2022), pp. 121–135. doi: 10.1177/13657127211070331.

25 Filipe Santos, 'Making Sense of the Story: The Dialogues between the Police and Forensic Laboratories in the Construction of DNA Evidence', *New Genetics and Society* 33:2 (2014), pp. 181–203.

doi: 10.1080/14636778.2014.916186; Susana Costa and Filipe Santos, 'The Social Life of Forensic Evidence and the Epistemic Sub-Cultures in an Inquisitorial Justice System: Analysis of Saltão Case', *Science and Justice* 59:5 (2019), pp. 471–479. doi: 10.1016/j.scijus.2019.06.003.
26 David L. Altheide, 'Moral Panic: From Sociological Concept to Public Discourse', *Crime, Media, Culture* 5:1 (2009), pp. 79–99. doi: 10.1177/1741659008102063.
27 Simon Cottle, 'Mediatized Public Crisis and Civil Society Renewal: The Racist Murder of Stephen Lawrence', *Crime, Media, Culture* 1:1 (2005), pp. 49–71. doi: 10.1177/1741659005050243.
28 Filipe Santos, *Do Meia Culpa a Madeleine McCann. Casos Mediáticos e Genética Forense Em Portugal* (Coimbra: Almedina, 2021).
29 Richard V. Ericson, Patricia Baranek, and Janet Chan, *Representing Order: Crime, Law, and Justice in the News Media* (Buckingham, Milton Keynes: Open University Press, 1991).
30 Colin Sparks, 'Introduction: The Panic over Tabloid News', in Colin Sparks, John Tulloch and Barbie Zelizer (eds), *Tabloid Tales: Global Debates over Media Standards* (New York: Rowman & Littlefield, 2000), pp. 1–40.
31 Richard V. Ericson, Patricia Baranek and Janet Chan, *Representing Order: Crime, Law, and Justice in the News Media* (Buckingham, Milton Keynes: Open University Press, 1991).
32 Pierre Bourdieu, 'L'emprise du journalisme', *Actes de La Recherche En Sciences Sociales* 101:1 (1994), pp. 3–9.
33 These distinctions were the subject of analysis in Helena Machado and Filipe Santos, 'Popular Press and Forensic Genetics in Portugal: Expectations and Disappointments Regarding Two Cases of Missing Children', *Public Understanding of Science* 20:3 (2011), pp. 303–318. doi: 10.1177/0963662509336710. While much has changed since then in terms of media outlets, the article contains information about the readership of the tabloid *Correio da Manhã*, which characterises it as being mainly constituted by comparatively lower socio-economic reading groups of the Portuguese population.
34 António de Oliveira Salazar, born in Santa Comba Dão, was the head of the fascist dictatorship that ruled Portugal from 1932 until he was substituted for health reasons in 1968, leading to the 1974 Carnation Revolution.
35 The authors argue that the: 'increased expectations of and demands for scientific evidence is more likely the result of much broader cultural influences related to modern technological advances, what we have chosen to call a "tech effect"' (p. 362). Shelton, Kim and Barak,

'A Study of Juror Expectations and Demands Concerning Scientific Evidence: Does the "CSI Effect" Exist?'.
36 José B. Amaro and Alexandra Campos, 'Detido incriminado pelos testes genéticos', *Público* July 2000.
37 This was an interesting development, particularly for the practices of forensic reporting, as the first DNA analyses stated that mixed samples found in the getaway car and in a bathroom were 'compatible' with Nuno (and others). The re-exam requested by Nuno's defence attorney, made in the same institution, but in another laboratory, stated that it was not possible to 'safely declare' that the mixed samples matched with Nuno. This illustrates an attempt to fit the evidence into the narrative that there was more than one offender. Subsequent forensic reports in other cases would be more accurately worded to prevent misinterpretation.
38 The *Público*'s news article briefly describes the discovery of identification through DNA profiles: 'As impressões digitais genéticas', *Público* (Porto, 27 April 1997).
39 António Lage, Leonete Botelho and Alfredo Leite, 'Os fios da meada', *Público*, April 1997.
40 Moira Peelo, 'Framing Homicide Narratives in Newspapers: Mediated Witness and the Construction of Virtual Victimhood', *Crime, Media, Culture* 2:2 (2006), pp. 159–175. doi: 10.1177/1741659006065404.
41 Richard V. Ericson, 'How Journalists Visualize Fact', *The ANNALS of the American Academy of Political and Social Science* 560:1 (1998), pp. 83–95. doi: 10.1177/0002716298560001007.
42 Monica Robbers, 'Blinded by Science: The Social Construction of Reality in Forensic Television Shows and its Effect on Criminal Jury Trials', *Criminal Justice Policy Review* 19:1 (2008), pp. 84–102.
43 Carlos Ferreira, 'Como a PJ apanhou o cabo', *Correio Da Manhã*, 27 January 2007.
44 Eduardo Dâmaso and Tânia Laranjo, 'Exames marcam morte de Maddie', *Correio Da Manhã*, 7 January 2008, www.cmjornal.xl.pt/exclusivos/detalhe/exames-marcam-morte-de-maddie.html.
45 Cavender and Deutsch, 'CSI and Moral Authority'.
46 The *Diário de Notícias* was first published in 1864 and is regarded as a quality newspaper. It belongs to the same media group as the *Jornal de Notícias*.
47 Duarte N. Vieira, 'Perícias não se compadecem com pressas', *Jornal de Notícias* (Porto, 2007), www.jn.pt/nacional/dossiers/o-caso-maddie-mccann/ponto-de-vista/pericias-nao-se-compadecem-com-pressas-664934.html.
48 José M. Fernandes, 'O fim do caso Maddie e o princípio de outros pecados', *Público*, 22 July 2008.

49 Umberto Eco, *Travels in Hyper Reality* (San Diego: First Harvest, 1990).
50 Santos, 'State, Wage Relations and Social Welfare'.
51 João Arriscado Nunes, 'As dinâmicas da(s) ciência(s) no perímetro do centro: Uma cultura científica de fronteira?', *Revista Crítica de Ciências Sociais*, 63:October (2002), pp. 189–198.
52 Tom R. Tyler, 'Viewing CSI and the Threshold of Guilt: Managing Truth and Justice in Reality and Fiction', *The Yale Law Journal* 115:5 (2006), pp. 1050–1085. doi: 10.2307/20455645.
53 Chris Greer and Eugene McLaughlin, ' "Trial by Media": Policing, the 24–7 News Mediasphere and the "Politics of Outrage" ', *Theoretical Criminology* 15:1 (2011), pp. 23–46. doi: 10.1177/1362480610387461.

Index

abortion 192
accountability 12, 17, 150, 151, 156, 157, 159, 163, 224–227, 233, 240, 241, 243, 244, 246–253, 256
accusatorial system 7
  see also adversarial system
acquittal 14, 54–56, 163, 171, 172, 174, 175, 176, 177, 178, 179, 183, 191, 197, 264, 275
Adam, Alison 4, 5, 169
admissible evidence 26, 28, 30, 36, 97
adultery 33, 42, 219, 224, 228, 231, 232
adversarial system 7, 18, 19, 28, 117, 119, 128, 184, 185, 243, 247, 263, 264, 265
agency 18
anthropology 217
  criminal anthropology 11, 15, 104, 147–165, 248
Austria 93, 100, 103, 106, 250
authoritarian regime 1, 11–12, 147–165, 191–207, 227–228, 229–234, 235
autopsy 2, 9, 84, 132, 173, 181, 182, 183, 193, 195, 196, 197, 199, 200, 202, 203, 204, 205, 252

Bates, Victoria 27, 51, 63
Belgium 250
Bertillonage 95
blood 9, 268, 273
  blood test 2, 31, 34, 36, 39, 43
  blood typing 13, 25–44
body 9, 12, 13, 71, 93, 120, 150, 153, 160, 162, 165, 173, 174, 176, 179, 182, 183, 184, 195, 198, 203, 267, 268, 270, 271, 272
Buenos Aires 192, 199
Burney, Ian 4, 9, 50, 53, 70, 92, 118, 140

Carrara, Mario 15, 147–165
character 26, 31, 39, 41, 42, 43, 151, 231
children 25–44, 50, 51, 52, 53, 58–61, 80, 86, 97, 155, 169–185, 191–207, 247, 254, 267, 271, 272
civil law 20, 39
class 1, 5, 6, 18, 117, 120, 121, 128, 129, 136, 137, 138, 139, 140, 217, 221, 222, 227, 229, 231, 232
clothing 117–135
common law 97, 170, 176, 177, 228, 247

Index

confession 10, 15, 57, 62–63, 64, 65, 96, 232, 270, 271
consensus 240–256
coroner 11, 172, 173, 178, 183
court 18, 25, 29, 31, 33, 34, 43, 61, 118, 122, 123, 127, 139, 140, 164, 171, 172, 173, 174, 176, 178, 179, 180, 184, 193, 195, 197, 198, 199, 201, 202, 205, 224, 225, 228, 231, 242, 243, 244, 247, 248, 249, 251, 252, 253, 255, 256, 264, 265
courtroom 1, 2, 12, 13, 16, 18, 63, 117–135, 152, 156, 158, 162, 163, 164, 165, 173, 177, 224, 265
crime 83, 84, 95, 108, 109, 157, 159, 163, 216–235, 248, 254, 261–276
crime of passion 12, 16, 216–235
crime scene 3, 9, 92, 94, 104, 105, 133, 268, 274
crime scene photography 53, 95
criminal law 12, 20, 39, 55, 57, 95, 100, 163, 165, 177, 178, 184, 191, 193, 207, 219, 225, 227, 228, 229, 230, 231, 232, 234, 241, 242, 246, 247, 248, 249, 250, 255, 256
criminalistics 2, 8, 9, 15, 53, 57, 65, 92–111
criminology 76, 147–165, 219, 220, 221, 222, 223, 225, 242, 243, 248
CSI effect 14, 261–276
cultural turn 2, 3
culture 3, 4, 5, 26, 44, 136, 138, 150, 165, 172, 178, 240
culture of testimony 16, 49, 65

dangerous criminal/individual 150, 151, 157, 159, 193, 207, 219, 221, 225, 230, 232, 234, 242, 253, 254, 255, 256
Daston, Lorraine 2

defence lawyer *see* lawyer
degeneration 154, 155, 159, 160, 161, 162, 254
dismissal 17, 54–56
divorce 13, 25, 32, 34, 42
DNA 2, 9, 14, 261–276
doctors *see* physicians

education 92–111, 184, 195, 199, 218, 221, 231, 234, 235, 248
  legal education 15, 99, 101, 102, 105, 109
Eichmann trial 10
emotion 32, 62, 153, 155, 160, 216–235, 244, 245, 270, 272
  see also sympathy
England 17, 18, 27, 50, 92, 94, 117–135, 169–185, 191
epistemic virtues/values 6, 12–14, 17, 18, 117–135, 169–185, 193, 200, 202, 205, 240–256, 265
era of testimony 73
era of witness 10, 73
evidence 1, 8–11, 13, 15, 17, 25–44, 49–65, 71–86, 95, 96, 99, 104, 118, 122, 123, 137, 140, 169–185, 191, 263, 264, 265, 270, 271, 272, 275
  see also admissible evidence
expert 3, 12, 13, 29, 63, 74, 118, 121, 122, 127, 136, 140, 248, 250, 251, 252, 254, 255, 256, 264, 265, 275
expert witness 1, 9, 10, 15, 29, 38, 95, 96, 104, 107, 117, 118, 119, 121, 122, 123, 128, 129, 137, 138, 139, 140, 147–165, 224, 244, 247
  see also forensic expert
expertise 1, 5, 84, 141, 240–256

fallibility 40
fashion *see* clothing
fatherhood 25–44, 33, 179
femicide 216, 217, 235

feminism 13, 54, 216
fiction 262, 263, 264, 265, 268, 269, 270, 273, 274, 275, 276
fingerprints 9, 29, 40, 43, 53, 83, 127, 268
forensic
  anthropology 9
  chemistry 9, 100, 105
  culture 3, 4, 5, 6–8, 13, 14, 15, 16, 17, 77, 92, 93, 94, 95–99, 107, 110, 117, 118, 141, 150, 151–153, 154, 156, 157, 164, 165, 173, 184, 193, 194, 200–206, 207, 227, 235, 242, 243, 246, 251, 252, 256, 261, 265
  expert 5, 7, 13, 17, 18, 27, 117–135, 147–165, 169–185, 191–207, 216–235, 246, 247, 248, 249, 251, 253, 254, 255
  expertise 2, 14, 27, 84, 111, 117, 132, 136, 191–207, 216–235, 240–256, 265
  medicine 11, 16, 17, 18, 27, 34, 43, 56–57, 73, 77, 85, 102, 104, 118, 122, 132, 140, 169–185, 191–207, 220, 241, 244, 245, 247, 249, 251, 252, 253, 255, 256, 274
  odontology 29
  patriotism 9, 95, 106–109
  practice 6, 14, 19, 20, 51, 53, 71, 72, 73, 75, 77, 78, 83, 92, 93, 95, 118, 119, 123, 126, 140, 141, 150
    see also legal practice
  psychiatry 11, 17, 53, 105, 147–165, 171, 172, 177, 178, 179, 180, 181, 183, 216–235, 240–256
  regime 15, 93, 110, 118, 119

science 9, 14, 53, 105, 107, 132, 134, 140, 261–276
  techniques 14, 71, 73, 74, 77
  textbooks 18, 52, 56, 150, 153, 154, 161, 162, 164, 165, 194, 195, 196
  theory 16
  turn 9, 10, 73
Foucault, Michel 12, 242
France 50, 64, 76, 93, 106, 151, 152, 178, 179, 191, 217, 218, 219, 220, 221, 222, 227, 234, 242, 250
Franco regime 8, 12, 13, 18, 191–207

Galison, Peter 2
gender 1, 5, 6, 13, 14, 25–44, 44, 52, 81, 117–135, 155, 157, 177, 178, 180, 191–207, 216–235
Germany 9, 50, 64, 72, 76, 78, 85, 92–111, 139, 151, 152, 179, 218, 220, 242, 243, 250, 251
  Imperial Germany 10, 15, 92–111
Gibson, Mary 12, 147, 163
Gross, Hans 53, 92–111
gynaecologists 197, 202, 204

Habermas, Rebekka 16, 217
Hamlin, Christopher 3, 96
history of medicine 1, 3
Holocaust 9
honour 16, 52, 217, 218, 219, 221, 222, 235
human rights law 9

identification 77, 78, 83, 84, 85, 105
ideology 6, 7, 10, 11–12, 65, 138, 205, 229, 231, 233, 267
impartiality 13, 18, 19, 117–135, 173, 205, 264, 270

Index 285

Imre v Mitchell case 34, 36, 39, 41, 42
infanticide 17, 18, 26, 27, 43, 169–185, 191–207
inquisitorial system 7, 96, 152, 220, 243, 264, 265, 275
insanity 153, 155, 156, 157, 158, 160, 161, 163, 177, 178, 179, 184, 185, 218, 219, 224, 233, 247, 254
institutionalisation 5, 8, 9, 14, 53, 79, 84, 92, 93, 94, 99, 103, 107, 110, 138, 225, 251, 265
international law 74, 75, 77
investigation *see* pre-trial investigation
Ireland 191
Italy 12, 15, 98, 103, 107, 110, 147–165, 198, 221, 222, 225, 234, 258

Jasanoff, Sheila 2, 139, 263
judge 17, 28, 29, 32, 33, 36, 37, 39, 41, 42, 50, 51, 52, 55, 58, 61, 62, 65, 95, 97, 98, 99, 105, 121, 151, 152, 153, 157, 161, 162, 163, 164, 165, 169, 170, 173, 175, 176, 177, 179, 181, 183, 184, 196, 198, 200, 201, 202, 204, 221, 222, 225, 226, 230, 231, 232, 246, 247, 249, 263, 264, 265
jurists 1, 61, 94, 97, 98, 99–103, 106, 107, 109, 128, 165, 193, 198, 201, 206, 216, 222, 229, 230, 232, 248
jury 11, 14, 27, 28, 97, 99, 118, 119, 123, 128, 139, 140, 148, 150, 151–153, 156–158, 161, 162, 164, 169–185, 219, 220, 221, 227, 247, 263, 264, 265, 275
justice 14, 15, 16, 17, 64, 71, 72, 74, 77, 92–111, 119, 140, 160, 170, 177, 191, 207, 216, 217, 224, 241, 261, 262, 263, 270

knowledge 1–6, 8, 14, 15, 19, 20, 40, 74, 85, 99–105, 109, 111, 118, 119, 120, 137, 138, 150, 151, 173, 176, 177, 184, 185, 199, 244, 245, 246, 251, 252, 254, 255, 256
see also transfer of knowledge
Kraepelin, Emil 154, 155, 156, 164
Kruze, Corinna 13

laboratory 2, 3, 9, 15, 28, 83, 94, 102, 104, 132, 133, 140, 264, 265, 269, 272, 273, 274
Latour, Bruno 2, 203
law 12, 35, 38, 172, 175, 177, 181, 216, 218, 220, 225, 227, 233, 243, 251
criminal law *see* criminal law
doing law 16, 216–235
lawyer 16, 17, 18, 37, 40, 41, 50, 64, 65, 76, 118, 127, 128, 152, 157, 169, 170, 172, 174, 175, 176, 180, 181, 183, 184, 197, 200, 201, 202, 205, 206, 218, 220, 221, 222, 224, 227, 235, 241, 264, 268
legal culture *see* culture
legal practice 1, 2, 4, 5, 6, 7, 11, 12, 13, 14, 16, 18, 19, 26, 51, 63, 64, 92, 97, 100, 128, 132, 151, 161, 165, 170, 179, 191, 192, 193, 195, 198, 201, 203, 205, 206, 217, 218, 219, 220, 224, 226, 227, 228, 229, 230, 231, 232, 233, 235, 241, 243, 251, 253, 255, 256, 262
legal scholars *see* jurists
legal system 2, 5, 6, 7, 17, 28, 65, 150, 191, 205, 218, 219, 220, 221, 225, 227, 235, 241, 242, 243, 251, 255, 264, 265
inquisitorial system *see* inquisitorial system

Liszt, Franz von 95, 102, 103, 241, 248
Lombroso, Cesare 12, 15, 147–165, 219, 233

Mant, Keith 80–85
manual *see* forensic textbooks
marriage 26
masculinity 13, 19, 117–135, 222
  see also gender
mass violence 9, 71–86, 240
material evidence *see* evidence
media 3, 4, 5, 6, 14, 17, 27, 117, 119, 133, 134, 139, 140, 163, 261–276
  see also newspapers
medical witnesses 4, 15, 56, 149, 157, 160, 163, 169–185, 244
Mexico 191
modernity 5, 6, 13, 14, 95, 105, 110, 118, 138, 191
mortuary 15, 84, 132
motherhood 13, 18, 25, 27, 32, 33, 169–185, 191–207
murder 29, 92, 129, 147–165, 169–185, 191–207, 216–235, 255, 267
  murder weapon 159

nation state 1, 6, 8, 95, 110
nationalism 9, 108, 221
Netherlands 12, 16, 49–65, 216–235, 242
newspapers 14, 65, 117, 119, 127, 133, 183, 220, 221, 222, 224, 227, 242, 261–276
Norway 17, 240–256
novels 178
Nuremberg trials 72, 73, 77, 81, 82, 83

objectivity 2, 4, 5, 13, 14, 18, 19, 26, 118, 138, 170, 171, 184, 243, 264, 265, 267

othering 16, 217, 222, 229, 234
Ottolenghi, Salvatore 98, 149

paternity 13, 25–44, 25
pathologist 9, 72, 79, 84, 85, 93, 105, 118, 132, 133, 139, 140, 179
pathology 18, 53, 132, 173, 203, 251, 252
Pemberton, Neil 9, 50, 53, 70, 92, 118, 140
performance 19, 27, 117, 119, 122, 123, 127, 128, 132, 136, 139, 140, 173, 204
performative turn 19
perpetrator 17, 20, 29, 58, 71, 205, 216–235
photography 267
physicians 8, 12, 56–57, 75, 77, 96, 117, 122, 126, 130, 136, 140, 191–207, 218, 220, 244, 245, 246, 247, 248, 249, 252, 253, 254
police 17, 56, 58, 59, 60, 62, 65, 98, 101, 103, 107, 110, 127, 147, 159, 183, 198, 248, 252, 262, 263, 264, 267, 268, 269, 270, 271, 273, 274, 276
  police handbook 52, 53
politics 5, 150, 158, 205, 229
Portugal 14, 250, 261–276
post-mortem *see* autopsy
practice *see* forensic practice, legal practice
pre-trial investigation 17, 151, 172, 173, 181, 182, 183, 184, 197, 264, 266, 269, 270, 272, 273, 274, 276
procedural law 2, 7, 11, 17, 55, 61, 64, 97, 150, 151, 152, 164, 165, 170, 201, 203, 206, 241, 247, 248, 264
professionalisation 6, 16, 137, 138, 191, 240–256

pronatalism 192, 193, 198, 199, 200, 206, 207
proof 26, 38, 39, 169, 175, 181, 184
prosecutor 17, 19, 51, 52, 54, 55, 58, 60, 63, 65, 72, 95, 99, 105, 118, 152, 171, 172, 175, 181, 196, 197, 198, 200, 202, 204, 205, 218, 220, 221, 222, 224, 227, 235, 247, 264, 265
psychiatry 2, 8, 9, 12, 16, 60, 171, 179, 216–235, 240–256
see also forensic psychiatry
psychology 9, 96, 97, 100, 102, 152, 160, 161, 223, 225
psychopathology 222, 223, 224, 227, 231
psychopathy 159, 218, 219, 233

race 5
rape 16, 26, 50, 52
rape myths 50, 65
see also sexual assault
Ravensbrück concentration camp 80–82
reliability 40, 43, 53, 55, 63, 96, 118
reliability of evidence 29, 38, 39
reliability of witnesses 13, 25, 27, 50, 51, 52–54, 58, 61, 64, 84, 97
respectability 26, 42, 43, 121
responsibility see accountability
Roman law 7
Russia see Soviet Russia
Ruxton case 129

scholarly persona 19, 120, 136, 138, 140
Science and Technology Studies (STS) 2, 139, 205
Scotland 7, 13, 25–44, 120, 203, 204
Second World War 9, 33, 71–86

serology 30, 34, 38
sexual assault 10, 16, 26, 43, 49–65, 254
see also rape
sexual revolution 13
silent witness 8, 10, 50, 65, 96
Simpson, Keith 132, 133, 139
Smith, Sydney 122, 133
solicitor see lawyer
Soviet Russia 12, 16, 216–235
Soviet Union see Soviet Russia
Spain 12, 18, 191–207, 250
Spilsbury, Bernard 127, 132, 139
surgeon 123, 173, 174, 176, 183
suspect 59, 60, 62, 196, 198, 199, 271, 275
Sweden 250
sympathy 43, 174, 176, 178, 180, 184, 223

Tammenoms Bakker, Symon 221, 222, 223, 226
Tanzi, Eugenio 154, 155, 156, 162, 163, 164
Tardieu, Ambroise 21, 195
technology 5, 14, 242, 261–276
see also forensic techniques
testimony 1, 10, 49–65, 71, 72, 73, 76, 80, 82, 84, 85, 96, 120, 122, 198
culture of testimony see culture of testimony
testimony of people 50
testimony of things 50, 53
totalitarian regime 5
toxicology 151, 251
transfer of knowledge 8, 19, 106, 109, 110
trial 51, 54, 57, 60, 62, 63, 72, 81, 84, 121, 147–165, 169–185, 197, 198, 204, 207, 221, 224, 240, 248, 255, 256, 263, 264, 265, 268, 272, 275
truth machine 14, 263

umbilical cord 18, 176, 191–207
unaccountability *see*
 accountability
uncertainty 13, 18, 169–185, 191, 203, 204
United Kingdom 11, 13, 25, 28
 see also England, Scotland and Wales
United States 9, 14, 31, 50, 139, 263, 264

victim 9, 13, 16, 17, 20, 27, 43, 49, 50, 51, 52–56, 57–61, 63, 71, 78, 80, 83, 84, 216, 217, 223, 224, 228, 232, 269, 270
Vogt, Ragnar 248, 249, 250, 252

Wales 27, 28, 32, 170
war crimes 1, 77, 82, 83
Watson, Katherine 169, 171, 175, 176, 184
Winge, Paul 244, 248, 249, 250, 251, 252, 253
witness 15, 19, 52–54, 72, 73, 76, 82, 96, 253, 265
 eye witness 57, 77
 speaking witness 50, 53
 witness psychology 16, 52, 58, 63, 64, 65, 95, 100
 witness testimony 49–65, 265
Wolffram, Heather 64

EU authorised representative for GPSR:
Easy Access System Europe, Mustamäe tee 50,
10621 Tallinn, Estonia
gpsr.requests@easproject.com

www.ingramcontent.com/pod-product-compliance
Ingram Content Group UK Ltd.
Pitfield, Milton Keynes, MK11 3LW, UK
UKHW021824140426
5217IPUK00004B/78